Epidemiology of Type 2 Diabetes

Edited By

Qing Qiao

Department of Public Health, Hjelt Institute, University of Helsinki, PL41, Mannerheimintie 172, 00014, Helsinki, Finland

Department of Chronic Disease Prevention, National Institute for Health and Welfare, Helsinki, Finland

eBooks End User License Agreement

CONTENTS

FOREWORD

In 1997, the American Diabetes Association decided to change the cut-points for glucose defining whether an individual had diabetes or not. This event triggered the development of an international research network within diabetes epidemiology - the Diabetes Epidemiology: Collaborative analysis of Diagnostic criteria in Europe (DECODE) and Asia (DECODA). Although the primary aim was to evaluate the impact of the revised diagnostic criteria from a public health perspective, this initiative proved to be an excellent platform for studies focusing on understanding the rationale for ethnic variability in susceptibility to diabetes and its complications. Such an insight can only be achieved through access to population-based data from different regions of the world. The DECODE and DECODA studies in combination with other initiatives like DETECT-2 have taught us, that well established risk factors for diabetes as obesity and age have very different impact in different populations. In a scientific community, dominated by data from Europe and North-America, our knowledge regarding risk factors and high risk groups stems from a small minority of the population of the world. Had we used this knowledge to develop prevention strategies in Asia and Africa, then our efforts would have had little effect. DECODE and DECODA taught us that although risk-factors may be the same, the cut-point for being at risk varies tremendously between populations. The International Diabetes Federation has taken the consequence of this, and developed region-specific cut-points for at-risk levels of obesity.

The present eBook is written by a group that has worked extensively on the DECODE and DECODA data. They have highlighted the importance of the variability within the species of Homo Sapiens when it comes to physiological responses to the external and internal environment. This eBook reviews the epidemiology of diabetes in this specific context, which has proven to be so helpful in diabetes and obesity epidemiology. It is my hope that in the future we will see similar trends in studies of human physiology and clinical medicine. Meanwhile, at least we can say that epidemiology showed us the way.

Knut Borch-Johnsen
Odense, Denmark

PREFACE

The idea of the eBook took shape in the editor's mind in 2010 when several co-authors of the eBook completed a series of doctorial theses covering a wide range of research topics on epidemiology of type 2 diabetes. Each of the theses comprises not only a comprehensive literature review and meta-analysis but also the author's own research results, which are mainly based on a well recognized large international collaborative study in Europe and Asia---the Diabetes Epidemiology: Collaborative analysis of Diagnostic criteria in Europe (DECODE) and Asia (DECODA) study. The authors, each at the forefront of his/her research field, have updated and dedicated their works to the eBook with aims to share their research outcomes with more people who are interested in doing epidemiological researches on diabetes, and to help the young researchers to understand easily the progress and the significant development in the relevant fields during the past decades.

This eBook consisting of eight chapters covers the frontiers of works on evolution of diagnostic criteria, prevalence of diabetes, screening programs and tools for early detection of type 2 diabetes, developing and evaluation of risk assessment algorithms, obesity and diabetes, anthropometric measures of obesity and its validity in predicting diabetes, comparison between central and general obesity, lipid levels in relation to glucose tolerance status, uric acid and diabetes, relationship of cancer with diabetes and non-diabetic hyperglycemia, cardiovascular disease in relation to diabetes and non-diabetic glycemic levels including outcomes from the recent randomized controlled clinical trials that have investigated the effect of intensive glycemic control on cardiovascular disease outcomes. The ethnic differences in the association of diabetes with obesity, dyslipidemia and other metabolic disorders have been extensively investigated in the DECODE/DECODA study and the interesting findings are included in this eBook, which are the most important original works of the authors.

Qing Qiao
University of Helsinki
Finland

List of Contributors

Gao, Weiguo[1,2,3]
E-mail: gwg1974@hotmail.com

Nan, Hairong[4]
E-mail: hnan@hku.hk

Ning, Feng[1]
E-mail: feng.ning@helsinki.fi

Nyamdorj, Regzedmaa[1]
E-mail: regzedmaa.nyamdorj@helsinki.fi

Qiao, Qing[1,2]
E-mail: qing.qiao@helsinki.fi

Zhang, Lei[1,2,3,5]
E-mail: diabetologist@126.com

Zhou, Xianghai[1,6]
E-mail: xianghaizhou@yahoo.com.cn

[1]*Department of Public Health, Hjelt Institute, University of Helsinki, Helsinki, Finland.*

[2]*Department of Chronic Disease Prevention, National Institute for Health and Welfare, Helsinki, Finland.*

[3]*Qingdao Endocrine & Diabetes Hospital, Qingdao, China.*

[4]*Department of Community Medicine, School of Public Health, The University of Hong Kong, Hong Kong, SAR, China.*

[5]*Department of Internal Medicine, Weifang Medical University, Weifang, China.*

[6]*Department of Endocrinology and Metabolism, Peking University People's Hospital, Beijing, China.*

2

CHAPTER 1

Evolution of Diagnostic Criteria for Type 2 Diabetes

Qing Qiao[*]

Department of Public Health, Hjelt Institute, University of Helsinki, Helsinki, Finland and Department of Chronic Disease Prevention, National Institute for Health and Welfare, Helsinki, Finland

Abstract: Type 2 diabetes has been diagnosed based on elevated glycemic levels that are quantified using different laboratory means in random, fasting or post-challenge status. The evolution of the diagnostic criteria for type 2 diabetes can be roughly divided into three different development stages according to the scientific basis upon which the criteria was developed. In 1950s to 1960s the diagnostic cut-off values were set solely on the basis of statistical estimate (mean±2SD). The reports of the bimodal distribution of fasting and 2h post-load glucose concentrations in certain populations and their relationships with retinopathy provided clinical evidence for making the diagnostic criteria for diabetes in 1979. On the basis of findings from studies on prevalence of retinopathy in 1990s the current diagnostic criteria was made based on either glucose or HbA1c levels. Although the definitions were evidence based, classifications of individuals with hyperglycemia based on different glycemic assays and criteria are not completely concordant. In this chapter the important scientific events and the milestones achieved during the evolution of the diagnostic criteria are traced back which may serve as a stimulus for the future research to improve the diagnostic criteria for diabetes.

Keywords: Type 2 diabetes, diagnostic criteria, evolution of the criteria, impaired glucose tolerance, impaired fasting glucose, HbA1c criteria.

1.1. INTRODUCTION

Type 2 diabetes is a non-communicable life-long health condition characterised by reduced insulin secretion by pancreas and impaired use of insulin by the body known as insulin resistance [1, 2]. Insulin is a hormone which regulates blood sugar levels in the body. As a results of the insulin deficiency and insulin resistance blood glucose level rises. Currently, a confirmative diagnosis of diabetes has been made absolutely based on the levels of glucose in the blood that exceeds certain diagnostic cut-off values. Different glycemic measures and diagnostic cut-off values have been applied in different historical periods, which reflects the development in science to understand the disease and in technology to quantify the glycemic levels.

A large number of type 2 diabetic patients do not have clinical manifestations during the early course of the disease, which adds additional difficulties to diagnose the disease early. About half of the asymptomatic diabetic individuals are unaware of their disease status unless a screening glucose test is performed. The disease is also associated with a number of micro-vascular complications such as diabetic retinopathy, nephropathy and neuropathy. Macro-vascular diseases such as Coronary Heart Disease (CHD) and stroke are the most common complications among diabetic patients. Before advent of chemical methods to determine sugar levels a diagnosis of diabetes was made purely based on observations of clinical manifestations, and thus only those with overt symptoms of diabetes could be diagnosed and often diabetes and long-term complications of diabetes were identified together.

The presence of hyperglycemia is often accompanied by glycosuria. Sweet taste of diabetic urine had been observed since ancient time. The detection of sugar in urine was facilitated by the development of chemical tests to detect the substance. Francis Home in 1780 proposed the yeast test for the detection of sugar in the

*Address correspondence to Qing Qiao: Department of Public Health, Hjelt Institute, University of Helsinki, Mannerheimintie 172, 00014 Helsinki, Finland. Email: qing.qiao@helsinki.fi

urine of diabetic patients. This test was superseded by the chemical test introduced by Hermann von Fehling in 1848 and eventually by that proposed in 1911 by the American chemist, Stanley Rossiter Benedict who proposed testing for the presence of reducing sugar using a special reagent containing blue copper sulphate, sodium carbonate and sodium citrate. With the development of glucose assays to measure glucose concentration in the blood, researchers found that in many individuals glycosuria is absence in the presence of high blood glucose levels due to the wide individual variation of renal threshold of glucose. The concept of a glucose challenge was introduced in 1913 by Dr. Jacobsen [3] with a aim to disclose diabetes early. He studied the effects of different food stuffs on the blood sugar and found that protein and fat have no influence on the blood sugar levels but that carbohydrate intake produces a rapid and often a marked hyperglycemia. Since then oral glucose tolerance test has been widely applied for diagnosis of diabetes but for a long time the definition of "abnormality" of glucose tolerance test was solely statistical. A glucose value greater than 2 Standard Deviations (SD) above the mean has been considered diagnostic of diabetes, which would define approximately 25% of the population [4].

1.2. STATISTICALLY (MEAN+2SD) ABNORMAL GLUCOSE TOLERANCE TEST

Based on a few studies of healthy and young individuals in early 1950s, diagnostic cut-off values for diabetes based on 2-hour whole blood glucose concentration after 100g glucose load have been set at 5.6 mmol/l [5, 6] to 6.7 mmol/l [7], and widely applied for many years. Obviously these criteria had over-diagnosed diabetes by the current standard. In 1957 based on a non-diabetic population of 20 to 59 years old, Unger [8] found that glucose levels increased with age, the diagnostic value (mean+2SD) for plasma glucose was 12.5 mmol/l. This was much higher than 6.7 mmol/l of the whole blood glucose at 2-hour, even taking into account the fact that plasma glucose concentration is approximately 15% higher than those of whole blood [9]. Results similar to Unger's have been published subsequently in 1960s [10-12], and a 2-hour value exceed 11.1 mmol/l to 12.2 mmol/l has been then accepted as abnormal glucose tolerance.

1.3. BIMODAL DISTRIBUTION OF GLUCOSE LEVELS AND MICROVASCULAR DISEASES

In most populations the frequency distributions of glucose is continuous and unimodal. The bimodality of 2-hour plasma glucose concentration after 75 glucose load was first reported in 1971 in adult Pima Indians who reside in central Arizona [13, 14], and soon the bimodality of fasting glucose concentration was also reported for Pima Indians [15]. Bimodality of glucose distribution was subsequently reported in other populations too including Mexican-American [16], Micronesians [17] and Polynesians [18]. The common characteristics of these populations are that they have extremely high prevalence of type 2 diabetes. In each of these populations the distribution was fitted better by a model of two overlapping normal distributions than by a single distribution, suggesting that subjects in the upper component of the frequency distribution may represent diabetes (Fig. **1**).

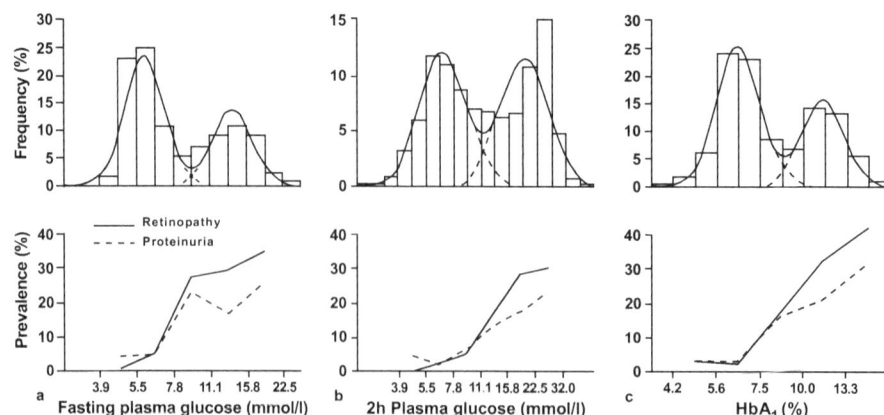

Figure 1: Upper panel: Bimodal distribution of glucose and HbA1 concentrations; Lower panel: Prevalence of retinopathy and heavy proteinuria in the same subjects. The figure was adapted from Pima Indian study in the U.S. among subjects aged 35 years or older regardless of previously diagnosed diabetes or hypoglycemic treatment [19].

The observed bimodal distribution suggests a logical separation between those with normal and high levels of glucose, and a possible diagnostic cut-off value for diabetes. This approach was further supported by both cross-sectional and longitudinal observations in Pima Indians [15, 20] and in the Whitehall and Bedford studies in the United Kingdom [21, 22]. These studies have shown that both retinopathy and nephropathy occurred almost exclusively among subjects with plasma glucose levels in the upper component (Fig. **1**). The development and progression of retinopathy over a 5-year period has been reported only in persons with 2-hour capillary blood glucose of 11.1 mmol/l and over after 50g glucose load, and there was no significant retinopathy identified in subject with baseline glucose level of 6.7-11.0 mmol/l [22]. These studies suggested that the diagnostic cut-off values for diabetes have been set too low previously and should be revised according to the findings on bimodal distribution of glucose concentration and the specific complications of diabetes. Thus, in 1979, the American National Diabetes Data Group (NDDG) [23] proposed a uniform definition for diabetes based on these findings. This was adopted by the WHO in 1980 with slight modification [24], and revised again in 1985 [25]. The diagnostic criteria for diabetes and Impaired Glucose Tolerance (IGT) based on Fasting Plasma Glucose (FPG) concentration after overnight fast and 2-hour plasma glucose (2hPG) concentration after 75g Oral Glucose Tolerance Test (OGTT) in the WHO 1985 definition [25] are shown in Table **1**.

Table 1: The WHO 1985 definition for diabetes

	Venous Plasma Glucose (mmol/l)	
	2hPG	FPG
Diabetes	≥11.1	≥7.8
IGT	7.8-11.0	<7.8

It was stated in the WHO 1985 recommendation that "for epidemiological or population screening purpose 2-hour value after 75g oral glucose load may be used alone or with the fasting value. The fasting value alone is considered less reliable since true fasting cannot be assured and spurious diagnosis of diabetes may more readily occur". This table was adapted from [25].

1.4. RATIONALE FOR DEFINITION OF IGT

The definition for IGT based on 2-hour glucose concentration after the 75g OGTT was introduced to replace the terms of borderline, chemical, subclinical, asymptomatic, and latent diabetes to avoid the psychological and socioeconomic stigma of the term diabetes [23]. The definition was made based on observations from long-term prospective studies carried out during 1960s to 1970s [22, 26-34] that found individuals within this category was not present with clinical manifestations of diabetes; the development of overt diabetic symptoms occurred at a rate of 1%-5% per year, and a large proportion of individuals with IGT showed reversion to normal glucose tolerance and the remainders stayed in the borderline category; they did not have clinically significant renal and retinal complications, but had an increased prevalence of arterial diseases and death, and IGT was present together with other known risk factors for cardiovascular disease such as hypertension, hyperlipidemia and adiposity. Thus, IGT may have prognostic implications and should not be ignored or taken lightly [23].

A number of long-term studies during the last three decades have now unequivocally shown that individuals with IGT have increased risk to develop diabetes, with annualized incidence of diabetes varied from 1.8% to 16.8%, approximately 2-10 times more likely to develop diabetes and 0.33 times as likely to be normoglycemic within 1 year compared to people without IGT (Figs. **2, 3**) [35]. Prevention or delay of onset of type 2 diabetes in people with IGT has been approved to be possible either by changes in lifestyle or by pharmacotherapy [36-41]. The relative risk reduction ranged from 28% in Indians [39] to 67% in Japanese [41]. A sustainable long-term effect of lifestyle intervention 20 years after trial in the Chinese Daqing Study [42] and 7 years after trial in the Finnish Diabetes Prevention Study [43] have also been reported, with an effect size of 43% for the both studies. Accumulative evidence have showed that IGT is also a risk predictor for future cardiovascular disease (details are discussed in Chapter **8**). Therefore, the definition of IGT has important prognostic and preventive implications.

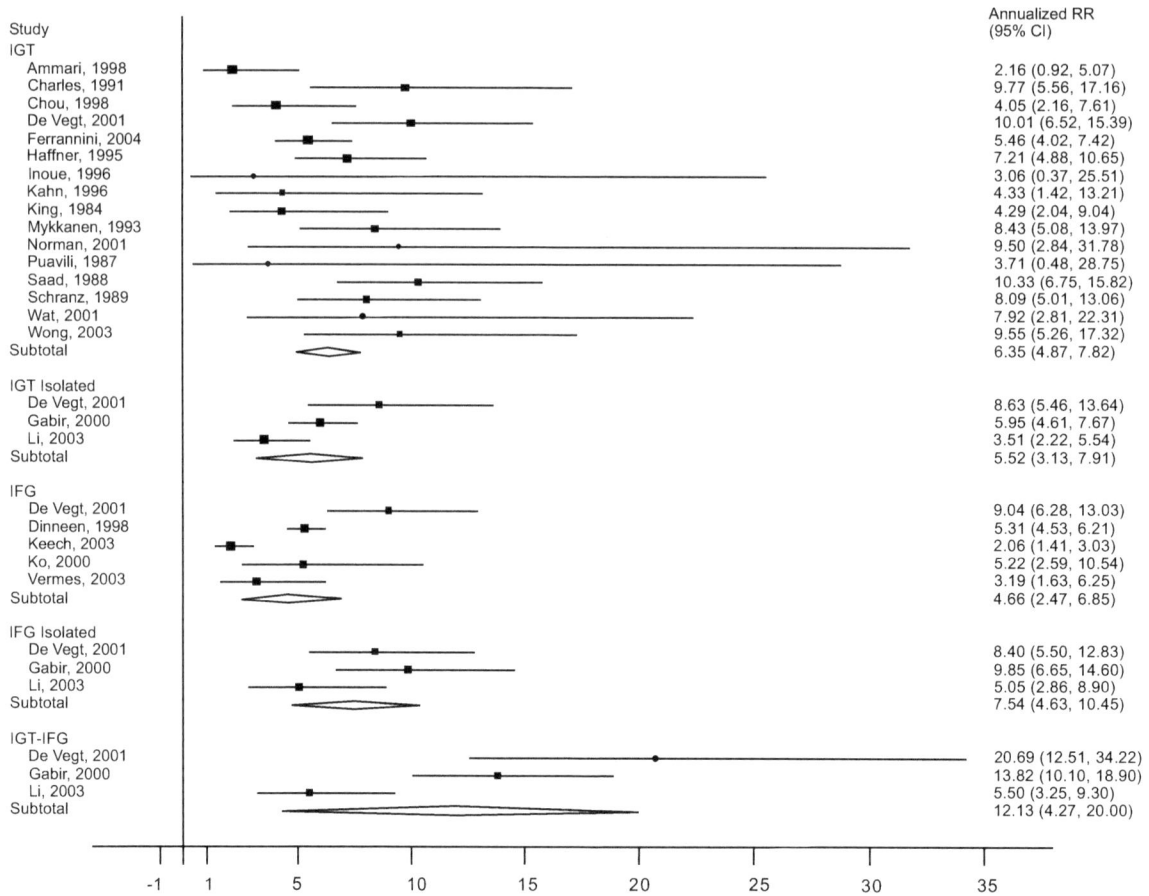

Figure 2: The annualized relative risks and meta-analyzed overall risks for diabetes in studies of people with IGT, isolated IGT, Impaired Fasting Glucose (IFG), isolated IFG, and both IGT and IFG [35].

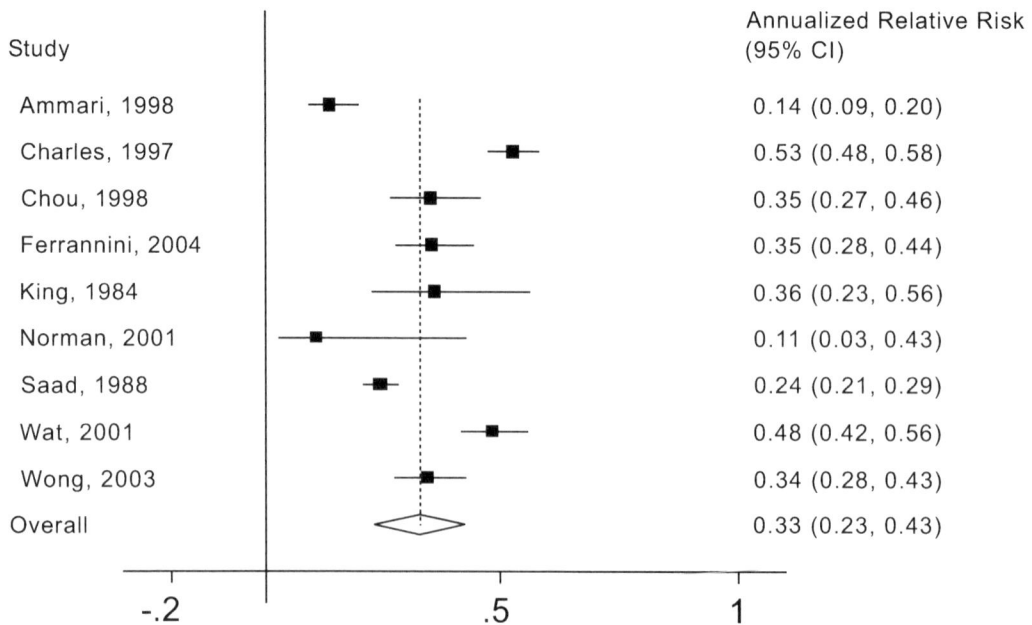

Figure 3: The annualized relative risks and meta-analyzed overall risks for regression to normoglycemia in studies of people with IGT [35].

1.5. CHANGES IN DIAGNOSTIC CRITERIA FOR DIABETES SINCE 1997

1.5.1. The Changes Made in 1997 by the American Diabetes Association (ADA)

The 1985 WHO diagnostic criteria for diabetes have been applied worldwide without changes until 1997. During the period the 2-hour 75g OGTT has been considered as a "gold standard" for diabetes, although the "gold standard" has been challenged with regard to its poor reproducibility, cost, time-consuming, labour intensive and uncomfortable for some patients [44]. Before the NDDG and the WHO 1985 criteria were put into effect enormous variations existed in diagnostic cut-off values for fasting and after glucose loading. The amount of the glucose load varied between 50g and 100g or was related to body weight, and the time after glucose loading was set from 30 minutes, 1 hour, 2 hours to 3 hours. The differences in assay methods used to determine glucose levels, glucose load and the time after loading have made the comparison between studies difficult. The universal application of the 2-hour 75g OGTT has created order out of the chaos and promoted researches on diabetes in the past decades worldwide.

In 1997 the ADA Expert Committee approved to revise the diagnostic criteria for diabetes [44]. The major change in the diagnostic criteria is related to FPG values. The ADA suggested to lower FPG from 7.8 mmol/l (140 mg/dl) to 7.0 mmol/l (126 mg/dl) for diagnosis of diabetes [44]. The positive diagnostic cut-off value for the 2hPG was remained unchanged, but the OGTT was not recommend for routine clinical use. If the OGTT will not be performed the classification of IGT will not exist. Thus, a new category of Impaired Fasting Glucose (IFG) based on the fasting plasma glucose level of 6.1-6.9 mmol/l (110-125 mg/dl) was introduced, an analogue of IGT based on the 2-hour value of 7.8-11.0 mmo/l. The choice of upper limit of normal FPG was somewhat arbitrary, but it is near the level above which acute phase insulin secretion is lost in response to intravenous administration of glucose and is associated with a progressively greater risk of developing micro-and macrovascular complications, as stated by the ADA in their Expert Committee report in 1997 [44].

The changes in diagnostic criteria have been made after careful consideration of the data, and rationale for what was accepted in 1979 by the NDDG group, along with emerging research findings since 1979. According to the ADA Expert Committee [44], the revision was made in order to 1) avoid the discrepancy between the FPG and the 2hPG cut-off values: almost all individuals with FPG≥140 mg/dl (7.8 mmol/l) have 2hPG≥200 mg/dl (11.1 mmol/l) if given an OGTT, whereas only about one-fourth of those with 2hPG≥200 mg/dl and without previously known diabetes have FPG≥140 mg/dl. Thus, the cut-off value of FPG≥140 mg/dl defined a greater degree of hyperglycemia than did the cut-off value of 2hPG≥200 mg/dl; 2) facilitate and encourage the use of a simple and equally accurate test, fasting plasma glucose, for diagnosis of diabetes: the OGTT has been performed infrequently in ordinary practice. The association of the FPG levels with the prevalence of retinopathy was also examined, and compared with that for the 2hPG in three studies of the Pima Indians in the U.S., among Egyptians, and in the Third National Health and Nutrition Examination Survey (NHANES III) in the U.S (Fig. **4a-4c**). Both the FPG and the 2hPG were equally associated with the prevalence of retinopathy, but, as noted by the ADA Expert Committee, the thresholds estimated in these studies could not be made more precise by using narrower glycemic intervals (*e.g.*, 20 instead of 10 shown in the Fig. **4a-4c**) because of the limited numbers of cases of retinopathy. "There were no absolute thresholds because some retinopathy occurred at all glucose levels, presumably because of measurement or disease variability and because of nondiabetic causes of retinopathy" as concluded by the ADA Expert Committee [44].

In 1999, the WHO accepted the new fasting glucose criteria for diabetes but retained the use of the 2-hour OGTT [9]. The classification of diabetes according to the 1999 WHO criteria is shown in Table **2**.

Following the revision of the diagnostic criteria for diabetes by the ADA in 1997, concerns and interest about the impact of the changes on prevalence of diabetes, reclassification of individuals and prognosis of individuals with different degrees of hyperglycemia, particularly the fasting *versus* the 2hPG criteria, have arisen. A number of data have been published to examine these concerns. Among these studies the **D**iabetes **E**pidemiology: **C**ollaborative analysis **O**f **D**iagnostic criteria in **E**urope (DECODE) study and its sister study in Asia, the DECODA study, have contributed greatly to the understanding of the issues.

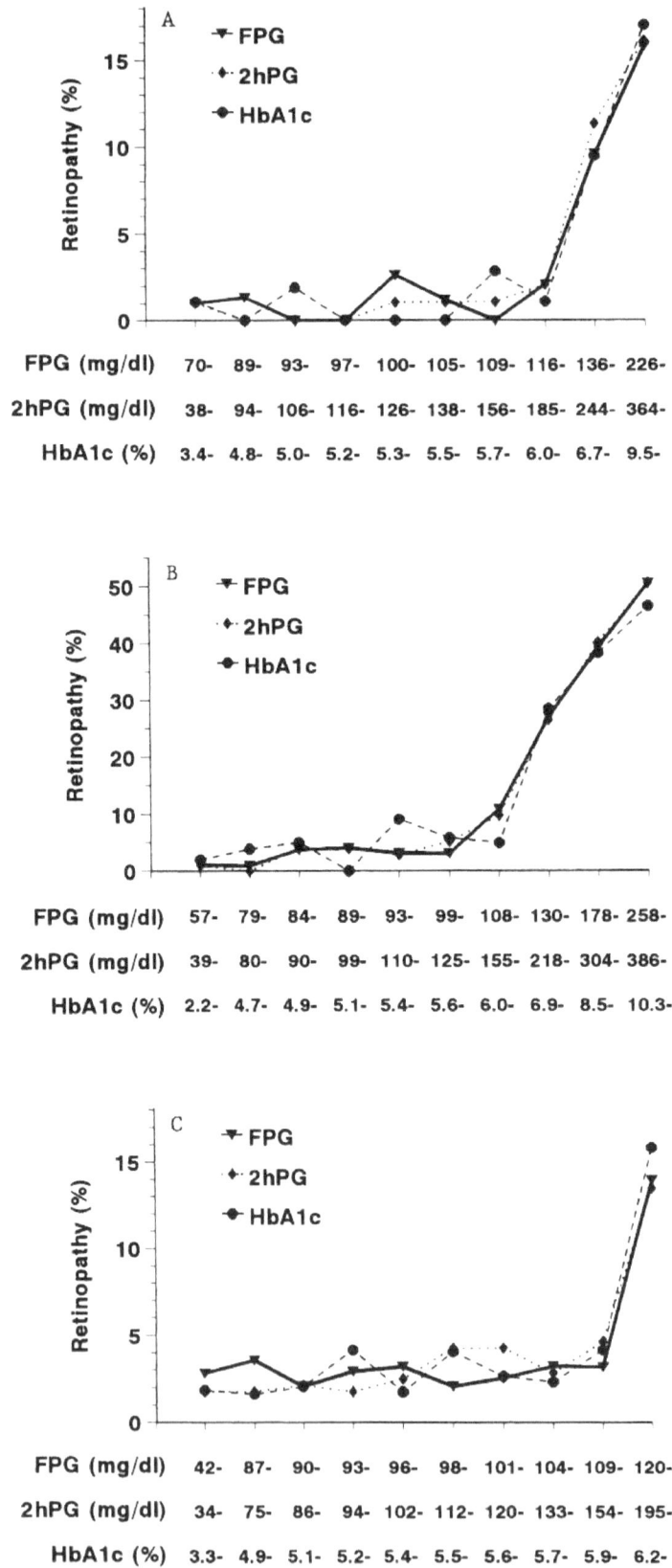

Figure 4: Prevalence of retinopathy by deciles of the distribution of FPG, 2hPG, and HbA1c in Pima Indians **(a)**, Egyptians **(b)** and in participants in NHANES III **(c)**. The figure was adapted from [44].

Table 2: The WHO 1999 definition for diabetes

	Venous plasma glucose (mmol/l)	
	FPG	**2hPG**
Diabetes	≥7.0	**or** ≥11.1
IGT	<7.0	**and** 7.8-11.0
IFG	6.1-6.9	**and** (if measured)<7.8

It was stated in the WHO 1999 recommendation that "for epidemiological or population screening purpose, the fasting or 2-hour value after 75g oral glucose load may be used alone. For clinical purpose, the diagnosis of diabetes should always be confirmed by repeating the test on another day unless there is unequivocal hyperglycemia with acute metabolic decompensation or obvious symptoms".This table was adapted from [9].

The prevalence of diabetes diagnosed using the FPG≥7.0 mmol/l criterion alone as compared with that using the 2hPG≥11.1 mmol/l criterion alone in 16 DECODE participating studies showed that in 7 studies the prevalence was lower with the FPG criterion but higher in the rest of the studies, with an overall change of 0.5% (95%CI 0.3%-0.8%) [45]. The changes in 18 Asian studies was, on the contrary, decreased in most of the studies with the FPG criterion, with an overall change of-1.8% (-2.3% to -1.4%) for population-based studies and -3.7% (-4.6% to -2.8%) in pre-selected hyperglycemic population [46]. There are marked discrepancies in reclassification of individuals between fasting and 2-hour glucose criteria. Among 1665 newly diagnosed diabetic European patients, diagnosed according to the 2-hour plasma glucose of ≥11.1 mmol/l and/or fasting plasma glucose of ≥7.0 mmol/l, only 489 (29%) diabetic individuals met the both criteria [47]. The concordance between IGT and IFG defined according to the fasting plasma glucose of 6.1-6.9 mmol/l [47] was even poorer, only 16%. Similar findings were also reported in the DECODA study [46]. The concordance between the two criteria was 37% for newly diagnosed diabetes; and 77% IGT individuals had a normal FPG value (<6.1 mmol/l) [46] (Table **3**). Therefore, diagnosis of diabetes based on the FPG criterion alone will miss individuals with diabetes and IGT based on the 2hPG values.

Table 3: Distribution of subjects according to the 2-h and the fasting glucose categories in people not previously diagnosed as diabetes from the DECODA population-based studies. Adapted from [46].

Fasting Glucose (mmol/l)	**2-h Glucose (mmol/l)**			
	<7.8	**7.8-11.0**	**≥11.1**	**Total**
<6.1	12443 (74.3)	1984 (11.9)	291 (1.7)	14718 (87.9)
6.1-6.9	621 (3.7)	476 (2.8)	255 (1.5)	1352 (8.1)
7.0-7.7	63 (0.4)	86 (0.5)	146 (0.9)	295 (1.8)
≥7.8	38 (0.2)	33 (0.2)	303 (1.8)	374 (2.2)
Total	13165 (78.6)	2579 (15.4)	995 (5.9)	16739 (100)

Figures are numbers (percentage of total).

In addition, the two studies have shown that post-load hyperglycemia increased more with aging, particularly in women [48, 49]. The prevalence of isolated post-load hyperglycemia (*i.e.,* 2-hour plasma glucose ≥11.1 mmol/l and fasting plasma glucose <7.0 mmol/l) was 0.7% in people who were 49 years of age or younger and 4.6% in those older than 70 years among Europeans. In contrast, the prevalence of isolated fasting hyperglycemia (*i.e.,* 2-hour plasma glucose <11.1 mmol/l and fasting plasma glucose ≥7.0 mmol/l) in these two age groups was 1.3% and 2.3%, respectively [50].

The prognosis of individuals with different degree of hyperglycemia was also widely investigated. Although the microvascular complications of diabetes cannot be equated with diabetes, they do represent a specific and relevant clinical endpoint. Intensive treatment to lower blood glucose levels in patients with diabetes has been approved to reduce the microvascular complications [51, 52]. However, most (about 50%) of the patients with type 2 diabetes died of CVD, primarily heart disease and stroke (http://www.who.int/mediacentre/factsheets/fs312/en/index.html). Studies that have examined the differences in CVD outcome and all-cause mortality in relation to fasting and 2h post-load hyperglycemia have unequivocally shown that post-load hyperglycemia could be of greater importance even in the non-diabetic ranges. In the DECODE study including 10 prospective European cohorts of 15388 men and 7126 women aged 30-89 years, with a median follow-up of 8.8 years, the researchers observed that the largest number of excess deaths was from individuals who had IGT but normal fasting glucose levels [53] (Fig. **5**). The DECODE study has also provided with convincing evidence showing that IGT is a better predictor for CVD mortality and morbidity than IFG [53-55] (Fig. **6**). Data from a Finnish study showed further that the prediction of the IGT to the future CHD was not explained by the development of diabetes during the follow-up [56]. In this Finnish study, 1234 men and 1386 women aged 45-64 years, who were free of diabetes at baseline examination, were followed up for 10 years. In subjects who had IGT at baseline and who did not progress to clinical diagnosed diabetes during the follow-up, the multivariate adjusted HR (95% CI) was 1.49 (0.95-2.34) for CHD incidence, 2.34 (1.42-3.85) for CVD mortality, and 1.65 (1.13-2.40) for all-cause mortality [56].

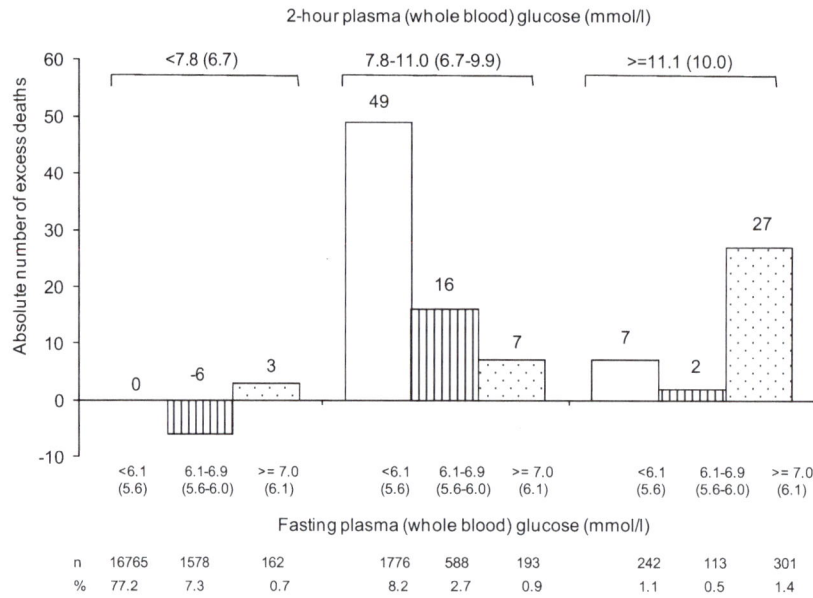

Figure 5: Estimated absolute number of excess cardiovascular deaths according to the duration of the follow-up, with reference to the fasting and the 2-hour glucose categories in subjects not previously known as diabetic. Number (n) and the total percentage of subjects in each glucose category are presented. Adapted from [53].

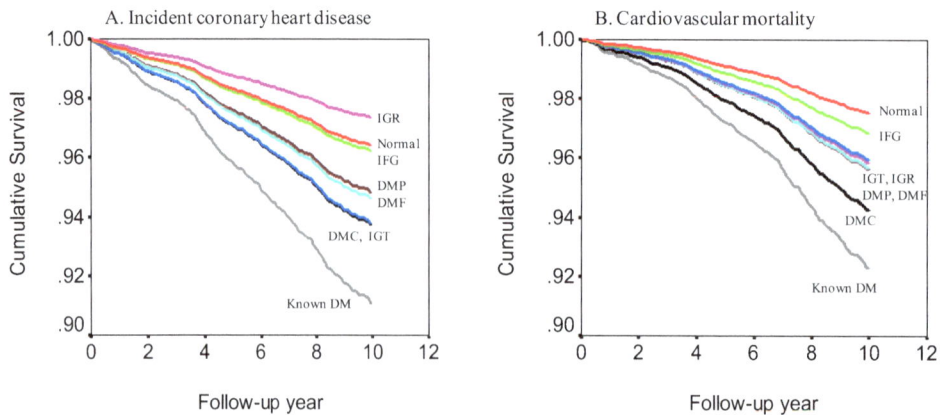

Figure 6: Cumulative survival curves for incidence of coronary heart disease **(A)** and for cardiovascular mortality **(B)** according to the glucose categories defined by both fasting and 2-h plasma glucose criteria. The cumulative survival is estimated from Cox proportional hazards models and adjusted for age, cohorts, sex, body mass index, blood pressure,

serum cholesterol and smoking. Normal=FPG <6.1 mmol/l and 2hPG<7.8 mmol/l; IFG=impaired fasting glucose only; IGT=impaired glucose tolerance only; IGR=impaired glucose regulation (IFG and IGT); DMF=undiagnosed diabetes by fasting glucose criteria alone (FPG≥7.0 mmol/l and 2hPG <11.1 mmol/l); DMP=undiagnosed diabetes by 2-h post-load glucose criteria alone (2hPG ≥11.1 mmol/l and FPG <7.0 mmol/l); DMC=undiagnosed diabetes by both fasting and 2-h glucose criteria combined (FPG ≥7.0 mmol/l and 2hPG ≥11.1 mmol/l); known DM=previously diagnosed diabetes. This figure was adapted from [56].

The relation between glucose levels and mortality of various causes was also investigated in details in the DECODE study [55]. Hazard ratio for all-cause mortality in individuals with newly diagnosed diabetes defined by the 2hPG criteria was 10% higher than in those diabetic defined according to the FPG criteria; individuals at upper range of the IGT had similar risk of death as those who met the FPG criteria for diabetes when both were compared with previous known diabetes (Fig. **7**). IFG did not convey an increased risk for various mortality. There was a J-shaped relation between mortality and glucose concentration for both FPG and 2hPG, except for the relation between 2hPG and CVD mortality (Fig. **8**). The risk of CVD death started to increase gradually far below the cut point for diabetes. There was no a threshold effect at which risk of death increase abruptly (Fig. **8**) [55].

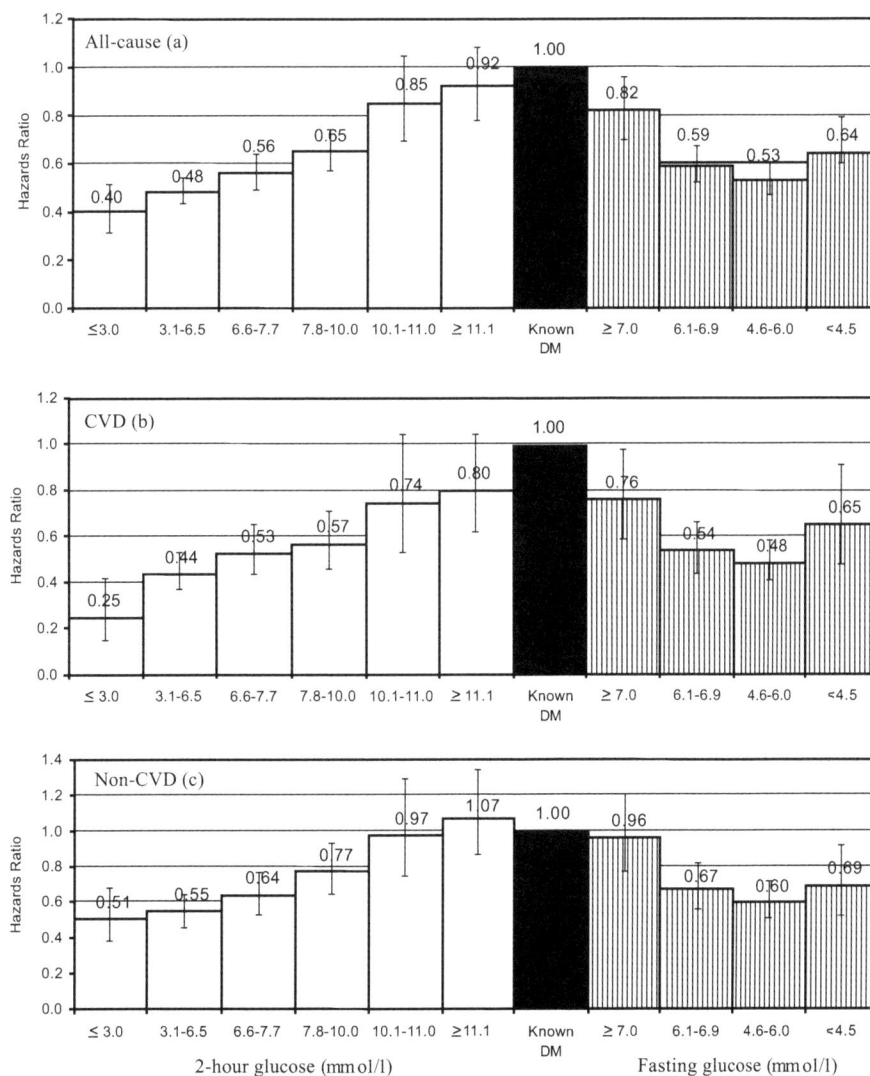

Figure 7: Hazard ratios (columns) and 95% CIs (vertical bars) for mortality from all causes **(a)**, CVD **(b)**, and non-CVD **(c)** for the FPG and 2hPG intervals using previously diagnosed diabetes as a common reference category, adjusted for age, sex, cohorts, BMI, systolic blood pressure, cholesterol, and smoking. Adapted from [55].

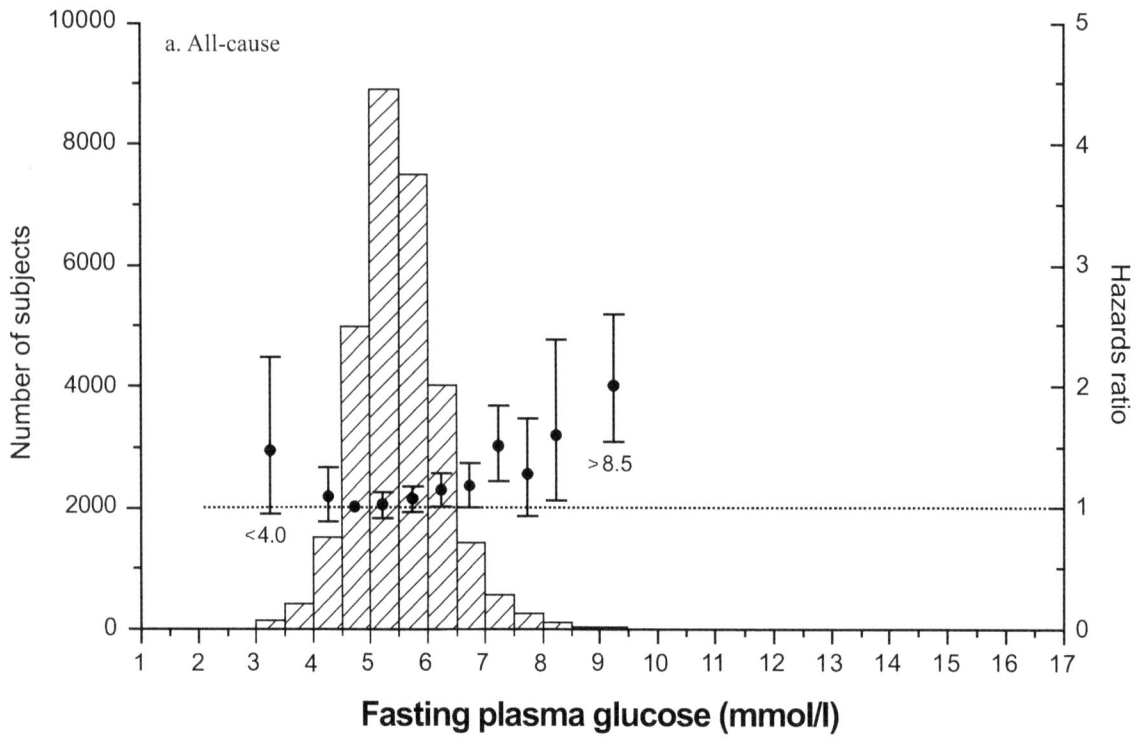

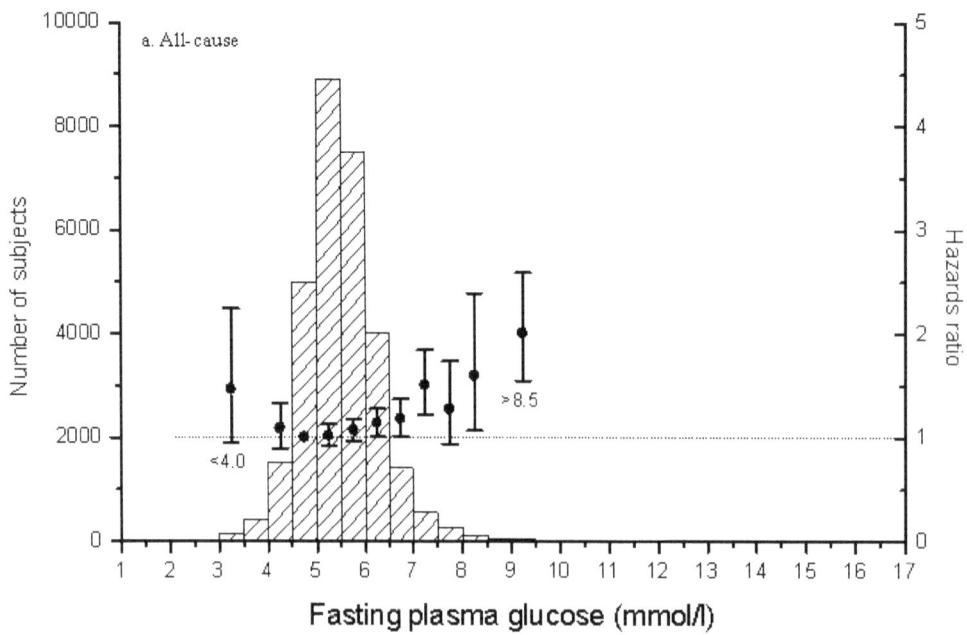

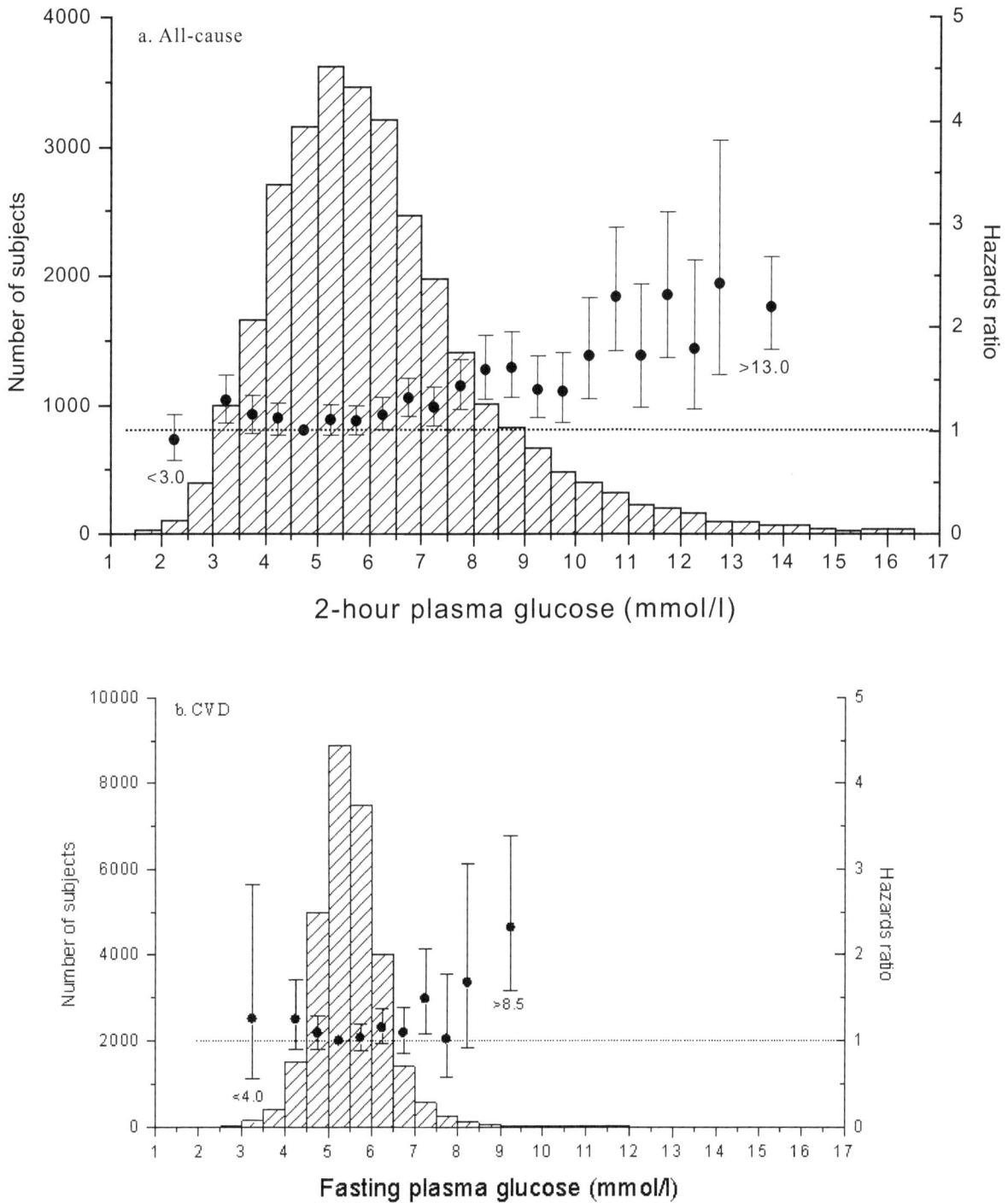

Figure 8: 2hPG and FPG distributions. Hazard ratios (dot) and 95% (vertical bars) for all-cause **(a)** and CVD **(b)** mortality according to glucose intervals of 0.5 mmol/l in subjects without previous history of diabetes, adjusted for age, sex, cohort, BMI, systolic blood pressure, cholesterol and smoking. This figure was adapted from [55].

In light of these findings and the reports from other studies since 1997, the ADA further revised the diagnostic criteria for diabetes in 2003 [57].

1.5.2. The Changes Made in 2003 by an ADA Expert Committee

The ADA Expert Committee recommended to remain the 1997 cut-off values for diagnosis of diabetes for both FPG and 2hPG, but to further lower the FPG cut-off value for IFG from 6.1-6.9 mmol/l to 5.6-6.9 mmol/l, in order to optimize its sensitivity for predicting future diabetes and to increase the proportion of those with IGT who can be identified by a FPG test [57]. The cut-off value for diagnosing IGT follows the previous definition. In addition, the Committee concludes that the FPG and 2hPG (but not the HbA1c test) remain the tests of choice for diagnosis of both their respective impaired states, as well as for the diagnosis of diabetes.

The ADA Expert Committee also acknowledged that to lower cut-off value for IFG will substantially increase the proportion of people with IFG, but the benefit of intervention targeting at these individuals is still not known, and need further researches. "There are obviously many aspects regarding the specific measurements of glycemia that are still unclear" [57].

The WHO and the International Diabetes Federation (IDF) subsequently organised a Consultation meeting in 2005 to reconsider the diagnostic criteria for diabetes. After careful review of the data the WHO/IDF Committee concluded to maintain the diagnostic criteria of the WHO 1999. The WHO/IDF Consultation Committee did not agree to lower FPG from 6.1 mmo/l to 5.6 mmol/l for IFG, because individuals identified by a lower FPG cut-off value have a more favourable CVD risk profiles and low risk of developing diabetes [58].

1.5.3. Diagnosis of Diabetes Based on the HbA1C Test-----ADA 2010 Position Statement

In 2008 an International Expert Committee, with members appointed by the ADA, the European Association for the Study of Diabetes (EASD), and the IDF, recommended the use of HbA1c assay for diagnosis of diabetes after review of both established and emerging epidemiological evidences that have led to the development of the diagnostic criteria for diabetes in the past decades. Several advantages of the HbA1c testing over the measurement of glucose have been identified including greater convenience, since fasting is not required, greater preanalytical stability, and less day-to-day perturbations during period of stress and illness, and a better marker of chronic glycemic exposure [59, 60]. The HbA1c test is, however, much more expensive, unavailable in certain regions of the developing world, less concordant with glucose results, and subject to measurement errors in the presence of certain forms of anemia and hemoglobinopathies, which may also have unique ethnic or geographic distributions [59, 60]. The HbA1c was not considered as a diagnostic test for diabetes previously in part due to lack of standardization of the assay. Considering the HbA1c assay has now been highly standardized, the International Expert Committee reached consensus to use of the HbA1c of ≥6.5% for the diagnosis of diabetes [59], and the ADA affirmed the decision in 2010 [60]. The diagnostic HbA1c cut-off value of 6.5% is associated with a change point for retinopathy prevalence, as are the diagnostic thresholds for FPG and 2hPG (Fig. **4**). This is also supported by the data from the DETECT-2 study (Evaluation of Screening and Early Detection Strategies for Type 2 Diabetes and Impaired Glucose Tolerance), a collaborative data analysis of 28 000 subjects from nine countries including the three presented in the Fig. **4** above [59]. In this study, the retinopathy was objectively assessed and graded by fundus photography. The data showed at the HbA1c of ≥6.5%, the prevalence of at least moderate retinopathy begins to rise (Fig. **9**) [59]. Among subjects who had HbA1c values <6.5%, moderate retinopathy was virtually nonexistent. The optimal cut-off value for detecting at least moderate retinopathy using the receive operating characteristic curve analysis of the same data was also at HbA1c of 6.5%.

In 2008, the International Expert Committee did not, however, define a category for intermediate hyperglycemia based on the HbA1c, which may bear an analogue to the categories of the IFG or IGT. In the ADA's 2010 Position Statement a category with HbA1c of 5.7%-6.4% has been introduced with an aim to identify individuals with high risk for future diabetes, and to initiate preventive intervention [60]. Although the definition was made somewhat arbitrarily because the risk of diabetes is a continuum, extending well into the normal ranges of the HbA1c, some evidences supporting the classification have been assembled by the ADA

[60]. Several prospective studies have shown that incidence of diabetes in people within the HbA1c range of 5.5-6.0% was three to eightfold higher than incidence in the U.S. population as a whole; data of the NHANES indicate that the HbA1c value that most accurately identifies people with IFG or IGT falls between 5.5% and 6.0%; and the evidence from the Diabetes Prevention Program (DPP) [38] has indirectly suggested that intervention targeting at people with HbA1c levels below or above 5.9% are effective because the mean HbA1c was 5.9% (SD 0.5%) among the DPP participants [60]. The ADA 2010 diagnostic criteria for diabetes and intermediate hyperglycemia are summarized below [60].

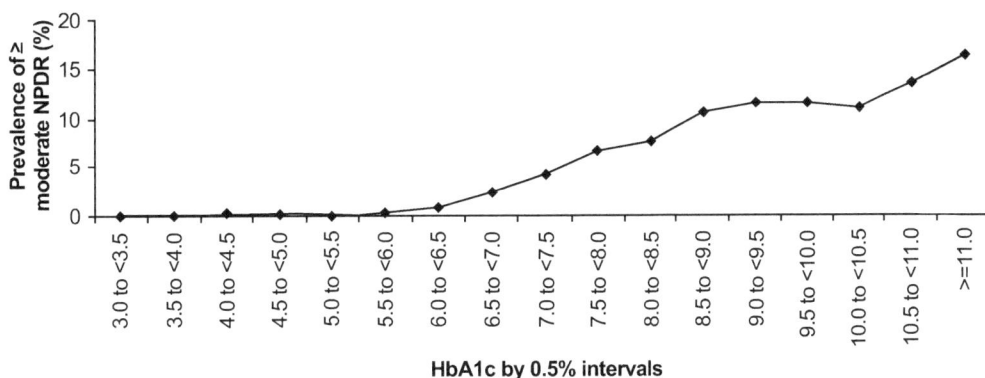

Figure 9: Prevalence of retinopathy by 0.5% intervals and severity of retinopathy in participants aged 20-79 years. NPDR, nonproliferative diabetic retinopathy. This figure was adapted from [59].

1.5.4. Criteria for the Diagnosis of Diabetes

1. HbA1c≥6.5%. The test should be performed in a laboratory using a method that is NGSP certified and standardized to the DCCT assay.*

   OR

2. FPG≥126 mg/dl (7.0 mmol/l). Fasting is defined as no caloric intake for at least 8 h. * OR

3. 2-h plasma glucose≥200 mg/dl (11.1 mmol/l) during an OGTT. The test should be performed as described by the World Health Organization, using a glucose load containing the equivalent of 75 g anhydrous glucose dissolved in water.*

   OR

4. In a patient with classic symptoms of hyperglycemia or hyperglycemic crisis, a random plasma glucose≥200 mg/dl (11.1 mmol/l).

1.5.5. Criteria for Categories of Increased Risk for Diabetes**

- FPG 100 mg/dl (5.6 mmol/l) to 125 mg/dl (6.9 mmol/l) (IFG).

- 2hPG in the 75-g OGTT 140 mg/dl (7.8 mmol/l) to 199 mg/dl (11.0 mmol/l)(IGT).

- HbA1c 5.7-6.4%.

Considering the discordance between the HbA1c and glucose tests, the ADA recommended the same test should be repeated for confirmation in patients who do not have a clinical symptom. In case two different

---

*In the absence of unequivocal hyperglycemia, criteria 1-3 should be confirmed by repeat testing.
NGSP, National Glycohemoglobin Standardization Program. DCCT, Diabetes Control and Complication Trial.
**For all three tests, risk is continuous, extending below the lower limit of the range and becoming disproportionately greater at higher ends of the range.

tests are available for one patient, if the two tests are both above the diagnostic threshold, a diagnosis of diabetes can be confirmed. When the results are discordant, the test whose result is above the diagnostic cut-off value should be repeated, and the diagnosis is made on the basis of the confirmed test [60]. As indicated by the ADA, further research is still needed to characterize patients whose glycemic status are categorised differently by two different tests (*e.g.,* glucose *vs.* HbA1c). The changes on the prevalence of diabetes in a population, and the clinical prognosis of the abnormal HbA1c categories (Diabetes and high risk category) as compared with those defined by the FPG or 2hPG criteria require further examination with prospective studies.

Following the publication of the ADA's Position Statement, an Expert Consultation Group was conveyed in 2010 by the WHO to consider the future means of diagnosis of diabetes. Diagnostic criteria based on plasma glucose values were reviewed in 2006 and were not revised in this update, and the recommendation for the HbA1c criteria was made (http://www.who.int/diabetes/publications/report-hba1c_2011.pdf).

"HbA1c can be used as a diagnostic test for diabetes providing that stringent quality assurance tests are in place and assays are standardised to criteria aligned to the international reference values, and there are no conditions present which preclude its accurate measurement.

An HbA1c of 6.5% is recommended as the cut point for diagnosing diabetes. A value of less than 6.5% does not exclude diabetes diagnosed using glucose tests.

Quality of evidence assessed by GRADE: moderate.

Strength of recommendation based on GRADE criteria: conditional".

The strength of the recommendation was based on the quality of evidence and feasibility and resource implications for low and middle-income countries. The strength of the recommendation is rated on a two-point scale:

- Weak/conditional: low/moderate/high quality of evidence and/or not applicable at population level in low-resource settings;

- Strong: high/moderate quality of evidence and applicable at population level in low-resource settings.

2. CLOSING WORDS

The diagnosis of type 2 diabetes has been proven to be difficult due to its heterogeneous nature, a long period of asymptomatic status and lack of a marker that denotes end-organ damage *per se*. All diagnostic criteria are made based on glycemic levels that are quantified using different assay methods. Hyperglycemia is a reflection of a complex dysfunctions in pancreases that results in insulin deficiency, and in liver and other tissues that impair the insulin action. Therefore, diabetes and intermediate hyperglycemia classified by different means are not completely concordant, and may have different clinical characteristics and prognostic implications. Future research is needed to improve the current means for diagnosis of diabetes.

REFERENCES

[1]   Kahn SE, Zraika S, Utzschneider KM, Hull RL. The beta cell lesion in type 2 diabetes: there has to be a primary functional abnormality. Diabetologia 2009; 52: 1003-12.
[2]   Mari A, Tura A, Natali A, *et al.* Impaired beta cell glucose sensitivity rather than inadequate compensation for insulin resistance is the dominant defect in glucose intolerance. Diabetologia 2010; 53: 749-56.
[3]   Jacobsen A. Untersuchungen iiber den Einfluss des Chloralhydrats auf experimentelle Hyperglykämieformen. Biochem Z 1913; 51: 443.

[4]　Klimt CR, Prout TE, Bradley RF, *et al.* Standardization of the oral glucose tolerance test. Report of the Committee on Statistics of the American Diabetes Association June 14, 1968. Diabetes 1969; 18: 299-307.

[5]　Mosenthal HO, Barry E. Criteria for and interpretation of normal glucose tolerance tests. Ann Intern Med 1950; 33: 1175-94.

[6]　Moyer JH, Womack CR. Glucose tolerance tests; relative validity of four different types of tests. Tex State J Med 1950; 46: 763-8.

[7]　Fajans SS, Conn JW. The early recognition of diabetes mellitus. Ann N Y Acad Sci 1959; 82: 208-18.

[8]　Unger RH. The standard two-hour oral glucose tolerance test in the diagnosis of diabetes mellitus in subjects without fasting hyperglycemia. Ann Intern Med 1957; 47: 1138-53.

[9]　Alberti KGMM, Aschner P, Assal JP, *et al.* WHO Consultation. Definition, diagnosis and classification of diabetes mellitus and its complications. Part 1: diagnosis and classification of diabetes mellitus. (Report No.: 99.2), World Health Organisation, Geneva: Switzerland 1999.

[10]　Hayner NS, Kjelsberg MO, Epstein FH, Francis T, Jr. Carbohydrate tolerance and diabetes in a total community, tecumseh, michigan. 1. Effects of age, sex, and test conditions on one-hour glucose tolerance in adults. Diabetes 1965;14:413-23.

[11]　Andres R. Relation of physiologic changes in aging to medical changes of disease in the aged. Mayo Clin Proc 1967; 42: 674-84.

[12]　Danowski TS, Aarons JH, Hydovitz JD, Wingert JP. Utility of equivocal glucose tolerances. Diabetes 1970; 19: 524-6.

[13]　Rushforth NB, Bennett PH, Steinberg AG, Burch TA, Miller M. Diabetes in the Pima Indians. Evidence of bimodality in glucose tolerance distributions. Diabetes 1971; 20: 756-65.

[14]　Bennett PH, Burch TA, Miller M. Diabetes mellitus in American (Pima) Indians. Lancet 1971; 298: 125-8.

[15]　Rushforth NB, Miller M, Bennett PH. Fasting and two-hour post-load glucose levels for the diagnosis of diabetes. The relationship between glucose levels and complications of diabetes in the Pima Indians. Diabetologia 1979; 16: 373-9.

[16]　Rosenthal M, McMahan CA, Stern MP, *et al.* Evidence of bimodality of two hour plasma glucose concentrations in Mexican Americans: results from the San Antonio Heart study. J Chronic Dis 1985; 38: 5-16.

[17]　Zimmet P, Whitehouse S. Bimodality of fasting and two-hour glucose tolerance distributions in a Micronesian population. Diabetes 1978; 27: 793-800.

[18]　Raper LR, Taylor R, Zimmet P, Milne B, Balkau B. Bimodality in glucose tolerance distributions in the urban Polynesian population of Western Samoa. Diabetes Res 1984; 1: 19-26.

[19]　Knowler WC, Pettitt DJ, Saad MF, Bennett PH. Diabetes mellitus in the Pima Indians: incidence, risk factors and pathogenesis. Diabetes Metab Rev 1990; 6: 1-27.

[20]　Pettitt DJ, Knowler WC, Lisse JR, Bennett PH. Development of retinopathy and proteinuria in relation to plasma-glucose concentrations in Pima Indians. Lancet 1980; 316: 1050-2.

[21]　Sayegh HA, Jarrett RJ. Oral glucose-tolerance tests and the diagnosis of diabetes: results of a prospective study based on the Whitehall survey. Lancet 1979; 314: 431-3.

[22]　Jarrett RJ, Keen H. Hyperglycemia and diabetes mellitus. Lancet 1976; 308: 1009-12.

[23]　National Diabetes Data Group. Classification and diagnosis of diabetes mellitus and other categories of glucose intolerance. National Diabetes Data Group. Diabetes 1979; 28: 1039-57.

[24]　WHO Expert Committee. WHO Expert Committee on Diabetes Mellitus: second report. World Health Organ Tech Rep Ser 1980; 646: 1-80.

[25]　Alberti KGMM, Assal JP, Baba S, *et al.* World Health Organisation. Diabetes Mellitus: Report of a Study Group. (Tech Rep Ser no. 727). World Health Organisation, Geneva: Switzerland 1985.

[26]　Bennett PH, Rushforth NB, Miller M, LeCompte PM. Epidemiologic studies of diabetes in the Pima Indians. Recent Prog Horm Res1976; 32: 333-76.

[27]　O'Sullivan JB, Mahan CM. Prospective study of 352 young patients with chemical diabetes. N Engl J Med 1968; 278: 1038-41.

[28]　Malins JM, FitzGerald MG, Gaddie R, *et al.* Birmingham Diabetes Survey Working Party. A diabetic survey: report of a working party appointed by the College of General Practitioners. Br Med J 1962;I:1497-503.

[29]　Crombie DL, Pike LA, Pinsent RJFH, *et al.* Birmingham Diabetes Survey Working Party. Five-year follow-up report on the Birmingham diabetes survey of 1962. Report by the Birmingham Diabetes Survey Working Party. Br Med J 1970; 3: 301-5.

[30]　Crombie DL, Pike LA, Malins JM, FitzGerald MG, Goodwin RP, Thompson J. Birmingham Diabetes Survey Working Party. Ten-year follow-up report on Birmingham Diabetes Survey of 1961. Report by the Birmingham Diabetes Survey Working Party. Br Med J 1976; 2: 35-7.

[31]   Jarrett RJ, Keen H. Diabetes and Atherosclerosis. In: Keen H, Jarrett RJ, editors. Complications of Diabetes. London: Edward Arnold 1976.

[32]   Keen H, Jarrett RJ. The effect of carbohydrate tolerance on plasma lipids and atherosclerosis in man. In: Jones RH, editor. Artherosclerosis, Proc II Symp. Berlin: Springer-Verlag; 1976.

[33]   Sharp CL, Butterfiled WJH, Keen H. Diabetes Survey in Bedford. Proc R Soc Med 1964; 57: 193.

[34]   Jarrett RJ, Keen H, Fuller JH, McCartney M. Worsening to diabetes in men with impaired glucose tolerance ("borderline diabetes"). Diabetologia 1979; 16: 25-30.

[35]   Gerstein HC, Santaguida P, Raina P, *et al.* Annual incidence and relative risk of diabetes in people with various categories of dysglycemia: A systematic overview and meta-analysis of prospective studies. Diabetes Res Clin Pract 2007; 78: 305-12.

[36]   Pan X, Li G, Hu Y, *et al.* Effects of diet and exercise in preventing NIDDM in people with impaired glucose tolerance. The Da Qing IGT and Diabetes Study. Diabetes Care 1997; 20: 537-44.

[37]   Tuomilehto J, Lindstrom J, Eriksson JG, *et al.* Prevention of type 2 diabetes mellitus by changes in lifestyle among subjects with impaired glucose tolerance. N Engl J Med 2001; 344: 1343-50.

[38]   Knowler WC, Barrett-Connor E, Fowler SE, *et al.* Diabetes prevention program research group. Reduction in the incidence of type 2 diabetes with lifestyle intervention or metformin. N Engl J Med 2002; 346: 393-403.

[39]   Ramachandran A, Snehalatha C, Mary S, Mukesh B, Bhaskar AD, Vijay V. The Indian Diabetes Prevention Programme shows that lifestyle modification and metformin prevent type 2 diabetes in Asian Indian subjects with impaired glucose tolerance (IDPP-1). Diabetologia 2006; 49: 289-97.

[40]   Eriksson KF, Lindgarde F. Prevention of type 2 (non-insulin-dependent) diabetes mellitus by diet and physical exercise. The 6-year Malmo feasibility study. Diabetologia 1991; 34: 891-8.

[41]   Kosaka K, Noda M, Kuzuya T. Prevention of type 2 diabetes by lifestyle intervention: a Japanese trial in IGT males. Diabetes Res Clin Pract 2005; 67: 152-62.

[42]   Li G, Zhang P, Wang J, *et al.* The long-term effect of lifestyle interventions to prevent diabetes in the China Da Qing Diabetes Prevention Study: a 20-year follow-up study. Lancet 2008; 371: 1783-9.

[43]   Lindstrom J, Ilanne-Parikka P, Peltonen M, *et al.* Sustained reduction in the incidence of type 2 diabetes by lifestyle intervention: follow-up of the Finnish Diabetes Prevention Study. Lancet 2006; 368: 1673-9.

[44]   Expert committee on the diagnosis and classification of diabetes mellitus. Report of the Expert committee on the diagnosis and classification of diabetes mellitus. Diabetes Care 1997; 20: 1183-97.

[45]   Borch-Johnsen K, Tuomilehto J, Balkau B, *et al.* The DECODE Study Group. Will new diagnostic criteria for diabetes mellitus change phenotype of patients with diabetes? Reanalysis of European epidemiological data. DECODE Study Group on behalf of the European Diabetes Epidemiology Study Group. BMJ 1998; 317: 371-5.

[46]   Qiao Q, Nakagami T, Tuomilehto J, *et al.* Comparison of the fasting and the 2-hour glucose criteria for diabetes in different Asian cohorts. Diabetologia 2000; 43: 1470-5.

[47]   Borch-Johnsen K, Tuomilehto J, Balkau B, Qiao Q. The DECODE Study Group. Is fasting glucose sufficient to define diabetes? Epidemiological data from 20 European studies. The DECODE-study group. European Diabetes Epidemiology Group. Diabetes Epidemiology: Collaborative analysis of Diagnostic Criteria in Europe. Diabetologia 1999; 42: 647-54.

[48]   Qiao Q, Hu G, Tuomilehto J, Eriksson J. The DECODE Study Group. Age-and Sex-Specific Prevalences of Diabetes and Impaired Glucose Regulation in 13 European Cohorts. Diabetes Care 2003; 26: 61-9.

[49]   Qiao Q, Hu G, Tuomilehto J, Nakagami T, *et al.* The DECODA Study Group. Age-and Sex-Specific Prevalences of Diabetes and Impaired Glucose Regulation in 11 Asian Cohorts. Diabetes Care 2003; 26: 1770-80.

[50]   Qiao Q, Tuomilehto J, Borch-Johnsen K. Post-challenge hyperglycemia is associated with premature death and macrovascular complications. Diabetologia 2003; 46 (Suppl1):M17-M21.

[51]   Shamoon H, Duffy H, FleischerN, *et al.* The diabetes control and complications trial research group. The effect of intensive treatment of diabetes on the development and progression of long-term complications in insulin-dependent diabetes mellitus. N Engl J Med 1993; 329: 977-86.

[52]   Turner R. UK Prospective Diabetes Study Group. Tight blood pressure control and risk of macrovascular and microvascular complications in type 2 diabetes: UKPDS 38. UK Prospective Diabetes Study Group. BMJ 1998; 317: 703-13.

[53]   Qiao Q, Tuomilehto J. The DECODE Study Group. Glucose tolerance and cardiovascular mortality: comparison of fasting and 2-hour diagnostic criteria. Arch Intern Med 2001; 161: 397-405.

[54]   Qiao Q, Pyorala K, Pyorala M, *et al.* Two-hour glucose is a better risk predictor for incident coronary heart disease and cardiovascular mortality than fasting glucose. Eur Heart J 2002; 23: 1267-75.

[55] Qiao Q, Tuomilehto J, Moltchanova E, Balkau B, Borch-Johnsen K. The DECODE Study Group. Is the current definition for diabetes relevant to mortality risk from all-cause, cardiovascular and non-cardiovascular disease? Diabetes Care 2003; 26: 688-96.

[56] Qiao Q, Jousilahti P, Eriksson J, Tuomilehto J. Predictive properties of impaired glucose tolerance for cardiovascular risk are not explained by the development of overt diabetes during follow-up. Diabetes Care 2003; 26: 2910-4.

[57] Genuth S, Alberti K.G.M.M., Bennett PH, *et al.* The expert committee on the diagnosis and classification of diabetes mellitus. Follow-up report on the diagnosis of diabetes mellitus. Diabetes Care 2003; 26: 3160-7.

[58] Alberti KGMM, Bennett PH, Borch-Johnsen K *et al.* World Health Organization and International Diabetes Federation. Definition and diagnosis of diabetes mellitus and intermediate hyperglycemia: report of a WHO/IDF consultation. Geneva: Switzerland 2006.

[59] Nathan DM, Balkau B, Bonora E, *et al.* International Expert Committee report on the role of the HbA1c assay in the diagnosis of diabetes. Diabetes Care 2009; 32: 1327-34.

[60] Inzucchi S, Bergenstal R, Fonseca V, *et al.* Diagnosis and classification of diabetes mellitus. Diabetes Care 2010; 33 (Suppl 1): S62-9.

CHAPTER 2

Prevalence of Type 2 Diabetes

Weiguo Gao[*]

Department of Public Health, Hjelt Institute, University of Helsinki, Helsinki, Finland; Department of Chronic Disease Prevention, National Institute for Health and Welfare, Helsinki, Finland and Qingdao Endocrine & Diabetes Hospital, Qingdao, China.

Abstract: Type 2 diabetes mellitus, with an increasing prevalence in both developing and developed countries, has become one of the major health threats to the human being. According to the International Diabetes Federation (IDF), the number of patients with diabetes is 285 million in the year of 2010 and will rise to 438 million in 2030. The greater increase will occur in the developing countries than in developed world. Most recent data have shown that the prevalence of diabetes increased about 9 folds from 1980 (1.0%) to 2008 (9.7%) in China. This explosive increase in prevalence of diabetes is mostly attributed to the increase in risk profiles at a population level including population aging, obesity, physically inactive and unhealthy diet. Diabetes prevention programs that target lifestyle intervention are urgently needed.

Keywords: Type 2 diabetes, prevalence, secular trend, risk factors.

2.1. PREVALENCE OF TYPE 2 DIABETES

Over the past decades, numerous studies have performed in different populations and regions all over the world to determine the prevalence of diabetes (WHO Global Infobase, https://apps.who.int/infobase/Indicators.aspx, accessed 26 July 2010). The results suggested that type 2 diabetes has become one of the major health threats globally. Although, currently, it is still lower than 4% in communities in traditional societies or in remote areas such as in a few African and Asian countries, the prevalence of diabetes was about 4%-10% in the adults aged 20-79 years in most regions of the worlds such as in Europe, Australia, most of the Asian and American countries (Fig. **1**) (prevalence of diabetes worldwide, http://www.who.int/diabetes/facts/world_figures/en/print.html, Accessed 21 July, 2010) [1-3]. In Bahrain, Saudi Arabia, United Arab Emirates, Singapore, Poland, Kirbati, and Nauru, the rate has reached 15%-30% [3, 4]. Globally, it was estimated that there are about 285 million adults (aged 20-79 years) with diabetes in the world in 2010, given a prevalence of 6.6% on average [3].

It is worthy of note that the proportion of undiagnosed diabetes is about 50% in most studies, conducted in either developed or developing regions. For example, it is about 40% in the United States [5], 54-60% in Indian [6, 7], 61% in China [8], and reached 80% in some African countries [9, 10]. Therefore, there is a need to organise screening programs to detect undiagnosed diabetes in order to provide with early treatment to reduce the diabetic complications.

2.2. INCREASING TREND IN PREVALENCE OF TYPE 2 DIABETES

There is an evident increasing trend in the prevalence of diabetes all over the world. As summarized in Table **1**, this increasing trend can be observed in either developed or developing countries. In the United State, for example, the National Health and Nutrition Examination Surveys (NHANES) revealed that the prevalence of diabetes was more than doubled from 1976-1980 (5.3%) to 2005-2006 (12.6%). In Greece and Mauritius, the prevalence rate increased almost 0.5% each year. Based on the current occurrence of the disease it has been estimated that the prevalence of diabetes will keep increasing and the number of diabetic patients will increase to 438 millions in 2030 in the world [3, 4, 11-13].

*Address correspondence to Weiguo Gao: Department of Public Health, Hjelt Institute, University of Helsinki, PL41, Mannerheimintie 172, 00014, Helsinki, Finland; Email: gwg1974@hotmail.com

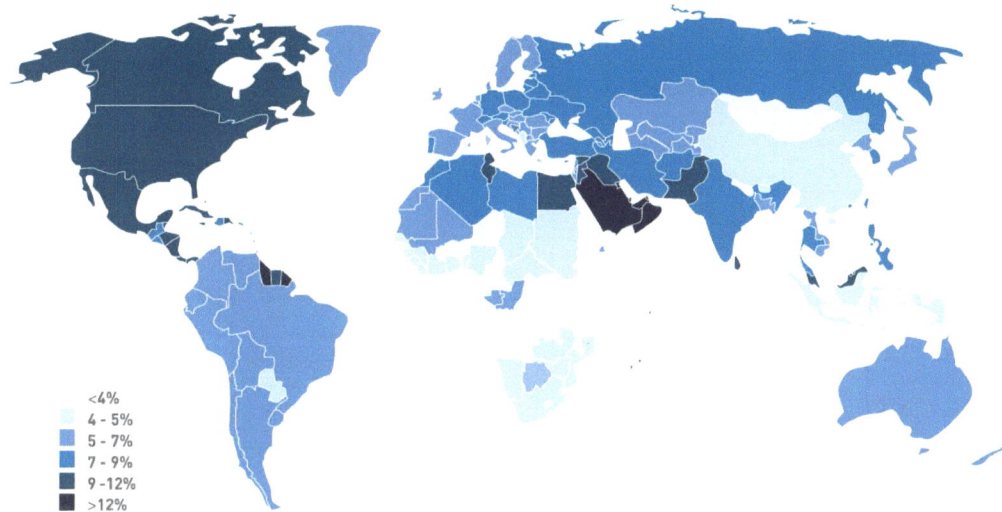

Figure 1: Prevalence estimates of diabetes (age 20-79 years), 2010. Adopted from Diabetes Atlas fourth edition [3].

Table 1: Secular increasing trend in prevalence of diabetes in different regions

Region	Age Range (years)	Prevalence (%)	Study Design	References
United States				
1976-1980	20-74	5.3	Series of cross-sectional population-based surveys	[14]
1988-1994	20-74	7.5		[5]
1999-2000	20-74	8.2		
2005-2006	20-74	12.6		
Western Samoa				
1978	25-74	7.2	Series of cross-sectional population-based surveys	[15]
1991	25-74	11.4		
Poole, United Kingdom				
1983	≥ 13	0.8	Series of surveys based on population-based diabetes registration	[16]
1988	≥ 13	0.9		
1996	≥ 13	1.5		
Netherlands				
1998	All ages	2.2	Series of surveys based on population-based diabetes registration	[17]
2000	All ages	2.9		
Nord-Trøndelag, Norway				
1984-1986	≥ 20	2.9	Series of whole population-based surveys	[18]
1995-1997	≥ 20	3.2		
Ontario, Canada				
1995	≥ 20	5.2	Series of surveys based on population-based diabetes registration	[19]
2005	≥ 20	8.8		
Skaraborg, Sweden				
From 1991 to 1995	All ages	Increased by 6%	Series of surveys based on population-based diabetes registration	[20]

		each year		
Laxå, Sweden				
1988-1992	35-79	2.8 in women 2.6 in men	Series of surveys based on population-based diabetes registration	[21]
1993-1997	35-79	4.5 in women 4.6 in men		
1998-2001	35-79	4.4 in women 4.5 in men		
Salamis, Greece				
2002	≥ 20	8.7	Series of cross-sectional population-based surveys	[22]
2006	≥ 20	10.3		
Mauritius				
1987	25-74	12.8	Series of cross-sectional population-based surveys	[23]
1992	25-74	15.2		
1998	25-74	17.9		
Singapore				
1992	18-69	8.6	Series of cross-sectional population-based surveys	[24]
1998	18-69	9.0		
Qingdao, China				
2001-2002	35-74	12.2	Series of cross-sectional population-based surveys	[25]
2006	35-74	18.8		

It has been recognized that the low- and middle-income countries face the greater increase of diabetes than developed countries. The Chennai Urban Rural Epidemiology Study (CURES) in India revealed that the prevalence of diabetes increased by 72.3% from 1989 (8.3%) to 2004 (14.3%) [7, 26-28]. Two population-based cross-sectional studies, conducted in Qingdao, China applying 2-hour 75g oral glucose tolerance test for diagnosis of diabetes, showed that the prevalence of diabetes increased from 12.2% to 18.8% within 5 years among people aged 35-74 years [25]. In spite of different criteria applied to diagnose diabetes among studies, the age standardized prevalence of diabetes has dramatically increased nationwide in China from 1980s to 2008 [8, 29-34] (Fig. **2**). As predicted by King H *et al.*, the number of diabetes will have a 170% increase in the developing countries, while 42% increase in the developed countries from 1995 to 2025 [35].

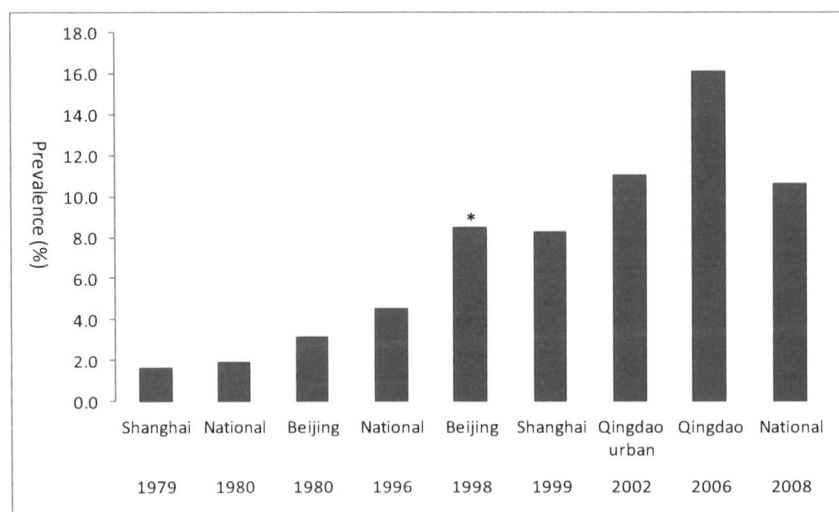

Figure 2: The age-standardized prevalence of diabetes in Chinese adults (aged 30 - 74 years old) from the early 1980s to 2008 in different regions. * The age of the subjects was 40 - 74 years old. Diabetes was defined according to FPG $\geq$ 7.8 mmol/l and/or 2hPG $\geq$ 11.1 mmol/l in the surveys made before 1998; and FPG $\geq$ 7.0 mmol/l and/or 2hPG $\geq$ 11.1 mmol/l for the surveys made since 1998.

2.3. RISK FACTORS ASSOCIATED WITH THE EPIDEMIC OF TYPE 2 DIABETES

As a multi-causes disorder, many kinds of environmental and lifestyle factors have contributed to the development of diabetes in addition to the genetic background. Population aging, the increasing trend in obesity, physical inactivity, and unhealthy diet are considered as the major contributor to the increasing prevalence of diabetes.

2.3.1. Non-Diabetic Hyperglycemia

Individuals with non-diabetic hyperglycemia, particularly those with Impaired Glucose Tolerance (IGT) and Impaired Fasting Glucose (IFG) are at increased risk to develop diabetes. About 5-12% of individuals with IGT develop diabetes per year [36]; the annual risk to progress from IFG or IGT to diabetes was 5 to 6-folds higher compared with the individuals without both the conditions [37]. The prevalence of non-diabetic hyperglycemia was also increasing worldwide. In Australia the prevalence of IGT increased from 2.9% in 1981 to 6.0% in 1992 and to 10.6% in 2000. In Qingdao, a city of China, the prevalence of IFG/IGT was doubled from 2001 (15.4%) to 2006 (28.7%) [25]. According to the IDF Altas, the global prevalence of IGT was estimated to be 7.9% in 2010, which will increase continuously to 8.4% in 2030 [3]. If this increasing trend continues the number of individuals with diabetes will certainly rise.

2.3.2. Obesity Epidemic

Type 2 diabetes is strongly associated with obesity and weight gain. The measurements of obesity, such as Body Mass Index (BMI), waist circumference, waist to hip ratio, whole or visceral fat mass *etc.*, have been reported to be positively associated with both prevalence and incidence of diabetes in numerous studies [38-43]. Weight gain during the follow-up and the duration of obesity was significantly related to an increased risk of incident diabetes in Pima Indians, in American Nurses Study and in a British prospective study in middle-aged men [44-49]. Strong evidences from the clinical trials have confirmed that the weight reduction can prevent or delay the onset of diabetes [50-52] among individuals with the IGT.

According to the WHO Consultation on Obesity, the global prevalence of obesity has been increasing rapidly since 1990s. The data from the US NHANES showed that the prevalence of obesity increased from 22.9% in 1988-1994 to 30.5% in 1998-2002, and most recently 33.8% [53-54]. In Finland, the mean level of BMI in men has been continuously increasing from 26.0 kg/m^2 in 1972 to 27.6 kg/m^2 in 2007 [55]; and in Chinese, who were considered as lean population, the proportion of overweight (BMI of 25-29kg/m^2) adults increased by 39% between 1992 and 2002, and the prevalence of obesity (BMI $\geq$ 30 kg/m^2) doubled [56].

2.3.3. Physical Inactivity

People with sedentary lifestyle have been consistently reported to have a high risk for diabetes in different populations [57-60]. Prolonged television watching, as a surrogate of sedentary lifestyle, was reported to be positively associated with diabetes risk [61-63]. The risk of developing diabetes among American men watching TV > 40 hour per week was 187% higher than among those spending 0-1 hour per week [61]; while in women, every 2 hour per day increment in television watching was associated with a 14% increase in risk of diabetes [62]. On the contrary, a higher level of physical activity was associated with a lower risk for developing diabetes [64-73]. Moreover, the clinical trials among Chinese, Europeans, Indians have shown that moderate physical activity reduced the progression of IGT to diabetes by 30-58% [50-52, 74-77]. There's no doubt that physical inactivity is an important modifiable risk factor of type 2 diabetes.

According to the WHO, 17% adults is physically inactive, and 31%-51% of the people do not have sufficient physical activity (< 2.5 hours per week of moderate activity) (Global Strategy on Diet, Physical Activity and Health, http://www.who.int/dietphysicalactivity/publications/facts/pa/en/. Accessed 12 August 2010). Physical inactivity is now also common in developing countries. The total physical activity decreased by 32% between 1991 and 2006 in Chinese adults, and currently there is only about 10% of Chinese adults reporting to be physically active in their leisure time [78-80].

2.3.4. Unhealthy Diet

Excess caloric intake, which results in a positive energy balance, promotes the onset of both obesity and diabetes. The westernized dietary pattern, which is rich in saturated fat and simple carbohydrate, and scarce in fibres, was suggested to be associated with a high risk of type 2 diabetes [81-84]. On the contrary, a low risk for diabetes was observed in people consuming high amount of vegetables, fruits, whole grain products, and fish, which are characterized by low energy density and low glycemic index but high fibre and unsaturated fat acid [85-90]. The antioxidant such as vitamin C and E, unsaturated fat acid, flavonoid, might also have protective effect [87, 91-93]. Dietary intervention, plus moderate or intensive physical activity have been proved to be effective on the prevention of diabetes [50-52].

Globally, food supply is becoming increasingly energy-dense, sweet, much processed, and fat-rich but fibre-short. In developed countries such as in the USA, increased portion sizes, fasting food, snacks, sweetened beverages are eating pattern shifts [94-99]. In China, the unhealthy diet transition has been reported to be increased consumption of edible oils and animal-source foods, accompanied with decreased intake of vegetable and/or fruit [100, 101].

In conclusion, the prevalence of type 2 diabetes, which casts a devastating effect on human health and social-economic development, is already high in some regions and will continue to increase all over the world. Although it is difficult to determine how much of each risk factor contributing to the increment in the prevalence of diabetes, it is clear that the increased prevalence of diabetes is associated with the rising risk profile at the population level. Lifestyle intervention program, which aims at controlling obesity, increasing consumption of healthy food and physical activity, is urgently needed to prevent the epidemic of diabetes.

REFERENCES

[1]   Qiao Q, Hu G, Tuomilehto J, *et al.* for The DECODE Study Group. Age-and sex-specific prevalences of diabetes and impaired glucose regulation in 13 European cohorts. Diabetes Care 2003; 26: 61-9.

[2]   Qiao Q, Hu G, Nakagami T, *et al.* for the DECODA Study Group. Age-and sex-specific prevalence of diabetes and impaired glucose regulation in 11 Asian cohorts. Diabetes Care 2003; 26: 1770-80.

[3]   Unwin N, Whiting D, Gan D, *et al.* International Diabetes Federation. IDF Diabetes Atlas Fourth Edition. International Diabetes Federation. Brussels: Belgium 2009.

[4]   Mbanya JC, Gan D, Allgot B, *et al.* International Diabetes Federation. Diabetes Atlas Third Edtion. International Diabetes Federation. Brussels: Belgium 2006.

[5]   Cowie CC, Rust KF, Ford ES, *et al.* Full accounting of diabetes and pre-diabetes in the U.S. population in 1988-1994 and 2005-2006. Diabetes Care 2009; 32: 287-94.

[6]   Menon VU, Kumar KV, Gilchrist A, *et al.* Prevalence of known and undetected diabetes and associated risk factors in central Kerala--ADEPS. Diabetes Res Clin Pract 2006; 74: 289-94.

[7]   Mohan V, Deepa M, Deepa R, *et al.* Secular trends in the prevalence of diabetes and impaired glucose tolerance in urban South India--the Chennai Urban Rural Epidemiology Study (CURES-17). Diabetologia 2006; 49: 1175-8.

[8]   Yang W, Lu J, Weng J, *et al.* Prevalence of diabetes among men and women in China. N Engl J Med 2010; 362: 1090-101.

[9]   Aspray TJ, Mugusi F, Rashid S, *et al.* Rural and urban differences in diabetes prevalence in Tanzania: the role of obesity, physical inactivity and urban living. Trans R Soc Trop Med Hyg 2000; 94: 637-44.

[10]   Motala AA, Esterhuizen T, Gouws E, Pirie FJ, Omar MAK. Diabetes and other disorders of glycemia in a rural south african community. Diabetes Care 2008; 31: 1783-8.

[11]   McCarty DJ, Zimmet P. Diabetes 1994 to 2010:Global estimates and projections. Melbourne: International Diabetes Institute1994.

[12]   Amos AF, McCarty DJ, Zimmet P. The rising global burden of diabetes and its complications: estimates and projections to the year 2010. Diabet Med 1997; 14: S1-85.

[13]   Wild S, Roglic G, Green A, Sicree R, King H. Global prevalence of diabetes: estimates for the year 2000 and projections for 2030. Diabetes Care 2004; 27: 1047-53.

[14]   Gregg EW, Cadwell BL, Cheng YJ, *et al.* Trends in the prevalence and ratio of diagnosed to undiagnosed diabetes according to obesity levels in the U.S. Diabetes Care 2004;27:2806-12.

[15]   Collins VR, Dowse GK, Toelupe PM, *et al.* Increasing prevalence of NIDDM in the Pacific island population of Western Samoa over a 13-year period. Diabetes Care 1994; 17: 288-96.

[16]   Gatling W, Budd S, Walters D, *et al.* Evidence of an increasing prevalence of diagnosed diabetes mellitus in the Poole area from 1983 to 1996. Diabet Med 1998; 15: 1015-21.

[17]   Ubink-Veltmaat LJ, Bilo HJ, Groenier KH, *et al.* Prevalence, incidence and mortality of type 2 diabetes mellitus revisited: a prospective population-based study in The Netherlands (ZODIAC-1). Eur J Epidemiol 2003; 18: 793-800.

[18]   Midthjell K, Kruger O, Holmen J, *et al.* Rapid changes in the prevalence of obesity and known diabetes in an adult Norwegian population. The Nord-Trondelag Health Surveys: 1984-1986 and 1995-1997. Diabetes Care 1999; 22: 1813-20.

[19]   Lipscombe LL, Hux JE. Trends in diabetes prevalence, incidence, and mortality in Ontario, Canada 1995-2005: a population-based study. Lancet 2007; 369: 750-6.

[20]   Berger B, Stenstrom G, Sundkvist G. Incidence, prevalence, and mortality of diabetes in a large population. A report from the Skaraborg Diabetes Registry. Diabetes Care 1999; 22: 773-8.

[21]   Jansson SP, Andersson DK, Svardsudd K. Prevalence and incidence rate of diabetes mellitus in a Swedish community during 30 years of follow-up. Diabetologia 2007; 50: 703-10.

[22]   Gikas A, Sotiropoulos A, Panagiotakos D, *et al.* Rising prevalence of diabetes among Greek adults: findings from two consecutive surveys in the same target population. Diabetes Res Clin Pract 2008; 79: 325-9.

[23]   Soderberg S, Zimmet P, Tuomilehto J, *et al.* Increasing prevalence of Type 2 diabetes mellitus in all ethnic groups in Mauritius. Diabet Med 2005; 22: 61-8.

[24]   Lee WR. The changing demography of diabetes mellitus in Singapore. Diabetes Res Clin Pract 2000; 50 (Suppl 2): S35-9.

[25]   Gao WG, Dong YH, Pang ZC, *et al.* Increasing trend in the prevalence of Type 2 diabetes and pre-diabetes in the Chinese rural and urban population in Qingdao, China. Diabet Med 2009; 26: 1220-7.

[26]   Ramachandran A, Snehalatha C, Dharmaraj D, Viswanathan M. Prevalence of glucose intolerance in Asian Indians. Urban-rural difference and significance of upper body adiposity. Diabetes Care 1992; 15: 1348-55.

[27]   Ramachandran A, Snehalatha C, Latha E, Vijay V, Viswanathan M. Rising prevalence of NIDDM in an urban population in India. Diabetologia 1997; 40: 232-7.

[28]   Ramachandran A, Snehalatha C, Kapur A, *et al.* High prevalence of diabetes and impaired glucose tolerance in India: National Urban Diabetes Survey. Diabetologia 2001; 44: 1094-101.

[29]   Shanghai Diabetes Research Cooperative Group. A survey of Diabetes mellitus among the population in Shanghai. Natl Med J Chin 1980; 60: 323-9.

[30]   National Diabetes Co-operative Study Group. A mass survey of diabetes mellitus in a population of 300 000 in 14 provinces and municipalities in China. Zhonghua Nei Ke Za Zhi 1981; 20: 678-83.

[31]   Beijing Diabetes Research Cooperative Group. The prevalence of diabetes mellitus in 40, 000 population in Beijing with discussion on difference criteria of its diagnosis. Zhonghua Nei Ke Za Zhi 1982; 21: 85-7.

[32]   Pan XR, Yang WY, Li GW, Liu J. Prevalence of diabetes and its risk factors in China, 1994. National Diabetes Prevention and Control Cooperative Group. Diabetes Care 1997; 20: 1664-9.

[33]   Wang K, Li T, Xiang HD. Study on the epidemiolgical characteristics of diabetes mellitus and IGT in China. Zhonghua Liu Xing Bing Xue Za Zhi 1998; 19: 282-5.

[34]   Dong Y, Gao W, Nan H, *et al.* Prevalence of Type 2 diabetes in urban and rural Chinese populations in Qingdao, China. Diabet Med 2005; 22: 1427-33.

[35]   King H, Aubert RE, Herman WH. Global burden of diabetes, 1995-2025: prevalence, numerical estimates, and projections. Diabetes Care 1998; 21: 1414-31.

[36]   Alberti KGMM, Bennett PH, Borch-Johnsen K *et al.* WHO/IDF Consultation. Definition and diagnosis of diabetes mellitus and intermediate hyperglycemia: report of a WHO/IDF consultation. World Health Organisation/ International Diabetes Federation. Geneva: Switzerland 2006.

[37]   Santaguida PL, Balion C, Hunt D, *et al.* Diagnosis, prognosis, and treatment of impaired glucose tolerance and impaired fasting glucose. Evid Rep Technol Assess (Summ). 2005:1-11.

[38]   Ramachandran A, Snehalatha C, Viswanathan V, Viswanathan M, Haffner SM. Risk of noninsulin dependent diabetes mellitus conferred by obesity and central adiposity in different ethnic groups: a comparative analysis between Asian Indians, Mexican Americans and Whites. Diabetes Res Clin Pract 1997; 36: 121-5.

[39]   Haffner SM. Epidemiology of type 2 diabetes: risk factors. Diabetes Care 1998;21 (Suppl 3):C3-6.

[40]   Chang CJ, Wu CH, Lu FH, *et al.* Discriminating glucose tolerance status by regions of interest of dual-energy X-ray absorptiometry. Clinical implications of body fat distribution. Diabetes Care 1999; 22: 1938-43.

[41]   Goodpaster BH, Krishnaswami S, Resnick H, *et al.* Association between regional adipose tissue distribution and both type 2 diabetes and impaired glucose tolerance in elderly men and women. Diabetes Care 2003; 26: 372-9.

[42]   Ni Mhurchu C, Parag V, Nakamura M, *et al.* Body mass index and risk of diabetes mellitus in the Asia-Pacific region. Asia Pac J Clin Nutr 2006; 15: 127-33.

[43]   Meisinger C, Doring A, Thorand B, Heier M, Lowel H. Body fat distribution and risk of type 2 diabetes in the general population: are there differences between men and women? The MONICA/KORA Augsburg Cohort Study. Am J Clin Nutr 2006; 84: 483-9.

[44]   Everhart JE, Pettitt DJ, Bennett PH, Knowler WC. Duration of obesity increases the incidence of NIDDM. Diabetes 1992; 41: 235-40.

[45]   Colditz GA, Willett WC, Rotnitzky A, Manson JE. Weight gain as a risk factor for clinical diabetes mellitus in women. Ann Intern Med 1995; 122: 481-6.

[46]   Wannamethee SG, Shaper AG. Weight change and duration of overweight and obesity in the incidence of type 2 diabetes. Diabetes Care 1999; 22:1266-72.

[47]   Koh-Banerjee P, Wang Y, Hu FB, *et al.* Changes in body weight and body fat distribution as risk factors for clinical diabetes in US Men. Am J Epidemiol 2004; 159: 1150-9.

[48]   Wannamethee SG, Shaper AG, Walker M. Overweight and obesity and weight change in middle aged men: impact on cardiovascular disease and diabetes. J Epidemiol Community Health 2005; 59: 134-9.

[49]   Schienkiewitz A, Schulze MB, Hoffmann K, Kroke A, Boeing H. Body mass index history and risk of type 2 diabetes: results from the European Prospective Investigation into Cancer and Nutrition (EPIC)-Potsdam Study. Am J Clin Nutr 2006; 84: 427-33.

[50]   Tuomilehto J, Lindstrom J, Eriksson JG, *et al.* Prevention of type 2 diabetes mellitus by changes in lifestyle among subjects with impaired glucose tolerance. N Engl J Med 2001; 344: 1343-50.

[51]   Knowler WC, Barrett-Connor E, Fowler SE, *et al.* Reduction in the incidence of type 2 diabetes with lifestyle intervention or metformin. N Engl J Med 2002; 346: 393-403.

[52]   Li G, Zhang P, Wang J, *et al.* The long-term effect of lifestyle interventions to prevent diabetes in the China Da Qing Diabetes Prevention Study: a 20-year follow-up study. Lancet 2008; 371: 1783-9.

[53]   Flegal KM, Carroll MD, Ogden CL, Johnson CL. Prevalence and trends in obesity among US adults, 1999-2000. JAMA 2002; 288: 1723-7.

[54]   Flegal KM, Carroll MD, Ogden CL, Curtin LR. Prevalence and trends in obesity among US Adults, 1999-2008. JAMA 2010; 303: 235-41.

[55]   Vartiainen E, Laatikainen T, Peltonen M, *et al.* Thirty-five-year trends in cardiovascular risk factors in Finland. Int J Epidemiol 2010; 39: 504-18.

[56]   Wu Y, Huxley R, Li M, Ma J. The growing burden of overweight and obesity in contemporary China. CVD Prevention and Control 2009; 4: 19-26.

[57]   Villegas R, Shu X-O, Li H, *et al.* Physical activity and the incidence of type 2 diabetes in the Shanghai women's health study. Int J Epidemiol 2006; 35: 1553-62.

[58]   Jeon CY, Lokken RP, Hu FB, van Dam RM. Physical activity of moderate intensity and risk of type 2 diabetes: a systematic review. Diabetes Care 2007; 30: 744-52.

[59]   Gimeno D, Elovainio M, Jokela M, *et al.* Association between passive jobs and low levels of leisure-time physical activity: the Whitehall II cohort study. Occup Environ Med 2009; 66: 772-6.

[60]   Chien KL, Chen MF, Hsu HC, Su TC, Lee YT. Sports activity and risk of type 2 diabetes in Chinese. Diabetes Res Clin Pract 2009; 84: 311-8.

[61]   Hu FB, Leitzmann MF, Stampfer MJ, *et al.* Physical activity and television watching in relation to risk for type 2 diabetes mellitus in men. Arch Intern Med 2001;161:1542-8.

[62]   Hu FB, Li TY, Colditz GA, Willett WC, Manson JE. Television watching and other sedentary behaviors in relation to risk of obesity and type 2 diabetes mellitus in women. JAMA 2003; 289:1785-91.

[63]   Krishnan S, Rosenberg L, Palmer JR. Physical activity and television watching in relation to risk of type 2 diabetes: the Black Women's Health Study. Am J Epidemiol 2009; 169: 428-34.

[64]   Manson JE, Rimm EB, Stampfer MJ, *et al.* Physical activity and incidence of non-insulin-dependent diabetes mellitus in women. Lancet 1991; 338: 774-8.

[65]   Schranz A, Tuomilehto J, Marti B, *et al.* Low physical activity and worsening of glucose tolerance: results from a 2-year follow-up of a population sample in Malta. Diabetes Res Clin Pract 1991; 11: 127-36.

[66]   Helmrich SP, Ragland DR, Leung RW, Paffenbarger RS, Jr. Physical activity and reduced occurrence of non-insulin-dependent diabetes mellitus. N Engl J Med 1991; 325: 147-52.

[67] Manson JE, Nathan DM, Krolewski AS, *et al.* A prospective study of exercise and incidence of diabetes among US male physicians. JAMA 1992; 268: 63-7.

[68] Burchfiel CM, Sharp DS, Curb JD, *et al.* Physical activity and incidence of diabetes: the Honolulu Heart Program. Am J Epidemiol 1995; 141: 360-8.

[69] Lynch J, Helmrich SP, Lakka TA, *et al.* Moderately intense physical activities and high levels of cardiorespiratory fitness reduce the risk of non-insulin-dependent diabetes mellitus in middle-aged men. Arch Intern Med 1996; 156: 1307-14.

[70] Haapanen N, Miilunpalo S, Pasanen M, Oja P, Vuori I. Association between leisure time physical activity and 10-year body mass change among working-aged men and women. Int J Obes Relat Metab Disord 1997; 21: 288-96.

[71] Folsom AR, Kushi LH, Hong CP. Physical activity and incident diabetes mellitus in postmenopausal women. Am J Public Health 2000; 90: 134-8.

[72] Fretts AM, Howard BV, Kriska AM, *et al.* Physical activity and incident diabetes in american indians: The strong heart study. Am J Epidemiol 2009; 170: 632-9.

[73] Hu FB, Sigal RJ, Rich-Edwards JW, *et al.* Walking Compared With Vigorous Physical Activity and Risk of Type 2 Diabetes in Women. JAMA 1999; 282: 1433-9.

[74] Eriksson KF, Lindgarde F. Prevention of type 2 (non-insulin-dependent) diabetes mellitus by diet and physical exercise. The 6-year Malmo feasibility study. Diabetologia 1991; 34: 891-8.

[75] Pan XR, Li GW, Hu YH, *et al.* Effects of diet and exercise in preventing NIDDM in people with impaired glucose tolerance. The Da Qing IGT and Diabetes Study. Diabetes Care 1997; 20: 537-44.

[76] Yamaoka K, Tango T. Efficacy of lifestyle education to prevent type 2 diabetes: a meta-analysis of randomized controlled trials. Diabetes Care 2005; 28: 2780-6.

[77] Ramachandran A, Snehalatha C, Mary S, *et al.* The indian diabetes prevention programme shows that lifestyle modification and metformin prevent type 2 diabetes in Asian Indian subjects with impaired glucose tolerance (IDPP-1). Diabetologia 2006; 49: 289-97.

[78] Ng SW, Norton EC, Popkin BM. Why have physical activity levels declined among Chinese adults? Findings from the 1991-2006 China Health and Nutrition Surveys. Soc Sci Med 2009; 68: 1305-14.

[79] Gao WG, Dong YH, Pang ZC, *et al.* A simple Chinese risk score for undiagnosed diabetes. Diabet Med 2010; 27: 274-82.

[80] Ning F, Pang ZC, Dong YH, *et al.* Risk factors associated with the dramatic increase in the prevalence of diabetes in the adult Chinese population in Qingdao, China. Diabet Med 2009; 26: 855-63.

[81] van Dam RM, Rimm EB, Willett WC, Stampfer MJ, Hu FB. Dietary patterns and risk for type 2 diabetes mellitus in U.S. men. Ann Intern Med 2002; 136: 201-9.

[82] Hodge AM, English DR, O'Dea K, Giles GG. Dietary patterns and diabetes incidence in the Melbourne Collaborative Cohort Study. Am J Epidemiol 2007; 165: 603-10.

[83] McNaughton SA, Mishra GD, Brunner EJ. Dietary patterns, insulin resistance, and incidence of type 2 diabetes in the Whitehall II Study. Diabetes Care 2008; 31: 1343-8.

[84] Liese AD, Weis KE, Schulz M, Tooze JA. Food intake patterns associated with incident type 2 diabetes: the Insulin Resistance Atherosclerosis Study. Diabetes Care 2009; 32: 263-8.

[85] Liu S, Serdula M, Janket SJ, *et al.* A prospective study of fruit and vegetable intake and the risk of type 2 diabetes in women. Diabetes Care 2004; 27: 2993-6.

[86] Hodge AM, English DR, O'Dea K, Giles GG. Glycemic index and dietary fiber and the risk of type 2 diabetes. Diabetes Care 2004; 27: 2701-6.

[87] Montonen J, Jarvinen R, Heliovaara M, *et al.* Food consumption and the incidence of type II diabetes mellitus. Eur J Clin Nutr 2005; 59: 441-8.

[88] de Munter JS, Hu FB, Spiegelman D, Franz M, van Dam RM. Whole grain, bran, and germ intake and risk of type 2 diabetes: a prospective cohort study and systematic review. PLoS Med 2007;4:e261.

[89] Villegas R, Shu XO, Gao YT, *et al.* Vegetable but not fruit consumption reduces the risk of type 2 diabetes in Chinese women. J Nutr 2008; 138: 574-80.

[90] Patel PS, Sharp SJ, Luben RN, *et al.* The association between type of dietary fish and seafood intake and the risk of incident type 2 diabetes: The EPIC-Norfolk cohort study. Diabetes Care 2009; 32: 1857-63.

[91] Harding AH, Wareham NJ, Bingham SA, *et al.* Plasma vitamin C level, fruit and vegetable consumption, and the risk of new-onset type 2 diabetes mellitus: the European prospective investigation of cancer--Norfolk prospective study. Arch Intern Med 2008; 168: 1493-9.

[92] Tuomilehto J, Hu G, Bidel S, Lindstrom J, Jousilahti P. Coffee consumption and risk of type 2 diabetes mellitus among middle-aged Finnish men and women. JAMA 2004; 291:1213-9.

[93]   Stote KS, Baer DJ. Tea consumption may improve biomarkers of insulin sensitivity and risk factors for diabetes. J Nutr 2008; 138: 1584S-8S.

[94]   Jahns L, Siega-Riz AM, Popkin BM. The increasing prevalence of snacking among US children from 1977 to 1996. J Pediatr 2001; 138: 493-8.

[95]   Popkin BM, Siega-Riz AM, Haines PS, Jahns L. Where's the fat? Trends in U.S. diets 1965-1996. Prev Med 2001; 32: 245-54.

[96]   Nielsen SJ, Siega-Riz AM, Popkin BM. Trends in food locations and sources among adolescents and young adults. Prev Med 2002; 35: 107-13.

[97]   Nielsen SJ, Siega-Riz AM, Popkin BM. Trends in energy intake in U.S. between 1977 and 1996: similar shifts seen across age groups. Obes Res 2002; 10: 370-8.

[98]   Nielsen SJ, Popkin BM. Patterns and trends in food portion sizes, 1977-1998. JAMA 2003; 289: 450-3.

[99]   Nielsen SJ, Popkin BM. Changes in beverage intake between 1977 and 2001. Am J Prev Med 2004; 27: 205-10.

[100]   Du S, Mroz TA, Zhai F, Popkin BM. Rapid income growth adversely affects diet quality in China--particularly for the poor! Soc Sci Med 2004; 59: 1505-15.

[101]   Zhai F, Wang H, Du S, *et al.* Prospective study on nutrition transition in China. Nutr Rev 2009; 67 (Suppl 1): S56-61.

CHAPTER 3

Screening for Type 2 Diabetes

Weiguo Gao[1,2,3]* and Qing Qiao[1,2]

[1]*Department of Public Health, Hjelt Institute, University of Helsinki, Helsinki, Finland;* [2]*Department of Chronic Disease Prevention, National Institute for Health and Welfare, Helsinki, Finland and* [3]*Qingdao Endocrine & Diabetes Hospital, Qingdao, China*

Abstract: Under increasing burden of diabetes and in the light of evidences it is clear that diabetes and its complication are preventable, screening for diabetes, which aims at early detecting and treating patients with diabetes to reduce the diabetic complications, and at the same time identifying individuals at high risk for diabetes to prevent or delay the onset of diabetes, has been recommended by several professional organizations such as the World Health Organization, the International Diabetes Federation, and the American Diabetes Association. Various screening programs have been developed and conducted by applying different screening tools including fasting or random capillary blood glucose tests, fasting and post challenge plasma glucose tests, HbA1c test, and a number of risk assessment questionnaires (or scores). The cost-effectiveness and the impact on the participants of these screening programs have not been fully evaluated, but the screening tests used in these programs have been validated in terms of discrimination, calibration and reclassification of individuals with and without the events.

Keywords: Diabetes screening, screening tests, diabetes risk score, discrimination, calibration, reclassification.

3.1. RATIONAL FOR SCREENING DIABETES

In the World Health Organization (WHO) guideline of Screening for Type 2 Diabetes, screening was defined as "the process of identifying those individuals who are at sufficiently high risk of a specific disorder to warrant further investigation or direct action" [1]. "It (screening) is systematically offered to a population of people who have not sought medical attention on account of symptoms of the disease for which screening is being offered and is normally initiated by medical authorities and not by a patient's request for help on account of a specific complaint".

Rationales to screen for asymptomatic type 2 diabetes include:

- Diabetes increases worldwide and has become one of the major threats to the human health. It casts devastating effects on the human health and social-economic development. According to the International Diabetes Federation (IDF) estimation, at least 376 billion US Dollars required to cover the global healthcare expenditures to treat and prevent diabetes and its complications [2]. And in the developing countries, such as in China and India, the economic development might be hindered by the heavy burden from diabetes.

- In the natural course of the development of diabetes, there is a long, latent, and asymptomatic period in which the disease may be detected [3, 4]. Early treatment and intensive control of hyperglymia have been reported to protect patients with diabetes from developing diabetic complication effectively [5-10].

- It has been unequivocally shown that risk to develop diabetes can be reduced by 40-60% through lifestyle intervention among individuals with Impaired Glucose Tolerance (IGT)

---

*Address correspondence to Weiguo Gao:** Department of Public Health, Hjelt Institute, University of Helsinki, PL41, Mannerheimintie 172, 00014, Helsinki, Finland. E-mail: gwg1974@hotmail.com

under controlled trail conditions [11-15]. Anti-diabetic drugs such as metformin, acarbose and rosiglitazone have also been shown to be able to reduce the progression from the IGT to diabetes by 25%-60% [13-17]. Accumulated evidence has shown that the diabetes prevention among high-risk individuals are cost-effective [18].

- The technique to determine the blood glucose or HbA1c, diagnostic test for diabetes and pre-diabetes, is well-developed and standardized. In addition, diabetes risk factors, such as obesity, physical inactivity, unhealthy diet, old age, family history of diabetes, have been well defined, and are not difficult to measure. Through identifying either single risk factor or an integrated risk assessment questionnaire or algorithm, individuals with a high risk for diabetes can be detected efficiently.

- In spite of the inconsistent findings, evidences have shown that screening for diabetes might be cost-effective [19-23].

3.2. EVALUATION OF SCREENING TOOLS

Performance of a screening test for diabetes is usually quantitatively evaluated against a "gold standard" test to assess its validity that is the ability of the test to correctly classify people with diabetes from those without in terms of sensitivity, specificity, Positive and Negative Predictive Values (PPV and NPV). A Receiver Operating Characteristic Curve (ROC) is drawn based on sensitivities and specificities calculated at different cut-off values of the screening test to predict diabetes defined based on a "gold standard" test. The area under a curve (AUC) for a test will be calculated and the larger the AUC the better the prediction of the screening test. In addition to the validity, a good screening test should be reliable to allow replication of the test result by other procedures, reproducible on repeat measures on the same individual, acceptable to the examinees and cost-effective. Other properties that need to be considered when choosing a screening test and implement a screening program is the psychosocial and psychologic impact on individuals having a positive or negative screening outcomes [1]. Recently the concept of the net reclassification improvement has been introduced to examine whether a new test, compared with an existing test, can improve the net reclassification of individuals with and without the disease. In this chapter, the commonly used statistic techniques to evaluate the screening tests are briefly introduced.

3.2.1. Validity of a Screening Test

Sensitivity measures the proportion of people with the disorder who test positive on the screening tests. The higher the sensitivity of a screening test, the more likely the disease of interest will be detected. A 100% of sensitivity means that the screening test identifies all people with the disease. Specificity measures the proportion of people who do not have the disorder who test negative on the screening test. A highly specific test is unlikely to misclassify non-diseased persons as having the disease. Theoretically, a perfect screening test will have both a high sensitivity and specificity. However, this is usually not possible in real practice since increasing one reduces the other.

Positive predictive value is the probability of the disorder in a person with a positive test result, and negative predictive value is the probability of a person not having the disorder when the test result is negative. The predicted probability may be a useful measure in a doctor's office when a patient present with a positive or negative testing results. The positive predictive value depends on the prevalence of the disease in the population being screened. A highly sensitive and specific test will have a high positive predictive value in a population with a high prevalence of the disorder. If the prevalence is low, the positive predictive value of the same test will be considerably lower. The 2×2 contingency table below illustrates how the sensitivity, specificity PPV and NPV are calculated (Table **1**).

Table 1: The 2×2 contingency table for calculation of sensitivity, specificity, Positive Predictive Value (PPV) and Negative Predictive Value (NPV)

	Disease defined by the gold standard test		PPV	NPV
Result of a screening test	Yes	No		
Positive	a (true positive)	b (false positive)	a/(a+b)	-
Negative	c (false negative)	d (true negative)	-	d/(c+d)
Sensitivity	a/(a+c)	-		
Specificity	-	d/(b+d)		

3.2.2. Receiver Operating Characteristic Curve (ROC)

ROC curve is commonly used to measure the ability of a screening test to discriminate individuals with the disease from those without. It is a plot of the true positive rate (sensitivity) on the vertical (y) axis against the false positive rate (1−specificity) on the horizontal (x) axis over a range of cut-off values. The AUC can be interpreted as the probability that when we randomly pick one positive and one negative example, the screening test will assign a higher score to the positive example than to the negative. A perfect test will have an AUC of 1.00 (100%), which means the test will separate correctly all individuals with the event of interest from those without; while an AUC of 0.50 (50%) indicates the test is uninformative. The ROC curve is useful to determine the optimal cut-off point, at which the sum of sensitivity and specificity is the maximum. To compare the discriminatory ability of different screening tests, it is possible to do with comparing their values of the AUCs.

3.2.3. Net Reclassification Improvement and Integrated Discrimination Improvement

Recently, Pencina MJ *et al.,* suggested two new measures: Net Reclassification Improvement (NRI) and Integrated Discrimination Improvement (IDI) [24]. NRI was suggested to compare two risk predicting models A and B, which share all risk factors except for one new marker included in the model B. After classification of the predicted probabilities from the two models into risk categories, the NRI is the proportion of times the model B correctly moves an individual with the event into a higher risk category or an individual without the event into a lower risk category, minus the proportion of times the new model incorrectly moves an individual with the event into a lower risk category or an individual without the event into a higher risk category. IDI is calculated by subtracting, for model A and B, the average probability of the event in the individuals without the event from the average probability of the event in the individuals with the event, and then calculating the difference in these two quantities. The values of NRI and IDI are both between 0 and 1 (or 0 and 100%). The higher the values are, the greater the improvement in performance of the new model is. It is also possible to test whether each statistic is significantly different from 0.

3.2.4. Calibration of Screening Tests

Currently, a number of diabetes screening tests are algorithms based on statistical risk predicting (or accessing) models. Calibration is the extent to which predicted risk from the risk predicting model equals the observed risk in the data. The Hosmer-Lemeshow Goodness of fit test is the most commonly used technique. Subjects were divided into ten equal sized groups by ordering the predicted probabilities of the event. The observed and expected numbers of individuals with the event within each group are then compared using a Chi-square statistic (with nine degrees of freedom if there are ten groups). A statistically non-significant result implies that the model is well calibrated; otherwise, it is poorly calibrated.

It should also keep in mind that the evaluation of screening tests is a dynamic research area. There are still some unresolved methodological issues concerning the development, validation and comparison of screening tests.

3.3. SCREENING TESTS FOR DIABETES AND THEIR PERFORMANCE

Various screening tests have been developed and evaluated in recent decades. Screening for diabetes have for a long time been carried out based on detecting glucose levels in either blood or urine. Due to its low agreement between the levels of the blood glucose and glycosuria, the glycosuria test is no longer used for screening of diabetes. Fasting blood glucose test, fasting or random capillary blood glucose test and hemoglobin A1c (HbA1c) test are commonly used screening tools for diabetes; some studies have administered 2-hour glucose test directly to the study populations. In addition to the glycemic test, more recently various risk assessment questionnaires or algorithms have been developed based on demographic, lifestyles, family history and anthropometric measures, some including glycemic measures as well. A few studies have added genetic makers into the risk assessment tools. In most of the previous studies the performance of these screening tools have been evaluated against the 2-hour post-load glucose criteria for diabetes the gold standard, but in other studies both fasting and/or 2-hour glucose criteria are considered as the gold standard.

3.3.1. Glycemic Tests

Urine glucose test is now not in use where the blood glucose tests are available. Although the specificity may be higher than 98%, the sensitivity of urine glucose test was only around 20% to 64% [25-27]. The renal threshold for re-absorption of glucose varies between individuals, and, the presence of glucose in the urine is more likely positive in individuals with a low threshold than those with a high threshold. Therefore, urine glucose test has its limitation as a tool for diabetes screening.

Fasting or Random finger capillary blood glucose assay is the easiest and simplest test to determine blood glucose levels. Most studies that have applied the capillary blood glucose test in their screening program showed high sensitivities of 80% at the optimal cut-off points and high specificities of 70%, but the optimal cut-off points varied from 5.0 mmol/l to 7.9 mmol/l in different studies (Table **2**). According to Engelgau *et al.*, different optimal cut-off points were required to account for the age and postprandial period [28]. Poor performance was, however, also reported, with a sensitivity of 40% in middle-aged Finnish women [29]. In addition, the accuracy of the glucose readings obtained from a portable blood glucose meter can be affected by calibration of the meter, ambient temperature and humidity, hematocrit, and, high blood triglyceride, *etc.,* [30].

Table 2: Sensitivity and specificity of a finger capillary blood glucose test in detecting diabetes

Studies	Metabolic State	Reference Test	Cut-Off Point (mmol/l)	Sensitivity (%)	Specificity (%)
Murphy *et al.,* [31]	Fasting	OGTTs	6.7	75.0	93.0
Bortheiry *et al.,*[32]	Fasting	OGTTs	5.6	89.4(men), 85.3(women)	67.7(men), 74.4(women)
Engelgau *et al.,* [28]	Random	2hPG	6.1-7.2, depending on age	76.0 - 81.0, depending on age	75.0 - 80.0, depending on age
Qiao *et al.,* [29]	Random	OGTTs	6.2	79.0(men), 40.0(women)	93.0(men), 92.0(women)
Husseini *et al.,* [33]	Fasting	OGTTs	5.0	83.3	79.0
Rolka *et al.,* [34]	Random	OGTTs	6.7	75.0	88.0
Herdzik *et al.,* [35]	Fasting	OGTTs	5.8	85.4	94.9
Zhang *et al.,* [36]	Random	OGTTs	6.7	68.0	89.0
Somannavar *et al.,* [37]	Random	OGTTs	7.9	78.6	83.9
Gao *et al.,* [38]	Fasting	OGTTs	6.3(men) 6.6 (women)	71.0(men) 65.9 (women)	69.7(men) 76.4(women)

Fasting plasma glucose (FPG) measures the concentration of plasma glucose at fasting condition. With $2hPG \geq 11.1mmol/l$ as a reference test, the sensitivity of FPG to screen diabetes varied from 32% to 95% at

FPG cut-off values ranging from 5.8-7.8 mmol/l; while the specificity was about 84-99% [27]. The ethnicity, age, sex and body mass index all influence the performance of FPG as a screening test for diabetes [39, 40]. The FPG was therefore considered as a specific but insensitive screening test for diabetes. It should be noticed that FPG is also one of the diagnostic tests for diabetes. A diagnosis of diabetes can be made if individuals had a FPG $\geq$ 7.0 mmol/l, with or without 2 hPG $\geq$ 11.1 mmol/l [41-43].

HbA1c reflects the mean blood glucose levels in 8-12 weeks preceding the test. At the HbA1c values of 5.3% and 6.5%, the sensitivity of HbA1c varied from 43% to 95%, and specificity from 67% to 99% in Chinese, Singaporean, Japanese and Non-Hispanic white adults [44-50]. However, it should be noticed that most of these studies were done in the preselected high-risk populations. In a population-based Chinese survey, the performance of HbA1c for screening diabetes is worse than the one of fasting capillary blood glucose (AUC 0.67 for HbA1c and 0.77 for fasting capillary blood glucose) [51]. It has also been reported that 60% of individuals with screen-detected diabetes based on FPG had a normal value of HbA1c [52, 53]. And the biology variation of hemoglobin limits the usage of the HbA1c test in certain situations such as women in pregnancy, individuals with anemia or with hemoglobinopathies. The assay of HbA1c is less standardized and also most expensive in low and middle income countries.

3.3.2. Genetic Markers

A genetic score, which adds up a number of genetic markers that are associated with the presence of diabetes, has been developed to predict the risk of diabetes in several studies recently. The genetic score may improve the performance over clinical predictors of prevalent diabetes in some studies [54-57]; but, the improvement was very limited, and was not detected in other studies [58, 59].

3.3.3. Risk Assessment Algorithms or Scores

Blood sampling is required for all the blood glucose tests and HbA1c assay. They are invasive, relatively expensive, time consuming, and not easy to apply in large population screening programs. Dozens of risk scores, risk predicting models or risk assessment questionnaires without biochemical measurements have been developed to serve as a first line screening tools for diabetes (Table **3**). Most of these risk assessment tools were developed and validated in the Caucasians, and a few in Indians, Chinese and other Asian populations. The AUCs of these risk assessment tools were moderate to high varying from 70% to 80%. The sensitivities of these risk assessment algorithms in predicting diabetes were above 70%; but, the specificities were relatively low or moderate, about 50-60% at the optimal cut-off points. As an example, a simple Chinese Diabetes Risk Score is shown in Table **4**. Individuals can easily apply the score to assess their risk of having diabetes without professional physical and biochemical measures.

Table 3: Risk assessment algorithms developed in different populations

Risk Assessment Algorithms (Ethnicity and Reference)	Risk Factors Included in the Model	Reference test	Optimal Cut-Off Point (Range)	AUC (95% CI), %	Sensitivity (95% CI) at the Optimal Cut-Off Point, %	Specificity (95% CI) at the Optimal Cut-Off Point, %
Cambridge risk model (British)[60]	Age, sex, drug-treated hypertension, corticosteroids treatment, family history of diabetes, BMI and smoking.	2h 75g OGTTs	0.199	80.0 (68.0-91.0)	77.3 (54.6-92.2)	72.0 (68.0-76.0)
Danish Risk score (Danish)[61]	Age, sex, BMI, known history of hypertension, diabetes in parents, physical activity at leisure time.	2h 75g OGTTs	29(0-60)	80.4 (76.5-83.8)	79.3 (71.4-86.3)	68.7 (67.1-70.3)
Indian risk score (Indian)[62]	Age, sex, family history of diabetes, BMI, waist circumference, physical activity.	2h Post load whole blood Glucose $\geq$ 11.1mmol/l	21(0-42)	73.2 (70.2-76.1)	76.6 (70.9-81.7)	59.9 (58.5-61.3)
Indian Diabetes	Age, waist circumference,	2hPG	60(0-100)	69.8 (66.3-	72.5	60.1

risk (Indian) score [63]	physical activity, family history of diabetes.			73.3)		
Rotterdam study (Dutch) [64]	Age, sex, drug-treated hypertension, BMI.	2h 75g OGTTs	6(0-22)	68.0 (64-72)	78.0	55.0
Finnish Risk Score (Finnish) [65]	Age, BMI, waist, drug-treated hypertension, physical inactivity, daily consuming vegetable, fruit, or berries.	Drug-treated diabetes	9(0-20)	85.0	78.0 (71.0-84.0)	77.0 (76.0-79.0)
DESIR Risk Score (French) [58]	Waist circumference, smoking, hypertension, family history of diabetes.	Clinical diagnosed diabetes or FPG	Not available (0-5)	73.3 in men. 83.9 in women	-	-
Thai Risk Score (Thai) [66]	Age, sex, BMI, waist circumference, hypertension, family history of diabetes.	2h 75g OGTTs	6 (0-17)	74.0 (71-78)	77.0	60.0
ADA recommendation (American) [67]	Delivery of a baby weighing > 9 pounds, diabetes in parents or siblings, BMI, age, physical activity.	2h 75g OGTTs	10(0-27)	71.0	80.0	34.6
QD Score (British) [68]	Age, BMI, family history of diabetes, smoking, history of treated hypertension, history of cardiovascular disease, use of corticosteroids, social deprivation, ethnicity.	Clinically diagnosed diabetes	-	85.3 (85.0-85.6) in women 83.4 (83.1-83.6) in men	-	-
Oman risk score (Arab) [69]	Age, waist circumference, BMI, family history of diabetes, hypertension.	2h post load serum glucose ≥ 11.1 mmol/l	10 (0-25)	76(74-79)	62.8(54.3-70.6)	78.2(75.8-80.4)
German risk score (German) [70]	Waist, height, age, hypertension, physical activity, smoking, consumption of red meat, whole-grain bread, coffee and moderate alcohol.	Self-reported diabetes	500(118-983)	82	94.4	66.7
SUNSET study (Surinamese and Dutch) [71]	Ethnicity, BMI, waist circumference, resting heart rate, family history of diabetes, hypertension, history of cardiovascular disease.	FPG	Not available (0-19)	74 (70-79) in Hindustani Surinamese, 79(76-85) in African Surinamese, 79 (75-87) in Dutch	79, 5(69.0-87.3) in Hindustani Surinamese, 78.1(66.6-86.6) in African Surinamese, 71.9(53.0-85.6) in Dutch	47.4(41.0-53.8) in Hindustani Surinamese, 60.7(56.3-65.0) in African Surinamese, 71.2(66.7-75.3) in Dutch
Canary Islands survey (Spanish) [72]	Age, waist/height ratio, family history of diabetes, systolic blood pressure, gestational diabetes.	FPG	100	83.7(80.3-87.1)in men 87.4(84.7-90.1) in women	93 in men 95 in women	54 in men 48 in women
ARIC study (American) [73]	Parental history of diabetes, hypertension, race, age, smoking, waist circumference, height, resting pulse, weight.	FPG, 2hPG or clinical diagnosis	38(0-100)	71(69-73)	69	64
A new risk score in U.S. (American) [74]	Age, sex, family history of diabetes, personal history of hypertension, obesity, and physical activity.	FPG	5(0-9)	79	79	67
Mauritian Indian risk score (Indian emigrantion) [75]	Age, sex, family history of diabetes, waist, body mass index.	2h 75g OGTTs	0.12(0.05-0.64)	62(56-68) in men 64(59-69) in women	72(71-74) in men 77(75-78) in women	47(45-49) in men 50(48-52) in women
Chinese risk score (Chinese) [38]	Age, sex, family history of diabetes, waist.	2h 75g OGTTs	14(3-32)	63.5(59.1-67.9) in men	85.6(83.9-87.4) in men	21.1(19.0-23.1) in men

					68.9(63.6-72.4) in women	75.5(73.8-77.2) in women	43.6(41.6-45.6) in women
AUSDRISK (Australian) [76]	Age, sex, ethnicity, parental history of diabetes, history of high blood glucose level, use of antihypertension medications, smoking, physical inactivity, waist circumference.	FPG, 2hPG or on treatment of diabetes	12(0-35)	78(76-81)	74.0	67.7	

Table 4: Chinese risk score based on the age, sex, waist girth and diabetes in parents or siblings

Waist (Chinese Chi *)			
Men	**Score**	**Women**	**Score**
≤2.3	1	≤2.0	1
2.4-2.6	4	2.1-2.3	3
2.7-2.9	8	2.4-2.6	6
≥3.0	12	≥2.7	9
Age (years)	**Score**		
≤35	1		
36-45	3		
46-55	6		
56-65	9		
≥65	12		
Diabetes in Parents and/or Siblings			**Score**
Negative			1
Positvie			8
Score (= score of waist + score of age + score of diabetes in parents and/or siblings)			( )

1 Chinese Chi ≈ 33 cm.This table was adapted from [38].

REFERENCES

[1]   Alberti KGMM, Colagiuri S, Goyder E, *et al.* World Health Orgnization. Screening for Type 2 Diabetes: Report of a World Health Organization and International Diabetes Federation meeting.WHO/IDF, Geneva:Switzerland 2003.

[2]   Mbanya JC, Gan D, Allgot B, *et al.* International Diabetes Federation. IDF Diabetes Atlas Fourth Edition. (Report No.: ISBN-13:978-2-930229-71-3) International Diabetes Federation, Brussels: Belgium 2009.

[3]   Harris MI, Klein R, Welborn TA, Knuiman MW. Onset of NIDDM occurs at least 4-7 years before clinical diagnosis. Diabetes Care 1992; 15: 815-9.

[4]   Thompson TJ, Engelgau MM, Hegazy M, *et al.* The onset of NIDDM and its relationship to clinical diagnosis in Egyptian adults. Diabet Med 1996; 13: 337-40.

[5]   Turner RC, Holman RR, Stratton IM, *et al.* United Kingdom Prospective Diabetes Study (UKPDS) Group. Effect of intensive blood-glucose control with metformin on complications in overweight patients with type 2 diabetes (UKPDS 34). Lancet 1998; 352: 854-65.

[6]   Turner RC, Holman RR, Cull CA, *et al.* United Kingdom Prospective Diabetes Study (UKPDS) Group. Intensive blood-glucose control with sulphonylureas or insulin compared with conventional treatment and risk of complications in patients with type 2 diabetes (UKPDS 33). Lancet 1998; 352: 837-53.

[7]   Gerstein HC, Miller ME, Byington RP, *et al.* Effects of intensive glucose lowering in type 2 diabetes. N Engl J Med 2008; 358: 2545-59.

[8]   Patel A, MacMahon S, Chalmers J, *et al.* Intensive blood glucose control and vascular outcomes in patients with type 2 diabetes. N Engl J Med 2008; 358: 2560-72.

[9]   Duckworth W, Abraira C, Moritz T, *et al.* Glucose control and vascular complications in veterans with type 2 diabetes. N Engl J Med 2009; 360: 129-39.

[10]   Turnbull FM, Abraira C, Anderson RJ, *et al.* Intensive glucose control and macrovascular outcomes in type 2 diabetes. Diabetologia 2009; 52: 2288-98.

[11]   Pan XR, Li GW, Hu YH, *et al.* Effects of diet and exercise in preventing NIDDM in people with impaired glucose tolerance. The Da Qing IGT and Diabetes Study. Diabetes Care 1997; 20: 537-44.

[12]   Tuomilehto J, Lindstrom J, Eriksson JG, *et al.* Prevention of type 2 diabetes mellitus by changes in lifestyle among subjects with impaired glucose tolerance. N Engl J Med 2001; 344: 1343-50.

[13]   Chiasson JL, Josse RG, Gomis R, *et al.* Acarbose for prevention of type 2 diabetes mellitus: the STOP-NIDDM randomised trial. Lancet 2002; 359: 2072-7.

[14]   Knowler WC, Barrett-Connor E, Fowler SE, *et al.* Reduction in the incidence of type 2 diabetes with lifestyle intervention or metformin. N Engl J Med 2002; 346: 393-403.

[15]   Ramachandran A, Snehalatha C, Mary S, *et al.* The indian diabetes prevention programme shows that lifestyle modification and metformin prevent type 2 diabetes in Asian Indian subjects with impaired glucose tolerance (IDPP-1). Diabetologia 2006; 49: 289-97.

[16]   Torgerson JS, Hauptman J, Boldrin MN, Sjöström L. XENical in the Prevention of Diabetes in Obese Subjects (XENDOS) Study. Diabetes Care 2004; 27: 155-61.

[17]   Gerstein HC, Yusuf S, Bosch J, *et al.* Effect of rosiglitazone on the frequency of diabetes in patients with impaired glucose tolerance or impaired fasting glucose: a randomised controlled trial. Lancet 2006; 368: 1096-105.

[18]   Li R, Zhang P, Barker LE, Chowdhury FM, Zhang X. Cost-effectiveness of interventions to prevent and control diabetes mellitus: a systematic review. Diabetes Care 2010; 33: 1872-94.

[19]   The CDC Diabetes Cost-Effectiveness Study Group. The Cost-effectiveness of Screening for Type 2 Diabetes. JAMA 1998; 280: 1757-63.

[20]   Chen TH, Yen MF, Tung TH. A computer simulation model for cost-effectiveness analysis of mass screening for Type 2 diabetes mellitus. Diabetes Res Clin Pract 2001; 54 (Suppl 1): S37-42.

[21]   Hoerger TJ, Harris R, Hicks KA, *et al.* Screening for Type 2 Diabetes Mellitus: A Cost-Effectiveness Analysis. Ann Intern Med 2004; 140: 689-99.

[22]   Hoerger TJ, Hicks KA, Sorensen SW, *et al.* Cost-effectiveness of screening for pre-diabetes among overweight and obese U.S. adults. Diabetes Care 2007; 30: 2874-9.

[23]   Gillies CL, Lambert PC, Abrams KR, *et al.* Different strategies for screening and prevention of type 2 diabetes in adults: cost effectiveness analysis. BMJ 2008; 336: 1180-5.

[24]   Pencina MJ, D'Agostino RB, Sr., D'Agostino RB, Jr., Vasan RS. Evaluating the added predictive ability of a new marker: from area under the ROC curve to reclassification and beyond. Stat Med 2008; 27: 157-72; discussion 207-12.

[25]   Davies MJ, Williams DR, Metcalfe J, Day JL. Community screening for non-insulin-dependent diabetes mellitus: self-testing for post-prandial glycosuria. Q J Med 1993; 86: 677-84.

[26]   Friderichsen B, Maunsbach M. Glycosuric tests should not be employed in population screenings for NIDDM. J Public Health 1997; 19: 55-60.

[27]   Engelgau MM, Narayan KM, Herman WH. Screening for type 2 diabetes. Diabetes Care 2000; 23: 1563-80.

[28]   Engelgau MM, Thompson TJ, Smith PJ, *et al.* Screening for diabetes mellitus in adults. The utility of random capillary blood glucose measurements. Diabetes Care 1995; 18: 463-6.

[29]   Qiao Q, Keinanen-Kiukaanniemi S, Rajala U, Uusimaki A, Kivela SL. Random capillary whole blood glucose test as a screening test for diabetes mellitus in a middle-aged population. Scand J Clin Lab Invest 1995; 55: 3-8.

[30]   Sacks DB, Bruns DE, Goldstein DE, *et al.* Guidelines and recommendations for laboratory analysis in the diagnosis and management of diabetes mellitus. Clin Chem 2002; 48: 436-72.

[31]   Murphy NJ, Boyko EJ, Schraer CD, Bulkow LR, Lanier AP. Use of a reflectance photometer as a diabetes mellitus screening tool under field conditions. Arctic Med Res 1993; 52: 170-4.

[32]   Bortheiry AL, Malerbi DA, Franco LJ. The ROC curve in the evaluation of fasting capillary blood glucose as a screening test for diabetes and IGT. Diabetes Care 1994;17:1269-72.

[33]   Husseini A, Abdul-Rahim H, Awartani F, *et al.* The utility of a single glucometer measurement of fasting capillary blood glucose in the prevalence determination of diabetes mellitus in an urban adult Palestinian population. Scand J Clin Lab Invest 2000; 60: 457-62.

[34]   Rolka DB, Narayan KM, Thompson TJ, *et al.* Performance of recommended screening tests for undiagnosed diabetes and dysglycemia. Diabetes Care 2001; 24: 1899-903.

[35]   Herdzik E, Safranow K, Ciechanowski K. Diagnostic value of fasting capillary glucose, fructosamine and glycosylated hemoglobin in detecting diabetes and other glucose tolerance abnormalities compared to oral glucose tolerance test. Acta Diabetol 2002; 39: 15-22.

[36]   Zhang P, Engelgau MM, Valdez R, *et al.* Efficient cutoff points for three screening tests for detecting undiagnosed diabetes and pre-diabetes: an economic analysis. Diabetes Care 2005; 28: 1321-5.

[37] Somannavar S, Ganesan A, Deepa M, Datta M, Mohan V. Random capillary blood glucose cut points for diabetes and pre-diabetes derived from community-based opportunistic screening in india. Diabetes Care 2009; 32: 641-3.

[38] Gao WG, Dong YH, Pang ZC, *et al.* A simple Chinese risk score for undiagnosed diabetes. Diabet Med 2010; 27: 274-82.

[39] Borch-Johnsen K, Tuomilehto J, Balkau B, Qiao Q. The DECODE Study Group. Is fasting glucose sufficient to define diabetes? Epidemiological data from 20 European studies. Diabetologia 1999; 42: 647-54.

[40] Nakagami T, Qiao Q, Tuomilehto J, *et al.* The fasting plasma glucose cut-point predicting a diabetic 2-h OGTT glucose level depends on the phenotype. Diabetes Res Clin Pract 2002; 55: 35-43.

[41] Expert committee on the diagnosis and classification of diabetes mellitus. Report of the Expert Committee on the Diagnosis and Classification of Diabetes Mellitus. Diabetes Care 1997; 20: 1183-97.

[42] Inzucchi S, Bergenstal R, Fonseca V, *et al.* American Diabetes Association. Diagnosis and Classification of Diabetes Mellitus. Diabetes Care 2010; 33: S62-S9.

[43] Alberti KGMM, Bennett PH, Borch-Johnsen K *et al.* WHO/IDF Consultation. Definition and diagnosis of diabetes mellitus and intermediate hyperglycemia: report of a WHO/IDF consultation, World Health Organisation/ International Diabetes Federation, Geneva: Switzerland 2006.

[44] Tavintharan S, Chew LS, Heng DM. A rational alternative for the diagnosis of diabetes mellitus in high risk individuals. Ann Acad Med Singapore 2000; 29: 213-8.

[45] Tanaka Y, Atsumi Y, Matsuoka K, *et al.* Usefulness of stable HbA(1c) for supportive marker to diagnose diabetes mellitus in Japanese subjects. Diabetes Res Clin Pract 2001; 53: 41-5.

[46] Bennett CM, Guo M, Dharmage SC. HbA(1c) as a screening tool for detection of Type 2 diabetes: a systematic review. Diabet Med 2007; 24: 333-43.

[47] Ko GT, Chan JC, Yeung VT, *et al.* Combined use of a fasting plasma glucose concentration and HbA1c or fructosamine predicts the likelihood of having diabetes in high-risk subjects. Diabetes Care 1998; 21: 1221-5.

[48] Colagiuri S, Hussain Z, Zimmet P, Cameron A, Shaw J. Screening for type 2 diabetes and impaired glucose metabolism: the Australian experience. Diabetes Care 2004; 27: 367-71.

[49] Bao Y, Ma X, Li H, *et al.* Glycated hemoglobin A1c for diagnosing diabetes in Chinese population: cross sectional epidemiological survey. BMJ 2010; 340: c2249.

[50] Olson DE, Rhee MK, Herrick K, *et al.* Screening for diabetes and pre-diabetes with proposed HbA1c-based diagnostic criteria. Diabetes Care 2010; 33: 2184-9.

[51] Zhou X, Pang Z, Gao W, *et al.* Performance of an HbA1c and fasting capillary blood glucose test for screening newly diagnosed diabetes and pre-diabetes defined by an oral glucose tolerance test in Qingdao, China. Diabetes Care 2010; 33: 545-50.

[52] Davidson MB, Schriger DL, Peters AL, Lorber B. Relationship between fasting plasma glucose and glycosylated hemoglobin: potential for false-positive diagnoses of type 2 diabetes using new diagnostic criteria. JAMA 1999; 281: 1203-10.

[53] Davidson MB, Schriger DL, Lorber B. HbA1c measurements do not improve the detection of type 2 diabetes in a randomly selected population. Diabetes Care 2001; 24: 2017-8.

[54] Meigs JB, Shrader P, Sullivan LM, *et al.* Genotype score in addition to common risk factors for prediction of Type 2 Diabetes. N Engl J Med 2008; 359: 2208-19.

[55] Lyssenko V, Jonsson A, Almgren P, *et al.* Clinical Risk Factors, DNA Variants, and the Development of Type 2 Diabetes. N Engl J Med 2008; 359: 2220-32.

[56] Lin X, Song K, Lim N, *et al.* Risk prediction of prevalent diabetes in a Swiss population using a weighted genetic score--the CoLaus Study. Diabetologia 2009; 52: 600-8.

[57] Cornelis MC, Qi L, Zhang C, *et al.* Joint effects of common genetic variants on the risk for type 2 diabetes in U.S. men and women of european ancestry. Ann Intern Med 2009; 150: 541-50.

[58] Balkau B, Lange C, Fezeu L, *et al.* Predicting diabetes: clinical, biological, and genetic approaches: data from the Epidemiological Study on the Insulin Resistance Syndrome (DESIR). Diabetes Care 2008; 31: 2056-61.

[59] Schulze MB, Weikert C, Pischon T, *et al.* Use of multiple metabolic and genetic markers to improve the prediction of Type 2 Diabetes: the EPIC-Potsdam Study. Diabetes Care 2009; 32: 2116-9.

[60] Griffin SJ, Little PS, Hales CN, Kinmonth AL, Wareham NJ. Diabetes risk score: towards earlier detection of type 2 diabetes in general practice. Diabetes Metab Res Rev 2000; 16: 164-71.

[61] Glumer C, Carstensen B, Sandbaek A, *et al.* A danish diabetes risk score for targeted screening: The Inter99 study. Diabetes Care 2004; 27: 727-33.

[62]   Ramachandran A, Snehalatha C, Vijay V, Wareham NJ, Colagiuri S. Derivation and validation of diabetes risk score for urban Asian Indians. Diabetes Res Clin Pract 2005; 70: 63-70.

[63]   Mohan V, Deepa R, Deepa M, Somannavar S, Datta M. A simplified Indian Diabetes Risk Score for screening for undiagnosed diabetic subjects. J Assoc Physicians India 2005; 53: 759-63.

[64]   Baan CA, Ruige JB, Stolk RP, *et al.* Performance of a predictive model to identify undiagnosed diabetes in a health care setting. Diabetes Care 1999; 22: 213-9.

[65]   Lindstrom J, Tuomilehto J. The diabetes risk score: a practical tool to predict type 2 diabetes risk. Diabetes Care 2003; 26: 725-31.

[66]   Aekplakorn W, Bunnag P, Woodward M, *et al.* A risk score for predicting incident diabetes in the Thai population. Diabetes Care 2006; 29: 1872-7.

[67]   American Diabetes Association. Screening for type 2 diabetes. Diabetes Care 2000; 23 (Suppl 1): S20-3.

[68]   Hippisley-Cox J, Coupland C, Robson J, Sheikh A, Brindle P. Predicting risk of type 2 diabetes in England and Wales: prospective derivation and validation of QDScore. BMJ 2009; 338: b880.

[69]   Al-Lawati JA, Tuomilehto J. Diabetes risk score in Oman: a tool to identify prevalent type 2 diabetes among Arabs of the Middle East. Diabetes Res Clin Pract 2007; 77: 438-44.

[70]   Schulze MB, Hoffmann K, Boeing H, *et al.* An accurate risk score based on anthropometric, dietary, and lifestyle factors to predict the development of type 2 diabetes. Diabetes Care 2007; 30: 510-5.

[71]   Bindraban NR, van Valkengoed IG, Mairuhu G, *et al.* Prevalence of diabetes mellitus and the performance of a risk score among Hindustani Surinamese, African Surinamese and ethnic Dutch: a cross-sectional population-based study. BMC Public Health 2008; 8: 271.

[72]   Cabrera de Leon A, Coello SD, Rodriguez Perez Mdel C, *et al.* A simple clinical score for type 2 diabetes mellitus screening in the Canary Islands. Diabetes Res Clin Pract 2008; 80:128-33.

[73]   Kahn HS, Cheng YJ, Thompson TJ, Imperatore G, Gregg EW. Two risk-scoring systems for predicting incident diabetes mellitus in U.S. adults age 45 to 64 years. Ann Intern Med 2009; 150:741-51.

[74]   Bang H, Edwards AM, Bomback AS, *et al.* Development and validation of a patient self-assessment score for diabetes risk. Ann Intern Med 2009; 151:775-83.

[75]   Gao WG, Qiao Q, Pitkaniemi J, *et al.* Risk prediction models for the development of diabetes in Mauritian Indians. Diabet Med 2009; 26: 996-1002.

[76]   Chen L, Magliano DJ, Balkau B, *et al.* AUSDRISK: an australian type 2 diabetes risk assessment tool based on demographic, lifestyle and simple anthropometric measures. Med J Aust 2010; 192: 197-202.

CHAPTER 4

Obesity and Type 2 Diabetes

Regzedmaa Nyamdorj[*]

Department of Public Health, Hjelt Institute, University of Helsinki, Helsinki, Finland

Abstract: Obesity is a well known major modifiable risk factor for type 2 diabetes and as many as 25 other chronic conditions. The prevalences of obesity and obesity-related metabolic disorders, such as type 2 diabetes and many others, are increasing in both the developed and the developing world. Public health programmes that encourage people at individual and community levels to adopt healthy lifestyle are urgently needed to tackle the globally felt burden imposed by obesity. Based on current evidence BMI or Waist Circumference (WC) or Waist-To-Hip Ratio (WHR) predict or are associated with type 2 diabetes independently. It remains an open question as to which of these obesity indicators is best at predicting type 2 diabetes. Therefore both BMI and WC can be used as surrogate measures of obesity. The fact that diabetes prevalence varies markedly among different ethnic groups for the same BMI or WC suggests uniform cutoff values can not be applied on a worldwide basis. Longitudinal studies are needed to clarify the mechanism by which body composition, body fat distribution, genetic, social, cultural and behavioural factors predispose individuals to type 2 diabetes.

Keywords: Type 2 diabetes, obesity, body mass index, waist circumference, ethnicity, cutoff values.

4.1. EPIDEMIOLOGY OF OBESITY

Currently obesity is one of the leading health threats in most countries across the world. Obesity is a modifiable risk factor for type 2 diabetes, hypertension and as many as 25 other chronic conditions [1-3]. Its prevalence is increasing in both the developed and the developing world, and is reaching epidemic proportions in some of the populations. This dramatic increase is probably due to unhealthy lifestyle changes that are associated with increased urbanization, westernization and rapid economic development. It has generally recognised that those developing countries that still have a substantial problem of undernutrition, are now simultaneously facing epidemics of obesity and undernutrition. There are more than 1.6 billion overweight adults worlwide of which at least 400 million are clinically obese, these totals have been predicted to increase further by 2015 (http://www.who.int/features/factfiles/obesity/facts/en/index1.html). Consequently, the prevalence of obesity-associated metabolic disorders, such as type 2 diabetes and many other chronic diseases, are increasing at an alarming rate. Overweight and obesity are also considered as the second most common cause of preventable death after smoking (at least 2.6 million deaths/year) (http://www.who.int/features/factfiles/obesity/en/).

4.1.1. Clinical Definition and Classification of Overweight and Obesity

Obesity is an excess of body fat accumulation in the body [4]. The classification of overweight and obesity in adults using surrogate anthropometric measures proposed by different organizations are shown in Table **1**.

The WHO classification categorises individuals into either being overweight or obesity based on the elevated BMI levels whereas the National Cholesterol Education Program (NCEP) [6] and the International Diabetes Federation (IDF) [7, 8] classify individuals as obese and non-obese according to the waist circumference levels with purpose to define the metabolic syndrome. Ethnic-specific waist circumference values of ≥ 94 cm for men and 80 cm for women for European, Eastern Mediterranean, Middle East (Arab) and Sub-Saharan Africans and of $\geq 90/80$ cm (men/women) for Chinese, Japanese, South Asians and South and Central American, have been proposed by the IDF [7]. Recently, a Joint Scientific Statement based on the consensus of many different

Address correspondence to Regzedmaa Nyamdorj: Department of Public Health, Hjelt Institute, University of Helsinki, PL41, Mannerheimintie 172, 00014, Helsinki, Finland .E-mail: regzedmaa.nyamdorj@helsinki.fi

international organizations recommended that the cutoff values to define central obesity using the IDF ethnic-specific waist circumference values for Non-Europeans of ≥ 90 cm in men and of 80 cm in women. The equivalent values for men and women of European origin were 94/80 cm as recommended by the IDF and > 102/88 cm by the American Heart Association/National Heart, Lung, and Blood Institutes [9].

Table 1: Classification of overweight and obesity by different international organizations

	WHO 2000 [4]	WHO 1995 [5]	NCEP 2001 [6]	IDF 2006 [7]	Joint Statement 2009 [9]
	BMI (kg/m^2)	Waist girth (cm)	Waist girth (cm)	Waist girth (cm)	Waist girth (cm)
Underweight	< 18.5				
Normal weight	18.5 - 24.9				
Overweight	25.0 - 29.9				
Obesity	≥ 30.0	≥94/80 men/women	>102/88 men/women	≥94/80 or ≥90/80 men/women	≥94/80 or ≥102/88 and ≥90/80 men/women

4.1.2. Increasing Prevalence of Obesity

According to a prediction by the WHO, there will be approximately 2.3 billion overweight adults of which 700 million will be clinically obese by 2015 (http://www.who.int/features/factfiles/obesity/facts/en/index1.html). The prevalence of obesity as defined by BMI of ≥30 kg/m^2 is shown in Fig. **1** for different ethnic groups around the world. It ranged from 0.3 - 3.4% in Indians, Filipinos, Japanese and Chinese [10] to 4.7 - 9.1% in Thais [11], Hong Kong Chinese [10] and Singaporeans [12]. The prevalence ranged between 6.0% and 9.3% in men and 12.0% and 25.0% in women among Africans [13], Mauritians [14], Brazilians [15] and Mongolians [16]. The prevalences of obesity were over 10.0% in Europe [17-24], Canada [25] and Mexico [26] with similar rates for men and women. In the USA, the prevalence of obesity was over 32.0%, with higher rates for Mexican Americans and African Americans than for Whites [27].

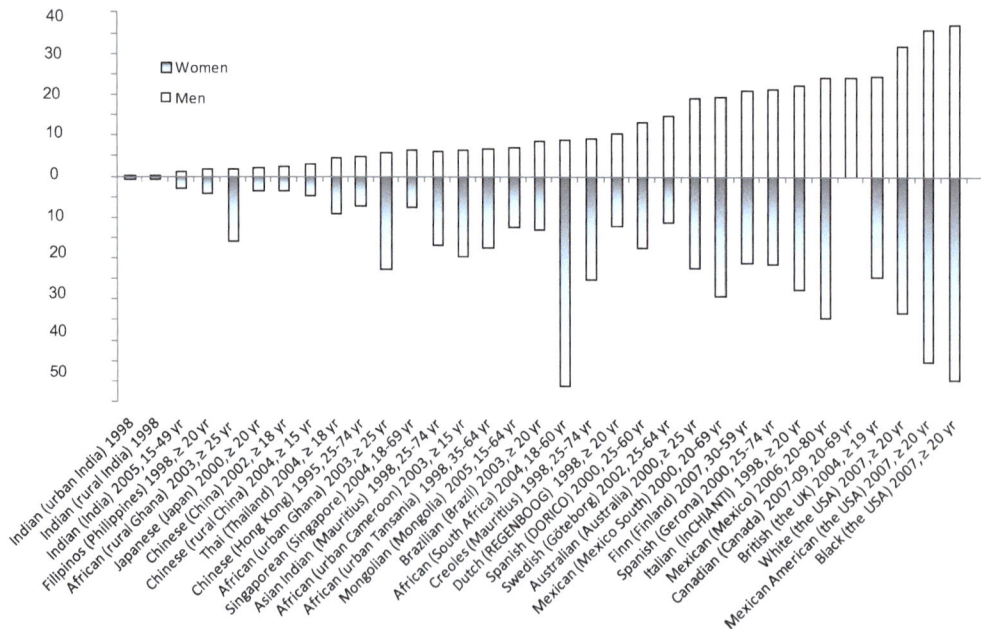

Figure 1: Adult prevalence (%) of obesity (BMI≥ 30 kg/m^2) measured by trained observers.

There is a similar increasing trend in the prevalence of obesity, in most of the populations based on national or population-based surveys, with a few exceptions (Table **2**). The prevalence has stabilized in India, Mongolia and the USA in the last decade but doubled in Brazil, China and Thailand.

Table 2: Increasing trend in the prevalence of obesity in different regions based on national or population-based surveys with random samples

Region	Prevalence (%)		Commnets
	Men	Women	
The USA			
1999-2000	27.5	33.4	NHANES cross-sectional studies, n = 22847, ≥ 20 years, [27]
2001-2002	27.8	33.3	
2003-2004	31.1	33.2	
2005-2006	33.3	35.3	
2007-2008	32.2	35.5	
Mexico			
2000	19.4	29.0	Mexican National Health Survey (South), [28]
2006	24.2	34.5	National Health and Nutrition Survey, ≥ 20 years, [26]
Brazil			National Surveys, n = 263734, ≥ 20 years, [15]
1975	2.7	7.4	National Study on Family Expenditure
1989	5.1	12.4	National Survey on Health and Nutrition
2003	8.8	13.0	National Household Budget Survey
England			
1993	13.6	16.9	Health Survey in England annually, n = 127876, ≥ 19 years, [23]
1994	14.4	17.7	
1995	15.6	18.0	
1996	16.9	19.2	
1997	17.0	20.4	
1998	17.6	21.7	
1999	19.3	21.6	
2000	21.5	21.8	
2001	21.3	24.1	
2002	22.5	23.7	
2003	23.2	24.2	
2004	24.0	24.4	
Spain (Girona)			
1995	15.4	15.4	Population-based cross-sectional surveys, n = 4918, 25-74 years, [21]
2000	21.9	21.4	
Sweden			
1985	6.4	7.2	WHO MONICA (Göteborg) and INTERGENE cohorts, n = 5622, 25-64 years, [18]
1990	9.1	9.8	
1995	11.5	9.8	
2002	14.8	11.0	
China			
Urban			China National Nutrition Survey 1992 and 2002, n=288553, ≥18 years, [29]
1992	4.9	7.5	
2002	8.7	8.0	
Rural			
1992	1.6	2.5	
2002	3.9	5.2	

India			
1993-1996	6.2	7.3	The Five City Study Group (urban), [30]
1998-1999		2.2	National Family Health surveys, n = 188900, 15-49 yers, [31]
2005-2006		2.8	
Mauritius			
Mauritian Indian			
1987	3.1	10.1	Mauritius Non-Communicable Disease Surveys,
1992	4.9	14.2	n = 5111, 25-74 years, [32]
Mauritian African			
1987	3.4	12.4	
1992	7.5	20.2	
Mongolia			
1999	13.8	24.6	National Survey, n = 2996, ≥ 35 years, [33]
2005	7.2	12.5	Mongolian STEPs Survey on NCD Risk Factors http://whqlibdoc.who.int/wpro/2007/9992998040_eng.pdf
Thailand			
1991	1.6	5.3	National Health Examination Surveys I-III, n = 69303, ≥ 18 years, [11]
1997	3.9	7.6	
2004	4.7	9.1	

Prevalence estimates were based on BMI ≥ 30 kg/ m^2 for all studies except the Chinese study.

BMI ≥ 28 kg/ m^2 was applied in the Chinese study.

4.1.3. Common/Shared Risk Factors for Obesity and Type 2 Diabetes

4.1.3.1. Gene and Family History

Since 2000, genomewide association studies have suggested a number of gene variants that are associated with a high risk for type 2 diabetes [34-36]. The FTO gene, first reported in 2007, predisposes individuals to diabetes through an associated effect of BMI which has subsequently been confirmed in many different ethnic groups [37-41]. Recently, new gene variants that are associated with population-level effects on BMI and waist circumference or WHR have been identified [42, 43]. It has been reported that some people are genetically predisposed to store more fat or have a higher prevalence of diabetes than others, particularly the Asian Indians [44-46]. Individuals with family histories of diabetes in their parents or siblings had from 2 to 6 times higher risk of diabetes than those with no familial background of type 2 diabetes [47-52].

4.1.3.2. Female Sex

In Central and Eastern Europe, Latin America, Asia and Africa, the prevalence of obesity was 1.5 to 2.0 times higher in women than in men [53, 54]. More recent estimates on the prevalence of obesity revealed an even higher (4-5 times) prevalence in women than in men in Ghana, Cameroon and South Africa [55-57]. This was most likely due to childhood deprivation (measured by the hunger index) and adult high socioeconomic status (measured by education and family income) in South Africa.

4.1.3.3. Age

Both diabetes [58, 59] and obesity [18, 23, 27, 29, 31, 54, 60-62] increase with age in men and women of all populations. However the age at which peak prevalence was reached is different across populations. The prevalence of diabetes was <10% in individuals younger than 60 years and was 10-20 % between the ages of 60-79 years, and continously increased with age up to 70s and 80s in 13 European cohorts [59]. In Asia, the prevalence of diabetes reached a peak at the age of 70-89 years in Chinese and Japanese whereas in Asian Indians the peak prevalence of diabetes occurred at the age of 60-69 years [58]. It has been reported that the age at the peak prevalence of obesity was also higher in developed countries (50-60 years) than in developing countries (40-50 years) [54].

4.1.3.4. Lifestyle Related and Other Environmental Risk Factors

4.1.3.4.1. Behavioural Factors

Pietraszek *et al.*, obtained J- or U-shaped associations between alcohol consumption and the incidence of type 2 diabetes, based on meta-analysis and cohort studies [63]. Compared with abstainers, moderate alcohol consumers had a 30% lower risk of diabetes. This phenomenon has been found to be due to an ethanol-mediated improvement in insulin sensitivity primarily observed in the obese individuals. In contrast heavy consumers had the same or higher risk of diabetes compared to abstainers [63]. In a Women's Health Study in the USA [64], it was reported that women who consumed a light to moderate amount of alcohol gained less weight and had a lower risk of becoming overweight and/or obese than abstainers. However, the effect of alcohol on obesity is still inconsistent among studies [65]. As for the association of smoking with type 2 diabetes, the results were inconsistent too. Some studies have shown that current smoking increased the risk of diabetes incidence by 44% [66] and 31% [67]. On the other hand another study reported a reduced risk of diabetes [68], which was probably due to weight reduction in heavy smokers.

4.1.3.4.2. Physical Inactivity

In modern society, a substantial proportion of the population is physically inactive due to the sedentary nature of their work, changing modes of transportation and increased urbanization. Prospective studies have reported a strong association between daily physical activity and a reduced risk of developing diabetes in different populations [69-74]. In those studies the relative risk reduction ranged from 15% to 60%. Clinical intervention trials that targeted lifestyle changes have clearly shown that weight reduction with a healthy diet in combination with physical activity can prevent or at least delay the onset of type 2 diabetes in individuals with impaired glucose tolerance in many ethnic groups around the world including Swedish [75], Chinese (Da Qing Study) [76], Finnish (Diabetes Prevention Study) [77], American (Diabetes Prevention Program, DPP) [78], Asian Indians [79] and Japanese [80]. The relative risk reduction for diabetes ranged from 28% for Asian Indians to 67% for Japanese undergoing intensive intervention regime as compared to the control group. Some of these studies have also demonstrated that the lifestyle intervention was as effective as that of metformin [78, 79, 81] or of pioglitazone [82] treatments. Weight reduction combined with a healthy diet and increased physical activity has played an important role in prevention of obesity-related conditions such as diabetes.

4.1.3.4.3. Socioeconomic Status

An individual's socioeconomic status (SES) defined by education level and income as determinant of obesity has been studied in different populations. Individuals, particularly women with low SES were more obese than those with high SES in highly developed countries [53, 61, 83, 84] in addition to Brazil [15]. In contrast women of high SES were more obese in the low- and middle-income countries [84] of Ghana [55], South Africa [57], Sub-Saharan Africa [85] and India [31]. A recent study from China found that low SES increased the risk for diabetes [86] in urban men only. On the other hand in another Chinese study, low SES lowered the risk in rural men living in Qingdao areas, which was mediated partly by obesity [87].

4.1.4. Anthropometric Measurements and Body Fatness

In epidemiological studies, a variety of surrogate anthropometric measures of obesity are used [88] as an indirect measures of obesity. BMI as a measure of general obesity, and waist circumference and WHR as measures of central obesity, have been proposed to define obesity [89]. The most common measure that has been used is the BMI. BMI is calculated as the individual's weight in kilograms divided by the square of individual's height in metres (kg/m^2). The concept of BMI dates back to 1869 as Quetelet's index [90], which was shown as a fairly good indicator of general fatness [4, 89, 91]. However, despite its common use in epidemiological and clinical studies, the degree of fatness for a given BMI varies by age, sex and ethnicity [92].

Since the early 1980s, waist-thigh-ratio or WHR has been considered to be more closely associated with abdominal visceral fat than BMI. Moreover, WHR is a better predictor of CVD or diabetes incidence than BMI [93-98]. In the 1990s, interest in waist circumferecne increased because it correlates more closely with abdominal visceral fat than with either WHR or BMI [5, 99-101]. Other measures, such as hip circumference [102-105], Waist-to-Height Ratio (WHtR) [106-109] and Waist-to-Stature Ratio (WSR) [110] may also be useful markers of central obesity. More precise and accurate methods such as dual-energy X-ray absorptiometry are also becoming available for large population studies.

4.1.4.1. Measurements of Waist and Hip Circumference

In the literature, there were as many as 14 different anatomical sites that have been used to measure waist circumference [111]. The most commonly used sites for measuring waist circumference in epidemiological studies are shown in Table 3.

Table 3: Anatomical sites for waist circumference measurement

Measurement Sites	Proposing Organization	References
Waist Circumference		
Immediately below the lowest rib		[111]
Narrowest or minimal waist	Anthropometric Standardization Reference Manual	[112]
Midpoint between the lowest rib and the iliac crest	WHO STEPS protocol	[113]
Umbilicus or navel level	NIH MESA protocol	[114]
Immediately above the iliac crest	NIH and NHANES III protocol	[115]
Hip Circumference		
The widest portions around the buttocks	WHO STEPS, MESA, and NHANES III protocols	[113-115]

According to the WHO Stepwise Approach to Surveillance (STEPS) protocol, the waist circumference should be measured at the midpoint between the top of the iliac crest (the uppermost part of the hip bone) and the lower margin of the last palpable rib [113], which is the method most commonly used. A second protocol, used by the National Institutes of Health (NIH) Multiethnic Study of Atherosclerosis (MESA) is to measure the waist circumference at the umbilicus or navel level [114]. A less frequently used method, described in the NIH manual [116] and the National Health and Nutrition Examination Survey III (NHANES III) [115] advises measuring the waist circumference from the top of the iliac crest. Because the waist circumferences measured at different anatomical sites of the same individual vary, the measurement protocol for the waist circumference needs to be unified and standardized worldwide in order to make the results comparable.

In contrast to the the situation for waist circumference, there is generally more consensus regarding the existing recommendations for measuring hip circumference around the widest portion of the buttocks [113-115].

4.1.4.2. Measurement Errors Related to BMI and Waist Circumference

Currently, there is no consensus regarding the optimal protocol for measurement of waist circumference and no scientific rationale that supports the measurement protocols identified. An important consideration in choosing an anthropometric measure of BMI or waist circumference as a screening tool is the measurement error. Some investigators have argued that measurement of the waist circumference is subject to less error because it entails only a single measurement, which favours the use of the waist circumference rather than the BMI. A study that has examined the measurement errors of different types of anthropometric measurements showed that weight and height were the most precise measurements, whereas waist circumference had strong inter-observer variation [117]. Two studies also showed a significantly higher inter-observer variability for waist circumference compared to BMI [118, 119]. Training, in the form of written instructions, eliminates random error but does not reduce the overall variation in waist circumference measurements between observers [119]. Although the various measurement protocols have no substantial influence on the association between waist circumference and health outcome [120], they will increase the difficulties in making direct comparisons between studies. Despite this, the measurement of waist circumference is still recommended due to its close association with unfavourable health consequences not because its measurement error is less than BMI. The advantages of anthropometric measures include low cost and less labour. However, there are also some potential disadvantages. For example, the ratios of WHR or BMI are difficult to interpret biologically. Further, the changes in body fat or visceral fat result in little or no change in the ration of WHR or BMI [121]. High correlations between these measures are another challenge [88].

4.2. OBESITY AND DIABETES

Since the blood glucose test is invasive, relatively expensive, time consuming and not easy to apply to mass screenings, the waist circumference and BMI measurements as indicators of obesity in combination with other non-invasive factors have often been included in various diabetes risk assessments. These assessments use algoritms that have been applied in screening programmes to serve as the first-line screening tool for diabetes and pre-diabetes in recent years [122-124].

4.2.1. General Obesity *Versus* Central Obesity in Relation to Type 2 Diabetes

Controversies exist as to which of these obesity measures, BMI or waist circumference, WHR or WSR are the most strongly associated with increased risk of type 2 diabetes.

During the 1990s, a number of epidemiological studies compared the performance of the BMI with waist circumference or WHR in assessing type 2 diabetes among different ethnic groups. A meta-analysis of 35 cohort studies that examined the association between different anthropometric measures of obesity and incident diabetes showed that the overall relative risk for diabetes incidence estimated based on BMI was not significantly different from those based on waist circumference or on WHR [125]. Another meta-analysis found a stronger association for diabetes risk for WSR than for BMI was observed in males only whereas there were no differences found between BMI, waist circumference, WHR, and WSR in females [126]. In the Obesity in Asia Collaboration study (OAC), prevalenc of diabetes was more strongly associated with waist circumference and WHR than with BMI in Asian and Caucasian women, but these measures did not differ in Caucasian men [127]. Results of a meta-analysis (Table 4) of 16 studies obtained from the DECODA collaboration showed that the Odds Ratios (ORs) for the BMI and central obesity indicators for prevalent diabetes in general did not differ in men nor women of any ethnic group. The two exceptions were for Filipino and Mauritian Indian men for whom the ORs for WSR were higher than for BMI [128]. For Filipino women, the ORs for the central obesity indicators were higher than for the BMI for prevalent diabetes.

Table 4: Paired homogeneity test results (*p*- values) comparing BMI with each of the central obesity indicators in their association with type 2 diabetes

Ethnicity	Diabetes Prevalence							
	Men				Women			
	No of subjects	WC	WHR	WSR	No of subjects	WC	WHR	WSR
Chinese	2980	0.246	0.604	0.081	3850	0.493	0.123	0.496
Filipino	1351	0.127	0.202	0.013*	2490	0.010*	0.011*	0.005*
Japanese	1040	0.620	0.623	0.377	1257	0.701	0.330	0.395
Native Indian	1232	0.783	0.625	0.684	1353	0.123	0.999	0.102
Mauritian Indian	1576	0.520	0.615	0.035*	1707	0.513	0.274	0.525
Mongolian	916	0.714	0.568	0.868	1075	0.560	0.801	0.603
	Diabetes Incidence							
	Men				Women			
Mauritian Indian	1345	0.207	0.922	0.122	1525	0.809	0.519	0.334
Mauritian African	496	0.283	0.831	0.120	579	0.697	0.625	0.536

*BMI is weaker otherwise there is no difference between the paired comparison.

When the same paired homogeneity tests were performed based on data where all ethnic groups were pooled, the OR for BMI did not differ from those for waist circumference or WHR, but were lower than those for WSR ($p = 0.001$) with undiagnosed diabetes in men (Fig. **2a**). In women the corresponding ORs were higher for waist circumference and WSR than for BMI (both $p < 0.05$) (Fig. **2b**). The same results were observed for individuals under 50 years of age. However, the ORs for these indicators did not differ for individuals aged 50 years and over (Fig. **2a** and **2b**). During the follow-up period from 1987-1998 of the Mauritius Non-communicable Disease Surveys (Table **4**), there was no difference found between BMI and each of the central obesity indicators for diabetes incidence for Mauritian Indians and Mauritian Africans, aged 25-74 years [129].

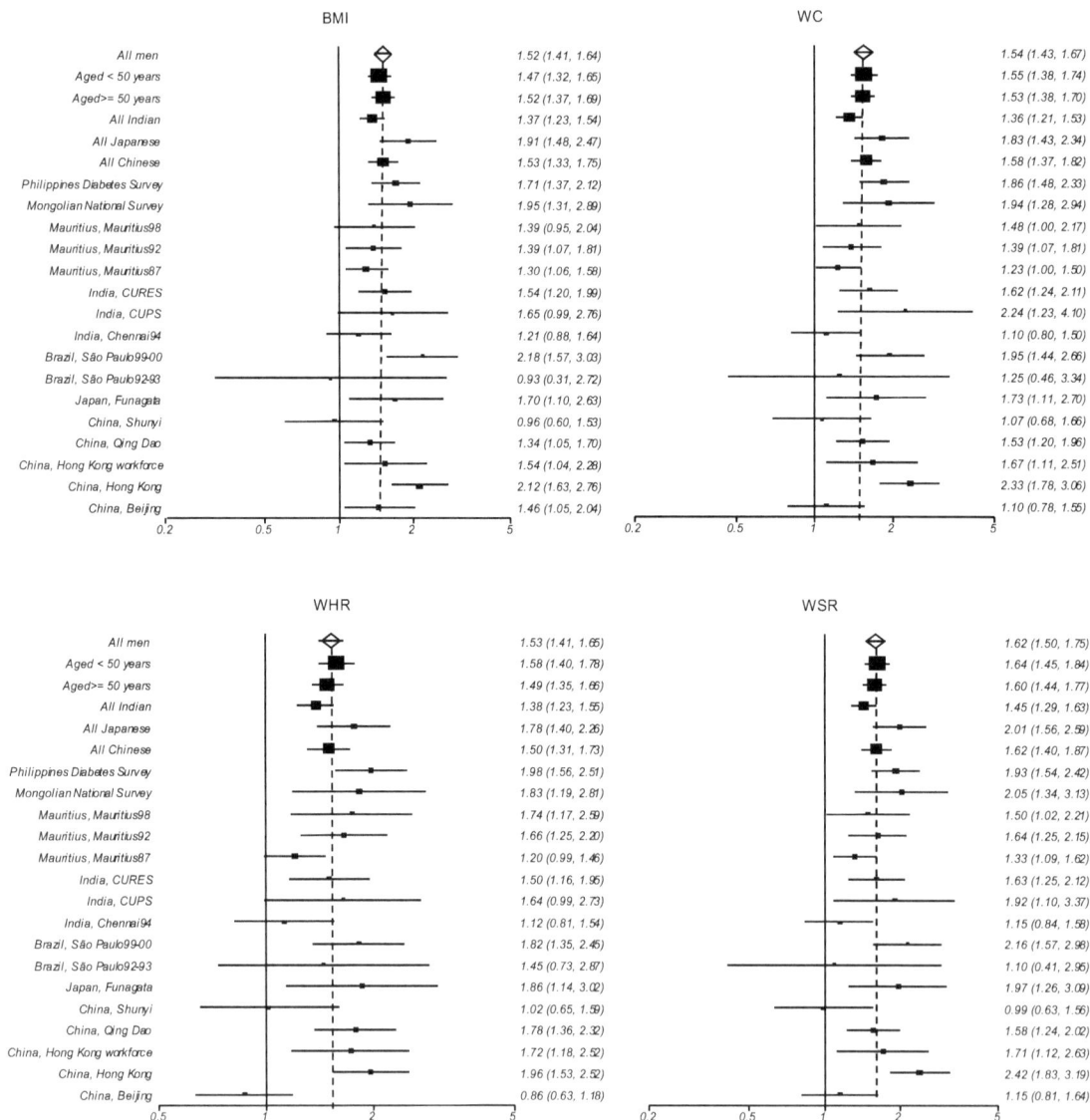

Figure 2a: Odds ratio (black diamond) and 95% CI (solid line) for diabetes corresponding to a one SD increase in BMI, WC, WHR and WSR in men [128].

Recently, we reviewed 17 prospective and 35 cross-sectional studies published from 1975 onwards that compared the performance of anthropometric measures in assessing diabetes incidence or prevalence by applying standard statistical approaches [130]. The results of the 17 prospective studies were inconsistent in that waist circumference was found to be the best predictor in Mexican Americans and African Americans, whereas the BMI was the best predictor in Pima Indians. Moreover, no differences were found in the

Diabetes Prevention Programme (DPP) study (Table **5**). Among 11 cross-sectional studies that used standard statistical testing on the data, most found a slightly higher OR or larger Area Under the Curve (AUC) for the Receiver-Operating Characteristics (ROC) for waist circumference than for BMI (Table **5**).

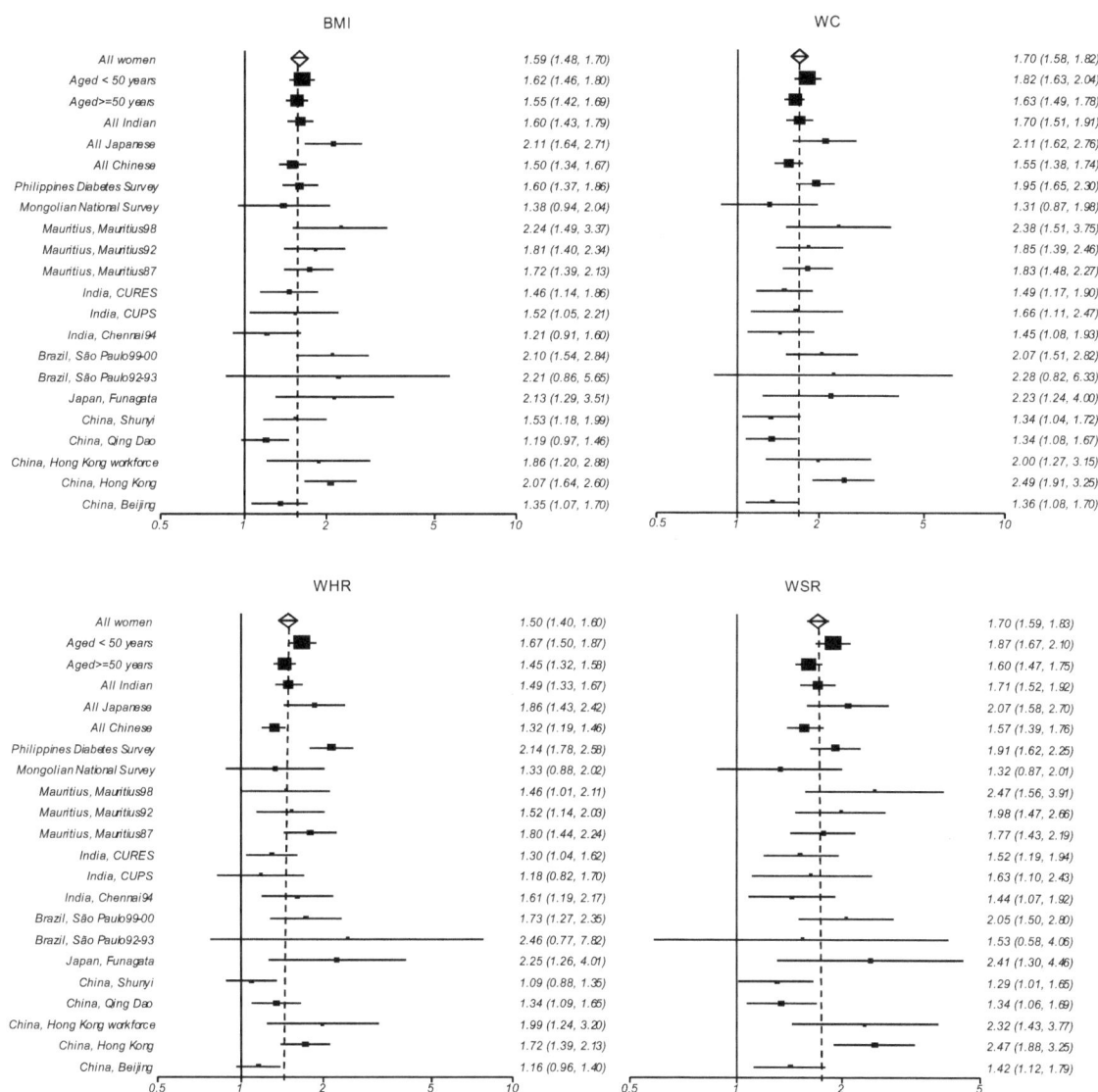

Figure 2b: Odds ratio (black diamond) and 95% CI (solid line) for diabetes corresponding to a one SD increase in BMI, WC, WHR and WSR in women [128].

All the reviewed studies showed that BMI, waist circumference, WHR and WSR predicted or were associated with type 2 diabetes independent of each other. These similarities are despite the controversial findings as to which of these obesity indicators is the most accurate predictor of type 2 diabets [130]. More recently, de Koning *et al.,* reported that a combination of BMI and WHR or a combination of waist circumference and hip circumference had a superior explanatory power for type 2 diabetes compared to those of BMI, waist circumference, WHR or hip circumference alone. Their findings were based on the EpiDREAM study from which they used the pooled data of Australian Aboriginals, Africans, Europeans, Latin American and South Asians [131]. The question as to which anthropometric measurement is the best predictor for type 2 diabetes needs to be clarified by more prospective studies in which the incidence of diabetes as an outcome.

Table 5: Difference between AUCs of the anthropometric measures tested using DeLong method, or difference in ORs tested applying paired homogeneity test as indicated.

Study	Ethnic Group	BMI	WC	WHR	WSR
Prospective Studies					
Wei 1997 [132]	Mexican (USA), 25-64 years				
n=721	Men	0.64*	*0.70*		
	Women	0.66*	*0.72*		
Tulloch-Reid 2003[133]	Pima Indian (USA), >18 years				
n = 1614	Men	*0.70*	0.68*	0.63*	0.69
	Women	*0.70*	0.69*	0.64*	0.70
DPP 2006 [134]	American (USA), 54 years				
n = 1070	Placebo, Men	*0.59*	0.61	0.60	0.60
	Placebo, Women	*0.58*	0.60	0.59	0.59
n = 1064	Metformin, Men	*0.57*	0.55	0.56	0.58
	Metformin, Women	*0.55*	0.56	0.57	0.57
n = 1067	Lifestyle, Men	*0.62*	0.62	0.67	0.63
	Lifestyle, Women	*0.63*	0.64	0.62	0.63
Stevens 2001 [135] n = 12814 ARIC Study	American (USA), 45-64 years				
	African men	**0.69**	0.70*	0.66	
	African women	**0.66**	0.69*	0.67	
	White men	**0.70**	0.70	0.67*	
	White women	**0.72**	0.73	0.72	
Cross-Sectional					
Wang 2004 [136]	Aboriginals (Australia), 18-74 years				
N = 915	Men	0.77 (0.71-0.83)	*0.80 (0.74-0.86)*	0.63 (0.55-0.70)*	
	Women	0.63 (0.57-0.69)*	*0.71 (0.66-0.77)*	0.67 (0.60-0.73)	
Foucan 2002 [137] n = 5149	African (Guadeloupe), 18-74 years	*0.70 (0.68-0.72)*	0.79 (0.77-0.81)*		
Stolk 2005 [138] n = 5302	Thai (Thailand) ≥ 35 years	*0.69*	0.75*	0.75*	
Hu 2007 [139] n = 15236	Chinese (China), 35-74 years	*0.62 (0.60-0.64)*	0.66 (0.64-0.68)*	0.67 (0.65-0.69)*	
Lorenzo 2007 [140]	Mexican and White, 35-64 years				
n = 1860	Mexican (USA) Men	*0.61*	0.66*	0.68*	0.67*
	Mexican (USA)	*0.71*	0.76*	0.75	0.77*

	Women				
n = 2233	Mexican (Mexico) Men	*0.56*	0.60*	0.64*	0.62*
	Mexican (Mexico) Women	*0.57*	0.61*	0.64*	0.63*
n = 2161	White (Spain) Men	*0.62*	0.63	0.65	0.58
	White (Spain) Women	*0.71*	0.72	0.69	0.73
n = 979	White (USA) Men	*0.73*	0.72	0.74	0.75
	White (USA) Women	*0.78*	0.81	0.78	0.81
Schneider 2007 [141]	Caucasian (German), ≥18 years				
n = 5377	Men	0.74 (0.72-0.77)*	0.75 (0.72-0.77)*	0.65 (0.62-0.68)*	*0.76 (0.74-0.79)*
	Women	0.69 (0.66-0.72)*	0.69 (0.66-0.72)*	0.61 (0.58-0.64)*	*0.72 (0.69-0.74)*
Diaz 2007	Bangladeshi n = 61				
Multi-ethinics ≥ 20 yr	Men Women	*0.67* *0.60*	0.73 0.65	0.75 0.65	
	Chinese n = 104				
	Men Women	*0.72* *0.79*	0.84 0.79	0.86 0.80	
	Indian n = 337				
	Men Women	*0.61* *0.63*	0.65 0.66	0.68* 0.69	
	Pakistan n = 134				
	Men Women	*0.57* *0.73*	0.51 0.83*	0.54 0.80	
	Black English n = 279				
	Men Women	*0.59* *0.59*	0.67* 0.68*	0.71* 0.70*	
	Black US n= 491				
	Men Women	*0.60* *0.61*	0.65* 0.69*	0.62 0.70*	
	Mexician American n =517				
	Men Women	*0.57* *0.64*	0.61 0.67	0.63* 0.68	
	White English n = 4488				
	Men Women	*0.67* *0.66*	0.68 0.72*	0.71* 0.74*	
	White US n = 1486				
	Men Women	*0.66* *0.65*	0.69 0.71*	0.71* 0.72*	
Pua 2005 [142]	Female Chinese, Malays, Indians, n = 566, 18-68 years	0.80*	0.86	0.85	*0.88*

Huxley 2008 [127]	OAC study, mean age 37-55 years	Paired Homogeneity Test for the ORs			
n = 263000	Asia men	*1.26*	1.35	1.47*	
	Asian women	*1.23*	1.40*	1.40*	
	Australian men	*1.39*	1.42	1.41	
	Australian women	*1.32*	1.50*	1.62*	

*indicating statistically significant difference (p<0.05) compared to reference measure (marked in bold).

4.2.2. Diagnostic Cutoff Values for Anthropometric Measurements in Assessing Type 2 Diabetes Risk

Currently, different values for obesity, using waist circumference has been proposed by different organizations for various populations. Central obesity, as measured by applying ethnic-specific waist circumference cutoff values has been defined by the IDF [9]. The recommended cutoff values of waist circumference and BMI for detecting diabetes differ among ethnic groups [9, 143-145], with lower values for Asians and higher for Europeans. Most studies that aimed at assessing BMI and waist circumference cutoff values almost exclusively used the ROC analysis approach. This approach detects optimal cutoff values at which the sum of the sensitivity and specificity is maximized [146].

There are marked variations in cutoff values for BMI and waist circumference among ethnic groups, as summarized in Table **6** [145]. A total of four prospective and 24 cross-sectional studies were reviewed. Among the ethnic groups, Tongans had the highest optimal cutoff values for BMI and waist circumference. This was followed by ethnic groups from the USA and the UK. The BMI and waist circumference cutoff values were higher for ethnic groups in the USA and the UK than in their counterparts in their original countries. The optimal cutoff values for BMI were 27 - 28 kg/m² in most studies of Caucasian men and women in Australia, Germany, men in France, the UK and the USA. The exceptions were for men in the NHANES III study who had a cutoff values of 30 kg/m² and for French women (25 kg/m²). The optimal cutoff values of BMI were 23 - 24 kg/m² in Chinese, Japanese and Thai and 22 - 23 kg/m² in Asian Indian men and women. The optimal waist circumference (WHR) cutoff values were 97 - 99 cm (0.95) for White/Caucasian men and 85 cm (0.83 - 0.85) for White/Caucasian women living outside the USA and the UK. The corresponding values for Chinese, Japanese, Indian and Thai men were 85 cm (0.90) and between 75 - 80 cm (0.79 - 0.85) for women of the same Asian ethnic groups. The values for other ethnic groups were between those for Whites/Caucasians and Asians. Men of European ancestry, Chinese, Japanese, Asian Indian and Bangladeshi had higher waist circumference values than women of the same ethnicity, but there was no gender difference among Thai, Iranian, Iraqi, Tunisian, Mexican, African and Tongan ethnic groups.

Table 6: Optimal BMI, waist circumference and WHR cutoff points (CP) for assessing risk of type 2 diabetes and sensitivity (Sen) (%) and specificity (Spe) (%) derived at the cutoff values.

Ethnicity	Men									Women								
	BMI (kg/m²)			WC (cm)			WHR			BMI (kg/m²)			WC (cm)			WHR		
	CP	Sen	Spe	CP	Sen	Spe	CP	Sen	Spe	CP	Sen	Spe	CP	Sen	Spe	CP	Sen	Spe
White (Others)	27-28	60-77	64-70	97-99	72	74	0.95	77	65	27-28	65-86	63-70	85	77	74	0.83-0.85	77	70
White (USA+UK)	28-30	60	70	101-6	61	67	0.97	69	58	27-28	65	69	95	67	68	0.91	69	64
Turkish (Turkey)				95	70	53							91	75	55			
Chinese	24	58-89	59-66	85	50-97	58-70	0.88-0.92	64-76	71-76	24	61-81	52-75	75-80	58-78	66-77	0.79-0.83	71-79	70-79
Chinese (USA+UK)	25			95						24			84					
Indian (India)	22-23	67-78	48-63	85-87	64-69	58-67	0.92	61	66	23	67-72	53-54	80-83	65-70	56-60	0.85	66	54
Indian	27			97						25			89					

(USA+UK)																	
Bangladeshi (USA+UK)	24			96						27			88					
Pakistani (USA+UK)	25			93						30			101					
Japanese (Japan)	24	59	59	85	62	62	0.92	71	71	23	67	67	73	70	70	0.81	78	78
Thai (Thailand)	23			85			0.91			25			85			0.88		
Iranian (Iran)																		
18-34 yr				86			0.88						82			0.82		
35-54 yr				91			0.94						93			0.87		
55-74 yr				92			0.96						95			0.91		
Iraqi (Iraq)	25	66	54	90	80	49	0.92	77	61	26	66	47	91	80	47	0.91	72	63
Tunisian (Tunisia)				85	71	63							85	76	67			
Tongan (Tonga)	32	66	68	103	63	64	0.93	69	71	35	62	61	103	65	63	0.86	69	71
Brazilian (Brazil)				88	69	68							84	67	66			
Mexican (Mexico)	27	56	56	90-95	47	47	0.90	57	57	28	59	59	85-97	53	53	0.86	62	62
Mexican (USA+UK)	28			100						30			104					
African American (USA)	28	61	68	99	61	71	0.94	62	60	30	63	60	101	62	68	0.92	61	66
African	25	71	71	88	71	79	0.87			29	62	65	85-89	62	65	0.90		
Black (USA+UK)	29-32			109-100						28			105-88					

The marked variations in the cutoff values within populations of the same ethnicity are probably due to differences in age range of the study participants or to the methods applied to identify cutoff values in different studies. Currently, consensus regarding the most appropriate approach for selecting waist circumference cutoff values has not been reached.

4.2.3. Anthropometric Measurement, Diabetes and Ethnicity

There are differences in the prevalence or incidence of diabetes and in the association of diabetes with different obesity measures between ethnic groups [125, 147-152]. However, a few studies have directly compared the strength of the association between obesity measures with the same level of obesity across ethnic groups. In comparison to Caucasians, non-Europeans (Australian Aboriginies, South Asians and Chinese in Canada), Aboriginies and Asians from different countries had higher levels of fasting glucose [153] or were at elevated risk of having diabetes [154] or had higher prevalences of diabetes [127] at any given level of BMI or waist circumference. Similarly, Filipino women living in the USA had a much higher risk of diabetes at every level of visceral adipose tissue compared with White/Caucasian or African American women. However, the high risk of the Filipino for diabetes was not explained by visceral adipose tissue [155]. The prevalence of undiagnosed diabetes at the same fixed values or over a range for BMI or waist circumference in the DECODA/DECODE studies was found to be highest in Asian Indians and lowest in Europeans and intermediate in other ethnic groups (Fig. **3**). The differences in prevalence of diabetes at each category of the BMI or waist circumference between ethnic groups were statistically significant ($p < 0.05$ for all BMI or waist circumference categories).

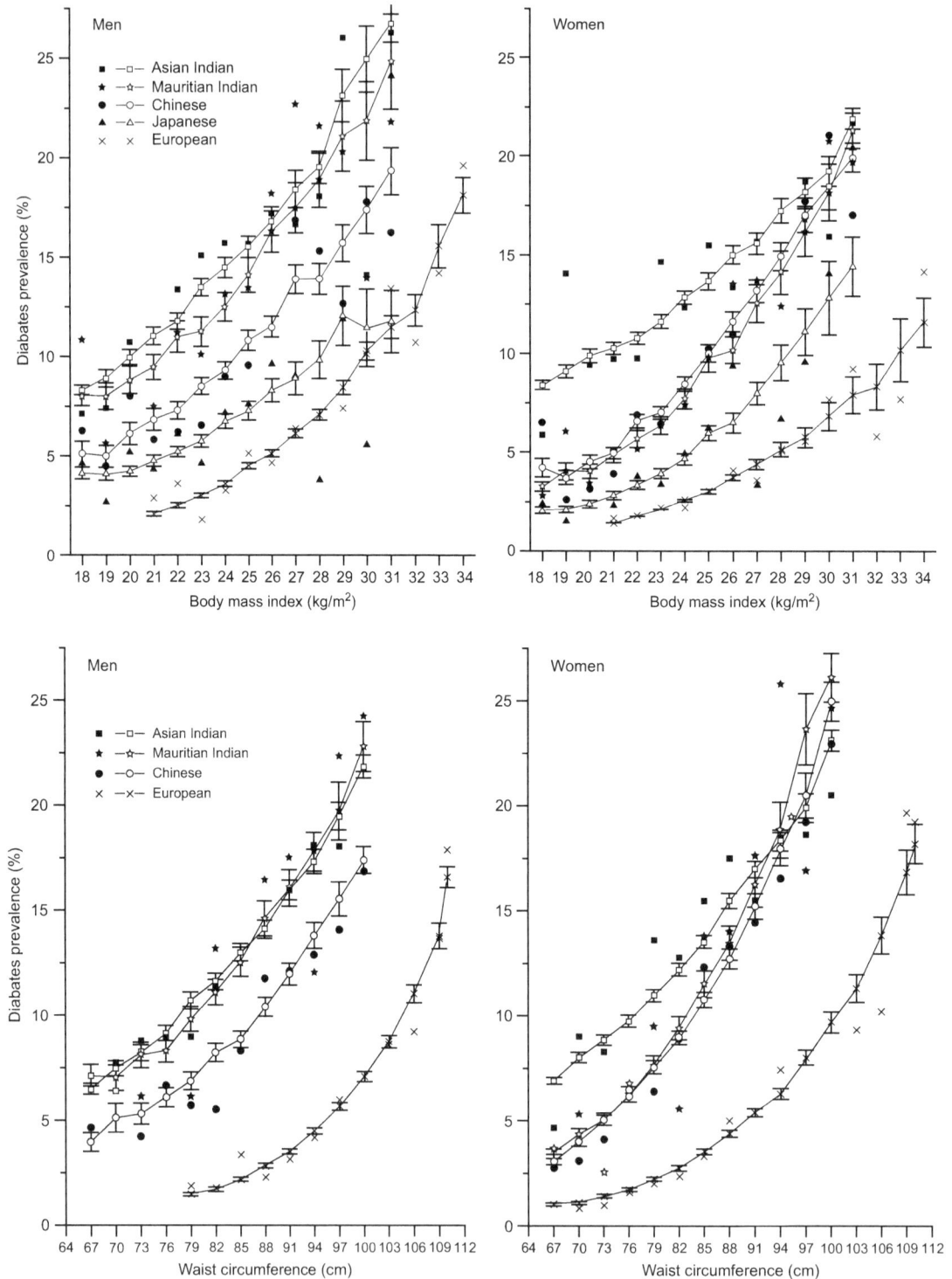

Figure 3: Crude (filled markers) and estimated (open markers) probability of undiagnosed diabetes according to BMI and waist circumference categories by ethnicity, the bars are 95% CIs [156].

The strength of the association of the anthropometric measures with diabetes incidence varies among different studies. The association between BMI and diabetes was reported to be stronger in Asians or Chinese than in Caucasians living in Australia [157] and the USA [158], but similar between Chinese and African Americans [158]. In other studies the association of diabetes with WHR or with BMI was found to be stronger in Caucasians/Whites than in Asians [125, 127]. In the DECODA/DECODE studies, the β coefficients for undiagnosed diabetes that corresponded to an increase in BMI or in waist circumference values of one standard deviation were not different among men of Asian Indian, Chinese, Japanese, Mauritian Indian and European (overall homogeneity test: $p > 0.05$ for both BMI and waist circumference) (Fig. **4a**) [156]. In contrast among women, the β coefficients that corresponded to an increase in BMI and waist circumference values of one standard deviation differed significantly among Asian Indian, Chinese, Mauritian Indian and European (overall homogeneity test: $p < 0.001$ for both BMI and waist circumference) (Fig. **4b**). Asian Indian women had lower β coefficients than women of other ethnic groups. More recently, de Koning *et al.*, obtained stronger associations between diabetes and BMI or hip circumference in Aborigines than in Africans and South Asians. Moreover, the weaker associations between diabetes and BMI in Africans compared to that in Europeans, was based on analysis by which men

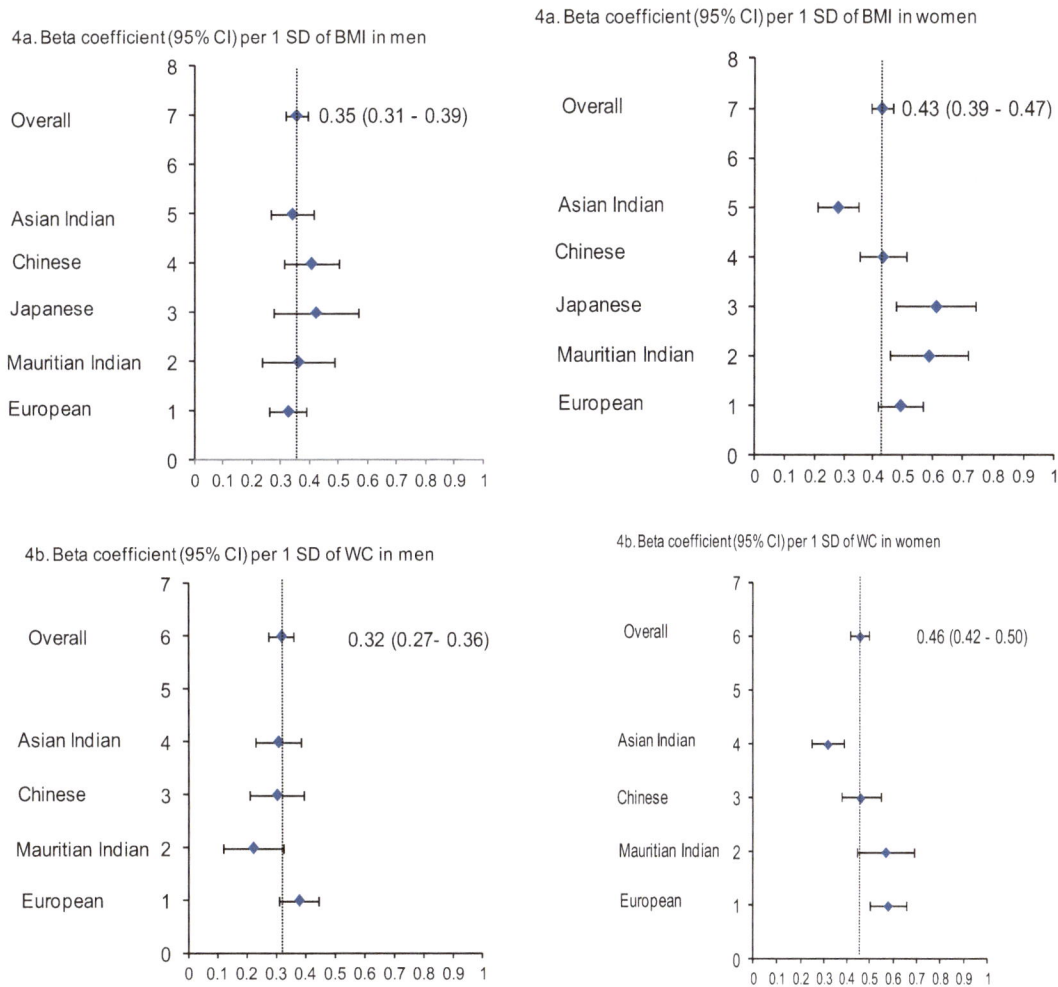

Figure 4: β coefficients corresponding to a one standard deviation (SD) increase in body mass index (BMI) (a) and waist circumference (WC) (b) for prevalence of undiagnosed diabetes [156].

and women of all five ethnic groups were pooled [131]. The evidence suggests that at any given level of the BMI, waist circumference, WHR or visceral adipose tissue accumulation, non-Europeans have a greater risk of developing diabetes than Europeans. An explanation for the higher susceptibility to diabetes in Asians compared to Europeans remains unclear. Possible factors are an increased genetic predisposition, changes in diet and lifestyle or the interaction of both. Longitudinal studies are needed to clarify the mechanism by which body composition, body fat distribution, or other genetic, social, cultural and behavioural factors predispose Asians to metabolic diseases.

4.2.4. Obesity in the Pathogenesis of Diabetes

Obesity as a major contributing factor in the pathogenesis of diabetes has been studied intensively in the last decade, but the underlying mechanism is still not clear. The hypothesised or candidate mechanisms of obesity in the pathogenesis of metabolic disorders are summarized in Fig. **5**.

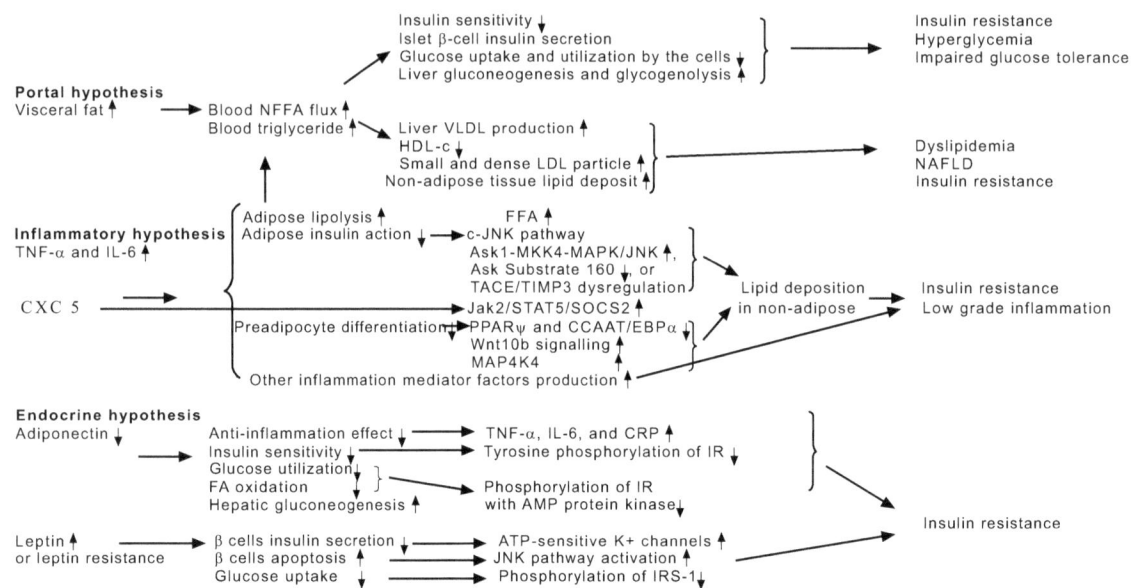

Figure 5: Role of obesity in insulin resistance or diabetes. AMP, Adenosine monophosphate; ATP, Adenosine-5'-triphosphate; CRP, C-reactive protein; FFA, free fatty acid; HDL-c, high density lipoprotein cholesterol; IR, insulin resistance; LDL, low density lipoprotein; IL-6, interleukin-6; NAFLD,non-alcoholic fatty liver disease; PAI,plasminogen activator inhibitor; TNF-α, tumor necrosis factor-alpha; VLDL, very low density lipoprotein cholesterol.

4.2.4.1. Abdominal/Visceral Obesity

Both abdominal visceral fat and subcutaneous fat contribute to obesity-related insulin resistance. Nonetheless, the data on the relative importance of these two fat depots are conflicting and require future investigation. A number of studies reported that visceral fat is more detrimental for the pathogenesis of type 2 diabetes than other fat depots [159-166]. This is due to more metabolic activity [167, 168] and high rates of lipolysis of the visceral fat [167, 169-171]. An alternative mechanism is the portal hypothesis. This hypothesis suggests an increased release of Nonesterified Fatty Acids (NEFAs) from the visceral fat through the portal circulation to the liver [169, 172, 173]. Others hypothesises that an increased release of NEFAs from subcutaneous fat into the systemic circulation [174-178] and/or inflammatory cytokines released from visceral fat [179] were considered as the link between visceral obesity and insulin resistance. A recent review by Taylor [180] suggested that gastric banding [181, 182] or bypass [181, 183] surgeries in extremely obese individuals improved or reversed insulin resistance and diabetes, due to visceral fat reduction [182]. This was also found in dogs [184].

4.2.4.2. Inflammatory Hypothesis

Overexpression of tumour necrosis factor alpha (TNF-α) in adipose tissue of rodents [185] and humans [186, 187] provided the first clear link between obesity, diabetes and chronic inflammation. In the inflammatory hypothesis [188-191], large adipocytes that are infiltrated by macrophages [192-195] produced TNF-α and interleukin-6 (IL-6) in obese individuals [192, 193]. These cytokines increased lipolysis of the adipose tissue [196], inhibited insulin receptor signalling through different pathways [197-206] and inhibited the differentiation of preadipocytes into mature adipocytes [207-211], all of which finally led to insulin resistance. The role played by these inflammatory cytokines in obesity-related insulin resistance is still under intensive investigation.

4.2.4.3. Endocrine Hypothesis

Adipocytes secrete adipokines such as leptin and adiponectin, which act at both the local and the systemic (endocrine) level [168, 196, 212, 213]. Current evidence for high leptin (or leptin resistance) and low adiponectin in obesity-related disorders is not clear, and consequently further investigations are needed. High leptin levels increased the risk of diabetes in men and women [214] or only in men [215, 216]. However, the increased risks in men and women were reduced after adjusting for body fat and inflammatory markers [214]. In the endocrine hypothesis, leptin inhibits insulin secretion [217-219] or impairs insulin-mediated glucose uptake in obese individuals [220]. Exposure of human islets of Langerhans to high levels of leptin and glucose resulted in β-cell apoptosis [219]. In contrast, an experimentally induced hyperinsulinemia had no effects on leptin [191].

Adiponectin levels were decreased in diabetes [221, 222] and obese individuals [222, 223], due to the inhibition of their synthesis by TNF-α and other cytokines. Low adiponectin levels decreased anti-inflammatory effects [224-226] and insulin sensitivity in skeletal muscle [227], liver [228] and also in the whole-body of Pima Indians [227], but it increased hepatic glucose production in mice [229]. It also inhibited glucose utilization and fatty acid oxidation [224, 229, 230]. In contrast, plasma adiponectin was not associated with fatty acid oxidation under resting conditions in nondiabetic Pima Indians and Whites/Caucasians [231].

REFERENCES

[1] Colditz GA, Willett WC, Rotnitzky A, Manson JE. Weight gain as a risk factor for clinical diabetes mellitus in women. Ann Intern Med 1995; 122: 481-6.

[2] Huang Z, Willett WC, Manson JE, *et al.* Body weight, weight change, and risk for hypertension in women. Ann Intern Med 1998; 128: 81-8.

[3] Zimmet P, Alberti KG, Shaw J. Global and societal implications of the diabetes epidemic. Nature 2001; 414: 782-7.

[4] WHO Consultation. Obesity: preventing and managing the global epidemic. Part 1: The problem of overweight and obesity.(Report No.: 894) World Health Organization, Geneva: Switzerland 2000 .

[5] Lean ME, Han TS, Morrison CE. Waist circumference as a measure for indicating need for weight management. BMJ 1995; 311: 158-61.

[6] Grundy SM, Becker D, Clark LT, *et al.* Expert panel on detection E, and treatment of high blood cholesterol in adults. Executive Summary of The Third Report of The National Cholesterol Education Program (NCEP) Expert Panel on Detection, Evaluation, And Treatment of High Blood Cholesterol In Adults (Adult Treatment Panel III). JAMA 2001; 285: 2486-97.

[7] Alberti KG, Zimmet P, Shaw J. Metabolic syndrome-a new world-wide definition. A Consensus Statement from the International Diabetes Federation. Diabet Med 2006; 23: 469-80.

[8] Alberti KG, Zimmet P, Shaw J. The metabolic syndrome-a new worldwide definition. Lancet 2005; 366: 1059-62.

[9] Alberti KG, Eckel RH, Grundy SM, *et al.* Harmonizing the metabolic syndrome: a joint interim statement of the International Diabetes Federation Task Force on Epidemiology and Prevention; National Heart, Lung, and Blood Institute; American Heart Association; World Heart Federation; International Atherosclerosis Society; and International Association for the Study of Obesity. Circulation 2009; 120: 1640-5.

[10] Lee C.M.Y, Martiniuk A.L.C, Woodward M, *et al.* Asia Pacific Cohort Study Collaboration. The burden of overweight and obesity in the Asia-Pacific region. Obes Rev 2007; 8: 191-6.

[11] Aekplakorn W, Mo-Suwan L. Prevalence of obesity in Thailand. Obes Rev 2009; 10: 589-92.

[12] Ministry of Health Singapore. National Health Survey 2004. 2005 [updated 2005; cited 2010 8 March 2010]; Available from: http: //www.moh.gov.sg/mohcorp/publicationsreports.aspx?id=2984.

[13] Bovet P, Ross AG, Gervasoni JP, *et al.* Distribution of blood pressure, body mass index and smoking habits in the urban population of Dar es Salaam, Tanzania, and associations with socioeconomic status. Int J Epidemiol 2002; 31: 240-7.

[14] International Obesity Task Force. Global Obesity prevalence in adults. [10 February 2010; cited 8 March 2010]; Available from: http: //www.iaso.org/site_media/uploads/Prevalence_of_Adult_Obesity_April_2011_New.pdf.

[15] Monteiro CA, Conde WL, Popkin BM. Income-specific trends in obesity in Brazil: 1975-2003. Am J Public Health 2007; 97: 1808-12.

[16] Bolormaa N, Narantuya L, De Courten M, Enkhtuya P, Tsegmed S. Dietary and lifestyle risk factors for noncommunicable disease among the Mongolian population. Asia Pac J Public Health 2008; 20 (Suppl): 23-30.

[17]   Aranceta J, Moreno B, Moya M, Anadon A. Prevention of overweight and obesity from a public health perspective. Nutr Rev 2009; 67 (Suppl 1): S83-8.

[18]   Berg C, Rosengren A, Aires N, *et al.* Trends in overweight and obesity from 1985 to 2002 in Goteborg, West Sweden. Int J Obes 2005; 29: 916-24.

[19]   Schokker DF, Visscher TL, Nooyens AC, van Baak MA, Seidell JC. Prevalence of overweight and obesity in the Netherlands. Obes Rev 2007; 8: 101-8.

[20]   Vartiainen E, Laatikainen T, Peltonen M, *et al.* Thirty-five-year trends in cardiovascular risk factors in Finland. Int J Epidemiol 2010; 39: 504-18.

[21]   Schroder H, Elosua R, Vila J, Marti H, Covas MI, Marrugat J. Secular trends of obesity and cardiovascular risk factors in a Mediterranean population. Obesity 2007; 15: 557-62.

[22]   Cameron AJ, Welborn TA, Zimmet PZ, *et al.* Overweight and obesity in Australia: the 1999-2000 Australian Diabetes, Obesity and Lifestyle Study (AusDiab). Med J Aust 2003; 178: 427-32.

[23]   Zaninotto P, Head J, Stamatakis E, Wardle H, Mindell J. Trends in obesity among adults in England from 1993 to 2004 by age and social class and projections of prevalence to 2012. J Epidemiol Community Health 2009; 63: 140-6.

[24]   Berghofer A, Pischon T, Reinhold T, Apovian CM, Sharma AM, Willich SN. Obesity prevalence from a European perspective: a systematic review. BMC Public Health 2008; 8: 200.

[25]   Shields M, Tremblay MS, Laviolette M, Craig CL, Janssen I, Gorber SC. Fitness of Canadian adults: results from the 2007-2009 Canadian Health Measures Survey. Health Rep 2010; 21: 21-35.

[26]   Malina RM, Reyes ME, Tan SK, Buschang PH, Little BB. Overweight and obesity in a rural Amerindian population in Oaxaca, Southern Mexico, 1968-2000. Am J Hum Biol 2007; 19: 711-21.

[27]   Flegal KM, Carroll MD, Ogden CL, Curtin LR. Prevalence and trends in obesity among US adults, 1999-2008. JAMA 2010; 303: 235-41.

[28]   Sanchez-Castillo CP, Velazquez-Monroy O, Berber A, Lara-Esqueda A, Tapia-Conyer R, James WP. Anthropometric cutoff points for predicting chronic diseases in the Mexican National Health Survey 2000. Obes Res 2003; 11: 442-51.

[29]   Wang Y, Mi J, Shan XY, Wang QJ, Ge KY. Is China facing an obesity epidemic and the consequences? The trends in obesity and chronic disease in China. Int J Obes 2007; 31: 177-88.

[30]   Singh RB, Pella D, Mechirova V, *et al.* Prevalence of obesity, physical inactivity and undernutrition, a triple burden of diseases during transition in a developing economy. The Five City Study Group. Acta Cardiol 2007; 62: 119-27.

[31]   Wang Y, Chen HJ, Shaikh S, Mathur P. Is obesity becoming a public health problem in India? Examine the shift from under- to overnutrition problems over time. Obes Rev 2009; 10: 456-74.

[32]   Hodge AM, Dowse GK, Gareeboo H, Tuomilehto J, Alberti KG, Zimmet PZ. Incidence, increasing prevalence, and predictors of change in obesity and fat distribution over 5 years in the rapidly developing population of Mauritius. Int J Obes Relat Metab Disord 1996; 20: 137-46.

[33]   Suvd J, Gerel B, Otgooloi H, *et al.* Glucose intolerance and associated factors in Mongolia: results of a national survey. Diabet Med 2002; 19: 502-8.

[34]   Prokopenko I, McCarthy MI, Lindgren CM. Type 2 diabetes: new genes, new understanding. Trends Genet 2008; 24: 613-21.

[35]   Florez JC. Genetic Susceptibility to Type 2 Diabetes and Implications for Therapy. J Diabetes Sci Technol 2009; 3: 690-6.

[36]   Dupuis J, Langenberg C, Prokopenko I, *et al.* New genetic loci implicated in fasting glucose homeostasis and their impact on type 2 diabetes risk. Nat Genet 2010; 42: 105-16.

[37]   Frayling TM, Timpson NJ, Weedon MN, *et al.* A common variant in the FTO gene is associated with body mass index and predisposes to childhood and adult obesity. Science 2007; 316: 889-94.

[38]   Liu Y, Liu Z, Song Y, *et al.* Meta-analysis Added Power to Identify Variants in FTO Associated With Type 2 Diabetes and Obesity in the Asian Population. Obesity 2010; 18: 1619-24.

[39]   Karasawa S, Daimon M, Sasaki S, *et al.* Association of the common fat mass and obesity associated (FTO) gene polymorphism with obesity in a Japanese population. Endocr J 2010; 57: 293-301.

[40]   Yajnik CS, Janipalli CS, Bhaskar S, *et al.* FTO gene variants are strongly associated with type 2 diabetes in South Asian Indians. Diabetologia 2009; 52: 247-52.

[41]   Wing MR, Ziegler J, Langefeld CD, *et al.* Analysis of FTO gene variants with measures of obesity and glucose homeostasis in the IRAS Family Study. Hum Genet 2009; 125: 615-26.

[42]   Lindgren CM, Heid IM, Randall JC, *et al.* Genome-wide association scan meta-analysis identifies three Loci influencing adiposity and fat distribution. PLoS Genet 2009; 5: e1000508.

[43]   Willer CJ, Speliotes EK, Loos RJ, *et al.* Six new loci associated with body mass index highlight a neuronal influence on body weight regulation. Nat Genet 2009; 41: 25-34.

[44]   Abate N, Carulli L, Cabo-Chan A, Jr., Chandalia M, Snell PG, Grundy SM. Genetic polymorphism PC-1 K121Q and ethnic susceptibility to insulin resistance. J Clin Endocrinol Metab 2003; 88: 5927-34.

[45]   Abate N, Chandalia M, Satija P, *et al.* ENPP1/PC-1 K121Q polymorphism and genetic susceptibility to type 2 diabetes. Diabetes 2005; 54: 1207-13.

[46]   Radha V, Vimaleswaran KS, Babu HN, *et al.* Role of genetic polymorphism peroxisome proliferator-activated receptor-gamma2 Pro12Ala on ethnic susceptibility to diabetes in South-Asian and Caucasian subjects: Evidence for heterogeneity. Diabetes Care 2006; 29: 1046-51.

[47]   Knowler WC, Pettitt DJ, Savage PJ, Bennett PH. Diabetes incidence in Pima indians: contributions of obesity and parental diabetes. Am J Epidemiol 1981; 113: 144-56.

[48]   Lin RS, Lee WC, Lee YT, Chou P, Fu CC. Maternal role in type 2 diabetes mellitus: indirect evidence for a mitochondrial inheritance. Int J Epidemiol 1994; 23: 886-90.

[49]   Sargeant LA, Wareham NJ, Khaw KT. Family history of diabetes identifies a group at increased risk for the metabolic consequences of obesity and physical inactivity in EPIC-Norfolk: a population-based study. The European Prospective Investigation into Cancer. Int J Obes Relat Metab Disord 2000; 24: 1333-9.

[50]   Harrison TA, Hindorff LA, Kim H, *et al.* Family history of diabetes as a potential public health tool. Am J Prev Med 2003; 24: 152-9.

[51]   Valdez R. Detecting Undiagnosed Type 2 Diabetes: Family History as a Risk Factor and Screening Tool. J Diabetes Sci Technol 2009; 3: 722-6.

[52]   Valdez R, Yoon PW, Liu T, Khoury MJ. Family history and prevalence of diabetes in the U.S. population: the 6-year results from the National Health and Nutrition Examination Survey (1999-2004). Diabetes Care 2007; 30: 2517-22.

[53]   Seidell JC. Epidemiology of obesity. Semin Vasc Med 2005; 5: 3-14.

[54]   Low S, Chin MC, Deurenberg-Yap M. Review on epidemic of obesity. Ann Acad Med Singapore 2009; 38: 57-9.

[55]   Amoah AG. Sociodemographic variations in obesity among Ghanaian adults. Public Health Nutr 2003; 6: 751-7.

[56]   Kamadjeu RM, Edwards R, Atanga JS, Kiawi EC, Unwin N, Mbanya JC. Anthropometry measures and prevalence of obesity in the urban adult population of Cameroon: an update from the Cameroon Burden of Diabetes Baseline Survey. BMC Public Health 2006; 6: 228.

[57]   Case A, Menendez A. Sex differences in obesity rates in poor countries: evidence from South Africa. Econ Hum Biol 2009; 7: 271-82.

[58]   Qiao Q, Hu G, Tuomilehto J, *et al.* Age- and sex-specific prevalence of diabetes and impaired glucose regulation in 11 Asian cohorts. Diabetes Care 2003; 26: 1770-80.

[59]   Qiao Q, Hu G, Tuomilehto J, Eriksson J. The DECODE Study Group. Age- and sex-specific prevalences of diabetes and impaired glucose regulation in 13 European cohorts. Diabetes Care 2003; 26: 61-9.

[60]   Lahti-Koski M, Jousilahti P, Pietinen P. Secular trends in body mass index by birth cohort in eastern Finland from 1972 to 1997. Int J Obes Relat Metab Disord 2001; 25: 727-34.

[61]   Lahti-Koski M, Seppanen-Nuijten E, Mannisto S, *et al.* Twenty-year changes in the prevalence of obesity among Finnish adults. Obes Rev 2010: 171-6.

[62]   Wang Y, Beydoun MA. The obesity epidemic in the United States-gender, age, socioeconomic, racial/ethnic, and geographic characteristics: a systematic review and meta-regression analysis. Epidemiol Rev 2007; 29: 6-28.

[63]   Pietraszek A, Gregersen S, Hermansen K. Alcohol and type 2 diabetes. A review. Nutr Metab Cardiovasc Dis 2010; 20: 366-75.

[64]   Wang L, Lee IM, Manson JE, Buring JE, Sesso HD. Alcohol consumption, weight gain, and risk of becoming overweight in middle-aged and older women. Arch Intern Med 2010; 170: 453-61.

[65]   Suter PM. Is alcohol consumption a risk factor for weight gain and obesity? Crit Rev Clin Lab Sci 2005; 42: 197-227.

[66]   Willi C, Bodenmann P, Ghali WA, Faris PD, Cornuz J. Active smoking and the risk of type 2 diabetes: a systematic review and meta-analysis. JAMA 2007; 298: 2654-64.

[67]   Yeh HC, Duncan BB, Schmidt MI, Wang NY, Brancati FL. Smoking, smoking cessation, and risk for type 2 diabetes mellitus: a cohort study. Ann Intern Med 2010; 152: 10-7.

[68]   Onat A, Ozhan H, Esen AM, *et al.* Prospective epidemiologic evidence of a "protective" effect of smoking on metabolic syndrome and diabetes among Turkish women-without associated overall health benefit. Atherosclerosis 2007; 193: 380-8.

[69]   Helmrich SP, Ragland DR, Leung RW, Paffenbarger RS, Jr. Physical activity and reduced occurrence of non-insulin-dependent diabetes mellitus. N Engl J Med 1991; 325: 147-52.

[70]   Hu FB, Sigal RJ, Rich-Edwards JW, *et al.* Walking compared with vigorous physical activity and risk of type 2 diabetes in women: a prospective study. JAMA 1999; 282: 1433-9.

[71]   Hu G, Lindstrom J, Valle TT, *et al.* Physical activity, body mass index, and risk of type 2 diabetes in patients with normal or impaired glucose regulation. Arch Intern Med 2004; 164: 892-6.

[72]   Meisinger C, Lowel H, Thorand B, Doring A. Leisure time physical activity and the risk of type 2 diabetes in men and women from the general population. The MONICA/KORA Augsburg Cohort Study. Diabetologia 2005; 48: 27-34.

[73]   Nakanishi N, Takatorige T, Suzuki K. Daily life activity and risk of developing impaired fasting glucose or type 2 diabetes in middle-aged Japanese men. Diabetologia 2004; 47: 1768-75.

[74]   Perry IJ, Wannamethee SG, Walker MK, Thomson AG, Whincup PH, Shaper AG. Prospective study of risk factors for development of non-insulin dependent diabetes in middle aged British men. BMJ 1995; 310: 560-4.

[75]   Eriksson KF, Lindgarde F. Prevention of type 2 (non-insulin-dependent) diabetes mellitus by diet and physical exercise. The 6-year Malmo feasibility study. Diabetologia 1991; 34: 891-8.

[76]   Pan X, Li G, Hu Y, *et al.* Effects of diet and exercise in preventing NIDDM in people with impaired glucose tolerance. The Da Qing IGT and Diabetes Study. Diabetes Care 1997; 20: 537-44.

[77]   Tuomilehto J, Lindstrom J, Eriksson JG, *et al.* Prevention of type 2 diabetes mellitus by changes in lifestyle among subjects with impaired glucose tolerance. N Engl J Med 2001; 344: 1343-50.

[78]   Knowler WC, Barrett-Connor E, Fowler SE, *et al.* Reduction in the incidence of type 2 diabetes with lifestyle intervention or metformin. N Engl J Med 2002; 346: 393-403.

[79]   Ramachandran A, Snehalatha C, Mary S, Mukesh B, Bhaskar AD, Vijay V. The Indian Diabetes Prevention Programme shows that lifestyle modification and metformin prevent type 2 diabetes in Asian Indian subjects with impaired glucose tolerance (IDPP-1). Diabetologia 2006; 49: 289-97.

[80]   Kosaka K, Noda M, Kuzuya T. Prevention of type 2 diabetes by lifestyle intervention: a Japanese trial in IGT males. Diabetes Res Clin Pract 2005; 67: 152-62.

[81]   Knowler WC, Fowler SE, Hamman RF, *et al.* 10-year follow-up of diabetes incidence and weight loss in the Diabetes Prevention Program Outcomes Study. Lancet 2009; 374: 1677-86.

[82]   Ramachandran A, Snehalatha C, Mary S, *et al.* Pioglitazone does not enhance the effectiveness of lifestyle modification in preventing conversion of impaired glucose tolerance to diabetes in Asian Indians: results of the Indian Diabetes Prevention Programme-2 (IDPP-2). Diabetologia 2009; 52: 1019-26.

[83]   Molarius A, Seidell JC, Sans S, Tuomilehto J, Kuulasmaa K. Educational level, relative body weight, and changes in their association over 10 years: an international perspective from the WHO MONICA Project. Am J Public Health 2000; 90: 1260-8.

[84]   McLaren L. Socioeconomic status and obesity. Epidemiol Rev 2007; 29: 29-48.

[85]   Martorell R, Khan LK, Hughes ML, Grummer-Strawn LM. Obesity in women from developing countries. Eur J Clin Nutr 2000; 54: 247-52.

[86]   Yang W, Lu J, Weng J, *et al.* Prevalence of Diabetes among Men and Women in China. N Engl J Med 2010; 362: 1090-101.

[87]   Ning F, Pang ZC, Dong YH, *et al.* Risk factors associated with the dramatic increase in the prevalence of diabetes in the adult Chinese population in Qingdao, China. Diabet Med 2009; 26: 855-63.

[88]   Molarius A, Seidell JC. Selection of anthropometric indicators for classification of abdominal fatness-a critical review. Int J Obes Relat Metab Disord 1998; 22: 719-27.

[89]   Seidell JC, Bjorntorp P, Sjostrom L, Sannerstedt R, Krotkiewski M, Kvist H. Regional distribution of muscle and fat mass in men-new insight into the risk of abdominal obesity using computed tomography. Int J Obes 1989; 13: 289-303.

[90]   Garrow JS, Webster J. Quetelet's index (W/H2) as a measure of fatness. Int J Obes 1985; 9: 147-53.

[91]   Onis MD, Habicht J-P, Himes J.H, *et al.* WHO Expert Commiittee. Physical status: the use and interpretation of anthropometry. Report of a WHO Expert Committee. World Health Organisation, Geneva: Switzerland 1995.

[92]   Deurenberg P, Deurenberg-Yap M, Guricci S. Asians are different from Caucasians and from each other in their body mass index/body fat per cent relationship. Obes Rev 2002; 3: 141-6.

[93]   Ashwell M, Chinn S, Stalley S, Garrow JS. Female fat distribution-a simple classification based on two circumference measurements. Int J Obes 1982; 6: 143-52.

[94]   Krotkiewski M, Bjorntorp P, Sjostrom L, Smith U. Impact of obesity on metabolism in men and women. Importance of regional adipose tissue distribution. J Clin Invest 1983; 72: 1150-62.

[95]   Larsson B, Svardsudd K, Welin L, Wilhelmsen L, Bjorntorp P, Tibblin G. Abdominal adipose tissue distribution, obesity, and risk of cardiovascular disease and death: 13 years follow up of participants in the study of men born in 1913. Br Med J 1984; 288: 1401-4.

[96]   Lapidus L, Bengtsson C, Larsson B, Pennert K, Rybo E, Sjostrom L. Distribution of adipose tissue and risk of cardiovascular disease and death: a 12 years follow up of participants in the population study of women in Gothenburg, Sweden. Br Med J 1984; 289: 1257-61.

[97]   Ashwell M, Cole TJ, Dixon AK. Obesity: new insight into the anthropometric classification of fat distribution shown by computed tomography. Br Med J 1985; 290: 1692-4.

[98]   Ohlson LO, Larsson B, Svardsudd K, *et al.* The influence of body fat distribution on the incidence of diabetes mellitus. 13.5 years of follow-up of the participants in the study of men born in 1913. Diabetes 1985; 34: 1055-8.

[99]   Pouliot MC, Despres JP, Lemieux S, *et al.* Waist circumference and abdominal sagittal diameter: best simple anthropometric indexes of abdominal visceral adipose tissue accumulation and related cardiovascular risk in men and women. Am J Cardiol 1994; 73: 460-8.

[100] Han TS, van Leer EM, Seidell JC, Lean ME. Waist circumference action levels in the identification of cardiovascular risk factors: prevalence study in a random sample. BMJ 1995; 311: 1401-5.

[101] Han TS, Feskens EJ, Lean ME, Seidell JC. Associations of body composition with type 2 diabetes mellitus. Diabet Med 1998; 15: 129-35.

[102] Lissner L, Bjorkelund C, Heitmann BL, Seidell JC, Bengtsson C. Larger hip circumference independently predicts health and longevity in a Swedish female cohort. Obes Res 2001; 9: 644-6.

[103] Seidell JC, Perusse L, Despres JP, Bouchard C. Waist and hip circumferences have independent and opposite effects on cardiovascular disease risk factors: the Quebec Family Study. Am J Clin Nutr 2001; 74: 315-21.

[104] Snijder MB, Dekker JM, Visser M, *et al.* Associations of hip and thigh circumferences independent of waist circumference with the incidence of type 2 diabetes: the Hoorn Study. Am J Clin Nutr 2003; 77: 1192-7.

[105] Snijder MB, Zimmet PZ, Visser M, Dekker JM, Seidell JC, Shaw JE. Independent and opposite assocations of waist and hip circumferences with diabetes, hypertension and dyslipidemia: the AusDiab Study. Int J Obes Relat Metab Disord 2004; 28: 402-9.

[106] Ashwell M, Cole TJ, Dixon AK. Ratio of waist circumference to height is strong predictor of intra-abdominal fat. BMJ 1996; 313: 559-60.

[107] Ashwell M, Lejeune S, McPherson K. Ratio of waist circumference to height may be better indicator of need for weight management. BMJ 1996; 312: 377.

[108] Ledoux M, Lambert J, Reeder BA, Despres JP. A comparative analysis of weight to height and waist to hip circumference indices as indicators of the presence of cardiovascular disease risk factors. Canadian Heart Health Surveys Research Group. CMAJ 1997; 157 (Suppl 1): S32-8.

[109] Hsieh SD, Muto T. The superiority of waist-to-height ratio as an anthropometric index to evaluate clustering of coronary risk factors among non-obese men and women. Prev Med 2005; 40: 216-20.

[110] Ho SY, Lam TH, Janus ED. Waist to stature ratio is more strongly associated with cardiovascular risk factors than other simple anthropometric indices. Ann Epidemiol 2003; 13: 683-91.

[111] Wang J, Thornton JC, Bari S, *et al.* Comparisons of waist circumferences measured at 4 sites. Am J Clin Nutr 2003; 77: 379-84.

[112] Lohman TG. Anthropometric standardization reference manual. Champaign, IL: Human Kinetiks; 1988.

[113] WHO. WHO STEPS Surveillance Manual: the WHO STEPwise Approach to Chronic Disease Risk Factor Surveillance. World Health Organisation, Geneva: Switzerland 2008.

[114] Devereux R, Manning WJ, Wexler L, *et al.* MESA Monitoring Board. Multi-Ethnic Study of Atherosclerosis (MESA) Protocol". National Institutes of Health. 2002 [updated 2002; cited]; Available from: http: //www.mesa-nhlbi.org/moreinfo.aspx.

[115] Westat I. The National Health and Nutrition Examination Survey III. 1988 [updated 1988; cited]; Available from: http: //www.cdc.gov/nchs/data/nhanes/nhanes3/cdrom/NCHS/MANUALS/ANTHRO.PDF.

[116] Pi-Sunyer FX, Becker DM, Bouchard C, *et al.* National Institute of Health. The Practical Guide; Identification, Evaluation, and Treatment of Overweight and Obesity in Adults. 2000 [updated 2000; cited]; Available from: http: //www.nhlbi.nih.gov/guidelines/obesity/prctgd_c.pdf.

[117] Ulijaszek SJ, Kerr DA. Anthropometric measurement error and the assessment of nutritional status. Br J Nutr 1999; 82: 165-77.

[118] Nadas J, Putz Z, Kolev G, Nagy S, Jermendy G. Intraobserver and interobserver variability of measuring waist circumference. Med Sci Monit 2008; 14: CR15-8.

[119] Panoulas VF, Ahmad N, Fazal AA, *et al.* The inter-operator variability in measuring waist circumference and its potential impact on the diagnosis of the metabolic syndrome. Postgrad Med J 2008; 84: 344-7.

[120]   Ross R, Berentzen T, Bradshaw AJ, *et al.* Does the relationship between waist circumference, morbidity and mortality depend on measurement protocol for waist circumference? Obes Rev 2008; 9: 312-25.

[121]   Bouchard C, Bray GA, Hubbard *vs.* Basic and clinical aspects of regional fat distribution. Am J Clin Nutr 1990; 52: 946-50.

[122]   Rolka DB, Narayan KM, Thompson TJ, *et al.* Performance of recommended screening tests for undiagnosed diabetes and dysglycemia. Diabetes Care 2001; 24: 1899-903.

[123]   Lindstrom J, Tuomilehto J. The diabetes risk score: a practical tool to predict type 2 diabetes risk. Diabetes Care 2003; 26: 725-31.

[124]   Schulze MB, Hoffmann K, Boeing H, *et al.* An accurate risk score based on anthropometric, dietary, and lifestyle factors to predict the development of type 2 diabetes. Diabetes Care 2007; 30: 510-5.

[125]   Vazquez G, Duval S, Jacobs DR, Jr., Silventoinen K. Comparison of body mass index, waist circumference, and waist/hip ratio in predicting incident diabetes: a meta-analysis. Epidemiol Rev 2007; 29: 115-28.

[126]   Lee CM, Huxley RR, Wildman RP, Woodward M. Indices of abdominal obesity are better discriminators of cardiovascular risk factors than BMI: a meta-analysis. J Clin Epidemiol 2008; 61: 646-53.

[127]   Huxley R, James WP, Barzi F, *et al.* Ethnic comparisons of the cross-sectional relationships between measures of body size with diabetes and hypertension. Obes Rev 2008; 9 (Suppl 1): 53-61.

[128]   Nyamdorj R, Qiao Q, Lam TH, *et al.* BMI compared with central obesity indicators in relation to diabetes and hypertension in Asians. Obesity (Silver Spring) 2008; 16: 1622-35.

[129]   Nyamdorj R, Qiao Q, Soderberg S, *et al.* BMI compared with central obesity indicators as a predictor of diabetes incidence in Mauritius. Obesity (Silver Spring) 2009; 17: 342-8.

[130]   Qiao Q, Nyamdorj R. Is the association of type II diabetes with waist circumference or waist-to-hip ratio stronger than that with body mass index? Eur J Clin Nutr 2010; 64: 30-4.

[131]   de Koning L, Gerstein HC, Bosch J, *et al.* Anthropometric measures and glucose levels in a large multi-ethnic cohort of individuals at risk of developing type 2 diabetes. Diabetologia 2010; 53: 1322-30.

[132]   Wei M, Gaskill SP, Haffner SM, Stern MP. Waist circumference as the best predictor of noninsulin dependent diabetes mellitus (NIDDM) compared to body mass index, waist/hip ratio and other anthropometric measurements in Mexican Americans-a 7-year prospective study. Obes Res 1997; 5: 16-23.

[133]   Tulloch-Reid MK, Williams DE, Looker HC, Hanson RL, Knowler WC. Do measures of body fat distribution provide information on the risk of type 2 diabetes in addition to measures of general obesity? Comparison of anthropometric predictors of type 2 diabetes in Pima Indians. Diabetes Care 2003; 26: 2556-61.

[134]   Diabetes Prevention Program Research Group. Relationship of body size and shape to the development of diabetes in the diabetes prevention program. Obesity 2006; 14: 2107-17.

[135]   Stevens J, Couper D, Pankow J, *et al.* Sensitivity and specificity of anthropometrics for the prediction of diabetes in a biracial cohort. Obes Res 2001; 9: 696-705.

[136]   Wang Z, Hoy WE. Body size measurements as predictors of type 2 diabetes in Aboriginal people. Int J Obes Relat Metab Disord 2004; 28: 1580-4.

[137]   Foucan L, Hanley J, Deloumeaux J, Suissa S. Body mass index (BMI) and waist circumference (WC) as screening tools for cardiovascular risk factors in Guadeloupean women. J Clin Epidemiol 2002; 55: 990-6.

[138]   Stolk RP, Suriyawongpaisal P, Aekplakorn W, Woodward M, Neal B. Fat distribution is strongly associated with plasma glucose levels and diabetes in Thai adults-the InterASIA study. Diabetologia 2005; 48: 657-60.

[139]   Hu D, Xie J, Fu P, *et al.* Central rather than overall obesity is related to diabetes in the Chinese population: the InterASIA study. Obesity (Silver Spring) 2007; 15: 2809-16.

[140]   Lorenzo C, Serrano-Rios M, Martinez-Larrad MT, *et al.* Which obesity index best explains prevalence differences in type 2 diabetes mellitus? Obesity (Silver Spring) 2007; 15: 1294-301.

[141]   Schneider HJ, Glaesmer H, Klotsche J, *et al.* Accuracy of anthropometric indicators of obesity to predict cardiovascular risk. J Clin Endocrinol Metab 2007; 92: 589-94.

[142]   Pua YH, Ong PH. Anthropometric indices as screening tools for cardiovascular risk factors in Singaporean women. Asia Pac J Clin Nutr 2005; 14: 74-9.

[143]   Regional Office for the Western Pacific of the World Health Organization, IASO and IOTF. The Asia-Pacific perspective: Redefining obesity and its treatment; 2000 [updated 2000; cited 10 October 2003]; Available from: www.diabetes.com/au/pdf/obesity-report.pdf.

[144]   Barba C, Cavalli-Sforza T, Cutter J, *et al.* WHO Expert Consultation. Appropriate body-mass index for Asian populations and its implications for policy and intervention strategies. Lancet 2004; 363: 157-63.

[145] Qiao Q, Nyamdorj R. The optimal cutoff values and their performance of waist circumference and waist-to-hip ratio for diagnosing type II diabetes. Eur J Clin Nutr 2010; 64: 23-9.

[146] Youden WJ. Index for rating diagnostic tests. Cancer 1950; 3: 32-5.

[147] Ramachandran A, Snehalatha C, Viswanathan V, Viswanathan M, Haffner SM. Risk of noninsulin dependent diabetes mellitus conferred by obesity and central adiposity in different ethnic groups: a comparative analysis between Asian Indians, Mexican Americans and Whites. Diabetes Res Clin Pract 1997; 36: 121-5.

[148] McBean AM, Li S, Gilbertson DT, Collins AJ. Differences in diabetes prevalence, incidence, and mortality among the elderly of four racial/ethnic groups: whites, blacks, hispanics, and asians. Diabetes Care 2004; 27: 2317-24.

[149] Lee CM, Huxley RR, Lam TH, *et al*. Prevalence of diabetes mellitus and population attributable fractions for coronary heart disease and stroke mortality in the WHO South-East Asia and Western Pacific regions. Asia Pac J Clin Nutr 2007; 16: 187-92.

[150] Sundborn G, Metcalf P, Scragg R, *et al*. Ethnic differences in the prevalence of new and known diabetes mellitus, impaired glucose tolerance, and impaired fasting glucose. Diabetes Heart and Health Survey (DHAH) 2002-2003, Auckland New Zealand. N Z Med J 2007; 120: U2607.

[151] Shai I, Jiang R, Manson JE, *et al*. Ethnicity, obesity, and risk of type 2 diabetes in women: a 20-years follow-up study. Diabetes Care 2006; 29: 1585-90.

[152] Signorello LB, Schlundt DG, Cohen SS, *et al*. Comparing diabetes prevalence between African Americans and Whites of similar socioeconomic status. Am J Public Health 2007; 97: 2260-7.

[153] Razak F, Anand S, Vuksan V, *et al*. Ethnic differences in the relationships between obesity and glucose-metabolic abnormalities: a cross-sectional population-based study. Int J Obes 2005; 29: 656-67.

[154] Kondalsamy-Chennakesavan S, Hoy WE, Wang Z, Shaw J. Quantifying the excess risk of type 2 diabetes by body habitus measurements among Australian aborigines living in remote areas. Diabetes Care 2008; 31: 585-6.

[155] Araneta MR, Barrett-Connor E. Ethnic differences in visceral adipose tissue and type 2 diabetes: Filipino, African-American, and white women. Obes Res 2005; 13: 1458-65.

[156] Nyamdorj R, Pitkaniemi J, Tuomilehto J, *et al*. Ethnic comparison of the association of undiagnosed diabetes with obesity. Int J Obes (Lond) 2010; 34: 332-9.

[157] Ni Mhurchu C, Parag V, Nakamura M, Patel A, Rodgers A, Lam TH. Body mass index and risk of diabetes mellitus in the Asia-Pacific region. Asia Pac J Clin Nutr 2006; 15: 127-33.

[158] Stevens J, Truesdale KP, Katz EG, Cai J. Impact of body mass index on incident hypertension and diabetes in Chinese Asians, American Whites, and American Blacks: the People's Republic of China Study and the Atherosclerosis Risk in Communities Study. Am J Epidemiol 2008; 167: 1365-74.

[159] Despres JP, Nadeau A, Tremblay A, *et al*. Role of deep abdominal fat in the association between regional adipose tissue distribution and glucose tolerance in obese women. Diabetes 1989; 38: 304-9.

[160] Lebovitz HE, Banerji MA. Point: visceral adiposity is causally related to insulin resistance. Diabetes Care 2005; 28: 2322-5.

[161] Fox CS, Massaro JM, Hoffmann U, *et al*. Abdominal visceral and subcutaneous adipose tissue compartments: association with metabolic risk factors in the Framingham Heart Study. Circulation 2007; 116: 39-48.

[162] Kuk JL, Kilpatrick K, Davidson LE, Hudson R, Ross R. Whole-body skeletal muscle mass is not related to glucose tolerance or insulin sensitivity in overweight and obese men and women. Appl Physiol Nutr Metab 2008; 33: 769-74.

[163] Lee JW, Lee HR, Shim JY, Im JA, Lee DC. Abdominal visceral fat reduction is associated with favorable changes of serum retinol binding protein-4 in nondiabetic subjects. Endocr J 2008; 55: 811-8.

[164] Hanley AJ, Wagenknecht LE, Norris JM, *et al*. Insulin resistance, beta cell dysfunction and visceral adiposity as predictors of incident diabetes: the Insulin Resistance Atherosclerosis Study (IRAS) Family study. Diabetologia 2009; 52: 2079-86.

[165] Gallagher D, Kelley DE, Yim JE, *et al*. Adipose tissue distribution is different in type 2 diabetes. Am J Clin Nutr 2009; 89: 807-14.

[166] Ledoux S, Coupaye M, Essig M, *et al*. Traditional anthropometric parameters still predict metabolic disorders in women with severe obesity. Obesity 2010; 18: 1026-32.

[167] Smith U. Regional differences in adipocyte metabolism and possible consequences *in vivo*. Int J Obes 1985; 9 (Suppl 1): 145-8.

[168] Trayhurn P, Beattie JH. Physiological role of adipose tissue: white adipose tissue as an endocrine and secretory organ. Proc Nutr Soc 2001; 60: 329-39.

[169] Bjorntorp P. "Portal" adipose tissue as a generator of risk factors for cardiovascular disease and diabetes. Arteriosclerosis 1990; 10: 493-6.

[170] Arner P. Insulin resistance in type 2 diabetes: role of fatty acids. Diabetes Metab Res Rev 2002; 18 (Suppl 2): S5-9.

[171] Yang YK, Chen M, Clements RH, Abrams GA, Aprahamian CJ, Harmon CM. Human mesenteric adipose tissue plays unique role *versus* subcutaneous and omental fat in obesity related diabetes. Cell Physiol Biochem 2008; 22: 531-8.

[172] Ferrannini E, Barrett EJ, Bevilacqua S, DeFronzo RA. Effect of fatty acids on glucose production and utilization in man. J Clin Invest 1983; 72: 1737-47.

[173] Gastaldelli A, Cusi K, Pettiti M, *et al.* Relationship between hepatic/visceral fat and hepatic insulin resistance in nondiabetic and type 2 diabetic subjects. Gastroenterology 2007; 133: 496-506.

[174] Abate N, Garg A, Peshock RM, Stray-Gundersen J, Grundy SM. Relationships of generalized and regional adiposity to insulin sensitivity in men. J Clin Invest 1995; 96: 88-98.

[175] Abate N, Garg A, Peshock RM, Stray-Gundersen J, Adams-Huet B, Grundy SM. Relationship of generalized and regional adiposity to insulin sensitivity in men with NIDDM. Diabetes 1996; 45: 1684-93.

[176] Goodpaster BH, Thaete FL, Simoneau JA, Kelley DE. Subcutaneous abdominal fat and thigh muscle composition predict insulin sensitivity independently of visceral fat. Diabetes 1997; 46: 1579-85.

[177] Frayn KN. Visceral fat and insulin resistance-causative or correlative? Br J Nutr 2000; 83 (Suppl 1): S71-7.

[178] Chandalia M, Lin P, Seenivasan T, *et al.* Insulin resistance and body fat distribution in South Asian men compared to Caucasian men. PLoS One 2007; 2: e812.

[179] Hyatt TC, Phadke RP, Hunter GR, Bush NC, Munoz AJ, Gower BA. Insulin sensitivity in African-American and white women: association with inflammation. Obesity 2009; 17: 276-82.

[180] Taylor R. Pathogenesis of type 2 diabetes: tracing the reverse route from cure to cause. Diabetologia 2008; 51: 1781-9.

[181] Sjostrom CD, Lissner L, Wedel H, Sjostrom L. Reduction in incidence of diabetes, hypertension and lipid disturbances after intentional weight loss induced by bariatric surgery: the SOS Intervention Study. Obes Res 1999; 7: 477-84.

[182] Carroll JF, Franks SF, Smith AB, Phelps DR. Visceral adipose tissue loss and insulin resistance 6 months after laparoscopic gastric banding surgery: a preliminary study. Obes Surg 2009; 19: 47-55.

[183] Dixon JB. Obesity and diabetes: the impact of bariatric surgery on type-2 diabetes. World J Surg 2009; 33: 2014-21.

[184] Lottati M, Kolka CM, Stefanovski D, Kirkman EL, Bergman RN. Greater omentectomy improves insulin sensitivity in nonobese dogs. Obesity 2009; 17: 674-80.

[185] Hotamisligil GS, Shargill NS, Spiegelman BM. Adipose expression of tumor necrosis factor-alpha: direct role in obesity-linked insulin resistance. Science 1993; 259: 87-91.

[186] Hotamisligil GS, Peraldi P, Budavari A, Ellis R, White MF, Spiegelman BM. IRS-1-mediated inhibition of insulin receptor tyrosine kinase activity in TNF-alpha- and obesity-induced insulin resistance. Science 1996; 271: 665-8.

[187] Hotamisligil GS, Johnson RS, Distel RJ, Ellis R, Papaioannou VE, Spiegelman BM. Uncoupling of obesity from insulin resistance through a targeted mutation in aP2, the adipocyte fatty acid binding protein. Science 1996; 274: 1377-9.

[188] Pickup JC, Mattock MB, Chusney GD, Burt D. NIDDM as a disease of the innate immune system: association of acute-phase reactants and interleukin-6 with metabolic syndrome X. Diabetologia 1997; 40: 1286-92.

[189] Pickup JC, Crook MA. Is type II diabetes mellitus a disease of the innate immune system? Diabetologia 1998; 41: 1241-8.

[190] Clement K, Viguerie N, Poitou C, *et al.* Weight loss regulates inflammation-related genes in white adipose tissue of obese subjects. FASEB J 2004; 18: 1657-69.

[191] Ruge T, Lockton JA, Renstrom F, *et al.* Acute hyperinsulinemia raises plasma interleukin-6 in both nondiabetic and type 2 diabetes mellitus subjects, and this effect is inversely associated with body mass index. Metabolism 2009; 58: 860-6.

[192] Xu H, Barnes GT, Yang Q, *et al.* Chronic inflammation in fat plays a crucial role in the development of obesity-related insulin resistance. J Clin Invest 2003; 112: 1821-30.

[193] Weisberg SP, McCann D, Desai M, Rosenbaum M, Leibel RL, Ferrante AW, Jr. Obesity is associated with macrophage accumulation in adipose tissue. J Clin Invest 2003; 112: 1796-808.

[194] Takahashi K, Mizuarai S, Araki H, *et al.* Adiposity elevates plasma MCP-1 levels leading to the increased CD11b-positive monocytes in mice. J Biol Chem 2003; 278: 46654-60.

[195] Lacasa D, Taleb S, Keophiphath M, Miranville A, Clement K. Macrophage-secreted factors impair human adipogenesis: involvement of proinflammatory state in preadipocytes. Endocrinology 2007; 148: 868-77.

[196] Goossens GH. The role of adipose tissue dysfunction in the pathogenesis of obesity-related insulin resistance. Physiol Behav 2008; 94: 206-18.

[197] Hirosumi J, Tuncman G, Chang L, *et al.* A central role for JNK in obesity and insulin resistance. Nature 2002; 420: 333-6.

[198] Ozcan U, Cao Q, Yilmaz E, *et al.* Endoplasmic reticulum stress links obesity, insulin action, and type 2 diabetes. Science 2004; 306: 457-61.

[199] Hotamisligil GS. Role of endoplasmic reticulum stress and c-Jun NH2-terminal kinase pathways in inflammation and origin of obesity and diabetes. Diabetes 2005; 54 (Suppl 2): S73-8.

[200] Gregor MF, Yang L, Fabbrini E, *et al.* Endoplasmic reticulum stress is reduced in tissues of obese subjects after weight loss. Diabetes 2009; 58: 693-700.

[201] Rask-Madsen C, Dominguez H, Ihlemann N, Hermann T, Kober L, Torp-Pedersen C. Tumor necrosis factor-alpha inhibits insulin's stimulating effect on glucose uptake and endothelium-dependent vasodilation in humans. Circulation 2003; 108: 1815-21.

[202] Plomgaard P, Bouzakri K, Krogh-Madsen R, Mittendorfer B, Zierath JR, Pedersen BK. Tumor necrosis factor-alpha induces skeletal muscle insulin resistance in healthy human subjects *via* inhibition of Akt substrate 160 phosphorylation. Diabetes 2005; 54: 2939-45.

[203] Krogh-Madsen R, Plomgaard P, Moller K, Mittendorfer B, Pedersen BK. Influence of TNF-alpha and IL-6 infusions on insulin sensitivity and expression of IL-18 in humans. Am J Physiol Endocrinol Metab 2006; 291: E108-14.

[204] Bluher M, Bashan N, Shai I, *et al.* Activated Ask1-MKK4-p38MAPK/JNK stress signaling pathway in human omental fat tissue may link macrophage infiltration to whole-body Insulin sensitivity. J Clin Endocrinol Metab 2009; 94: 2507-15.

[205] Monroy A, Kamath S, Chavez AO, *et al.* Impaired regulation of the TNF-alpha converting enzyme/tissue inhibitor of metalloproteinase 3 proteolytic system in skeletal muscle of obese type 2 diabetic patients: a new mechanism of insulin resistance in humans. Diabetologia 2009; 52: 2169-81.

[206] Chavey C, Lazennec G, Lagarrigue S, *et al.* CXC ligand 5 is an adipose-tissue derived factor that links obesity to insulin resistance. Cell Metab 2009; 9: 339-49.

[207] Hotamisligil GS. Inflammation and metabolic disorders. Nature 2006; 444: 860-7.

[208] Wu Z, Rosen ED, Brun R, *et al.* Cross-regulation of C/EBP alpha and PPAR gamma controls the transcriptional pathway of adipogenesis and insulin sensitivity. Mol Cell 1999; 3: 151-8.

[209] Rosen ED, MacDougald OA. Adipocyte differentiation from the inside out. Nat Rev Mol Cell Biol 2006; 7: 885-96.

[210] Gustafson B, Smith U. Cytokines promote Wnt signaling and inflammation and impair the normal differentiation and lipid accumulation in 3T3-L1 preadipocytes. J Biol Chem 2006; 281: 9507-16.

[211] Isakson P, Hammarstedt A, Gustafson B, Smith U. Impaired preadipocyte differentiation in human abdominal obesity: role of Wnt, tumor necrosis factor-alpha, and inflammation. Diabetes 2009; 58: 1550-7.

[212] Mohamed-Ali V, Pinkney JH, Coppack SW. Adipose tissue as an endocrine and paracrine organ. Int J Obes Relat Metab Disord 1998; 22: 1145-58.

[213] Karastergiou K, Mohamed-Ali V. The autocrine and paracrine roles of adipokines. Mol Cell Endocrinol 2010; 318: 69-78.

[214] Schmidt MI, Duncan BB, Vigo A, *et al.* Leptin and incident type 2 diabetes: risk or protection? Diabetologia 2006; 49: 2086-96.

[215] McNeely MJ, Boyko EJ, Weigle DS, *et al.* Association between baseline plasma leptin levels and subsequent development of diabetes in Japanese Americans. Diabetes Care 1999; 22: 65-70.

[216] Soderberg S, Zimmet P, Tuomilehto J, *et al.* Leptin predicts the development of diabetes in Mauritian men, but not women: a population-based study. Int J Obes 2007; 31: 1126-33.

[217] Emilsson V, Liu YL, Cawthorne MA, Morton NM, Davenport M. Expression of the functional leptin receptor mRNA in pancreatic islets and direct inhibitory action of leptin on insulin secretion. Diabetes 1997; 46: 313-6.

[218] Kieffer TJ, Heller RS, Leech CA, Holz GG, Habener JF. Leptin suppression of insulin secretion by the activation of ATP-sensitive K+ channels in pancreatic beta-cells. Diabetes 1997; 46: 1087-93.

[219] Maedler K, Schulthess FT, Bielman C, *et al.* Glucose and leptin induce apoptosis in human beta-cells and impair glucose-stimulated insulin secretion through activation of c-Jun N-terminal kinases. FASEB J 2008; 22: 1905-13.

[220] Hennige AM, Stefan N, Kapp K, *et al.* Leptin down-regulates insulin action through phosphorylation of serine-318 in insulin receptor substrate 1. FASEB J 2006; 20: 1206-8.

[221] Hotta K, Funahashi T, Arita Y, *et al.* Plasma concentrations of a novel, adipose-specific protein, adiponectin, in type 2 diabetic patients. Arterioscler Thromb Vasc Biol 2000; 20: 1595-9.

[222] Weyer C, Funahashi T, Tanaka S, *et al.* Hypoadiponectinemia in obesity and type 2 diabetes: close association with insulin resistance and hyperinsulinemia. J Clin Endocrinol Metab 2001; 86: 1930-5.

[223] Arita Y, Kihara S, Ouchi N, *et al.* Paradoxical decrease of an adipose-specific protein, adiponectin, in obesity. Biochem Biophys Res Commun 1999; 257: 79-83.

[224] Chandran M, Phillips SA, Ciaraldi T, Henry RR. Adiponectin: more than just another fat cell hormone? Diabetes Care 2003; 26: 2442-50.

[225] Devaraj S, Torok N, Dasu MR, Samols D, Jialal I. Adiponectin decreases C-reactive protein synthesis and secretion from endothelial cells: evidence for an adipose tissue-vascular loop. Arterioscler Thromb Vasc Biol 2008; 28: 1368-74.

[226] Ouchi N, Walsh K. A novel role for adiponectin in the regulation of inflammation. Arterioscler Thromb Vasc Biol 2008; 28: 1219-21.

[227] Stefan N, Vozarova B, Funahashi T, *et al.* Plasma adiponectin concentration is associated with skeletal muscle insulin receptor tyrosine phosphorylation, and low plasma concentration precedes a decrease in whole-body insulin sensitivity in humans. Diabetes 2002; 51: 1884-8.

[228] Stefan N, Stumvoll M, Vozarova B, *et al.* Plasma adiponectin and endogenous glucose production in humans. Diabetes Care 2003; 26: 3315-9.

[229] Yamauchi T, Kamon J, Minokoshi Y, *et al.* Adiponectin stimulates glucose utilization and fatty-acid oxidation by activating AMP-activated protein kinase. Nat Med 2002; 8: 1288-95.

[230] Redinger RN. The physiology of adiposity. J Ky Med Assoc 2008; 106: 53-62.

[231] Stefan N, Vozarova B, Funahashi T, *et al.* Plasma adiponectin levels are not associated with fat oxidation in humans. Obes Res 2002; 10: 1016-20.

CHAPTER 5

Lipid Levels and Glucose Intolerance

Lei Zhang[*]

Department of Public Health, Hjelt Institute, University of Helsinki, Helsinki, Finland; Department of Chronic Disease Prevention, National Institute for Health and Welfare, Helsinki, Finland; Qingdao Endocrine & Diabetes Hospital, Qingdao, China and Department of Internal Medicine, Weifang Medical University, Weifang, China

Abstract: Dyslipidemia is one of the major risk factors for Cardiovascular Disease (CVD) that coexists with diabetes. It plays an important role in the development and progress of atherosclerosis, the underlying pathogenesis of CVD. Hyperglycemia is associated with adverse lipid profiles. An atherogenic lipid profile, consisting of high Triglycerides (TG) and small dense Low-Density Lipoprotein Cholesterol (LDL-C) and low High-Density Lipoprotein Cholesterol (HDL-C), is common not only in patients with overt diabetes but also in individuals with prediabetes. The impact of dyslipidemia on risk of CVD in patients with hyperglycemia has been extensively studied. Reduced HDL-C is well documented as an independent predictor of CVD events, the role of TG as an independent risk factor for CVD is, however, controversial. Recently, the interest to use novel parameters such as total cholesterol (TC) to HDL ratio (TC/HDL-C), non-HDL-cholesterol (non-HDL-C), apolipoprotein B (apoB) and apolipoprotein A (apoA) to assess CVD risk has increased. This chapter provides a comprehensive review of the physiology, pathophysiology, prognosis and management of dyslipidemia in individuals with different glycemic levels. The ethnic differences in occurrence of dyslipidemia are also addressed.

Keywords: Lipid, glucose levels, cardiovascular mortality and mobidity, ethnicity.

5.1. LIPIDS IN RELATION TO GLUCOSE INTOLERANCE

5.1.1. Physiology of Lipid Metabolism

Lipids are fats that are either absorbed from food or synthesized by the liver. All lipids are hydrophobic and therefore they are transported associated with proteins as lipoproteins (Table **1**), which are hydrophilic and with spherical structures.

Table 1: Physical properties, lipid and apolipoprotein composition of human plasma lipoproteins

	Chylomicron	VLDL	IDL	LDL	HDL
Source	Intestine	Liver	Lipolysis of VLDL	Lipolysis of VLDL, *via* IDL	Liver, intestine;
Diameter (nm)	75-1200	30-80	25-35	18-25	5-12
Density (kg/l)	< 0.96	0.96-1.006	1.006-1.019	1.019-1.063	1.063-1.210
Composition (%)					
Triglycerides	86	55	23	6	5
Phospholipids	7	18	19	22	33
Cholesteryl esters	4	12	29	42	17
Free cholesterol	2	7	9	8	5
Protein	2	8	19	22	40-55
Apolipoproteins contained	A-I, A-IV, B-48, C, E	B-100, C, E	B-100, C, E	B-100	A-I, A-II, C, E

VLDL, very-low density lipoprotein; IDL, intermediate-density lipoprotein; LDL, low-density lipoprotein; HDL, high-density lipoprotein.

*Address correspondence to Lei Zhang: Department of Public Health, Hjelt Institute, University of Helsinki, PL41, Mannerheimintie 172, 00014, Helsinki, Finland and South Fuzhou Road 81, Qingdao Endocrine & Diabetes Hospital, 266071 Qingdao, China; E-mail: diabetologist@126.com

5.1.1.1. Exogenous Lipid Metabolism

Over 95% of dietary lipids are TG; the rest are phospholipids, Free Fatty Acids (FFA), cholesterol and fat-soluble vitamins. Dietary fats are digested in the stomach and duodenum into Monoglycerides (MGs) and FFAs by gastric lipase, pancreatic lipase and emulsification from vigorous stomach peristalsis (Fig. 1). Dietary cholesterol esters are de-esterified into Free Cholesterol (FC) by the same mechanisms. MGs, FFAs and FC are then solubilized in the intestine by bile acid micelles, which shuttle them to intestinal villi for absorption. They are reassembled into TGs and packaged with cholesterol into chylomicrons once absorbed into the enterocytes.

Chylomicrons, the largest lipoproteins, transport dietary TG and cholesterol from within enterocytes through lymphatics into the circulation. In the capillaries of adipose and muscle tissues, apolipoprotein C-II (apoC-II) on the chylomicron activates endothelial lipoprotein lipase (LPL) [1] to convert 90% of chylomicron TG to fatty acids and glycerol, which are taken up by adipocytes and muscle cells for energy use or storage (Fig. 1). Cholesterol-rich chylomicron remnants are then cleared rapidly from circulation by the liver through a process mediated by apolipoprotein E (apoE) [2].

5.1.1.2. Endogenous Lipid Metabolism

Lipoproteins synthesized by the liver transport endogenous TGs and cholesterol (Fig. 1). Lipoproteins circulate through the blood continuously until the TGs are taken up by peripheral tissues or the lipoproteins themselves are cleared by the liver. They become more cholesterol-rich by the loss of TGs. Therefore factors that stimulate hepatic lipoprotein synthesis generally lead to elevated plasma cholesterol.

Very-Low-Density Lipoproteins (VLDL) containing apoB-100, are synthesized in the liver, and transport TG and cholesterol to peripheral tissues. VLDL is the way the liver exports excess intrahepatic FFA, such is the case with high-fat diets and with release FFAs from excess adipose directly into the circulation (*e.g.*, in obesity, uncontrolled diabetes). ApoC-II on the VLDL surface activates endothelial LPL to hydrolyze TGs into FFAs and glycerol, which are taken up by cells.

Intermediate-Density Lipoproteins (IDL) are the product of LPL processing of VLDL and chylomicrons [3]. IDL are cholesterol-rich VLDL and chylomicron remnants that are either cleared by the liver or metabolized by hepatic lipase into LDL, which retains apoB [4, 5].

LDL, the products of VLDL and IDL catabolism, are the most cholesterol-rich of all lipoproteins. About 40-60% of all LDL are cleared by the liver in a process mediated by apoB and hepatic LDL receptors [6]; the rest are taken up by either non-hepatic LDL or non-hepatic scavenger receptors. Hepatic LDL receptors are down-regulated by delivery of cholesterol to the liver and by increased dietary saturated fat [7, 8]. Non-hepatic scavenger receptors, most notably on macrophages, take up excess oxidized LDL not processed by hepatic receptors. Monocytes rich in oxidized LDL migrate into the subendothelial space and become macrophages, which takes up more oxidized LDL and form foam cells within atherosclerotic plaques. There are 2 forms of LDL: large, buoyant and small, dense LDL [9, 10]. Small, dense LDL is especially rich in cholesterol esters, associated with metabolic disturbances such as hypertriglyceridemia, insulin resistance and atherogenesis [11, 12]. The increased atherogenicity of small, dense LDL derives from less efficient hepatic LDL receptor binding, leading to prolonged circulation and exposure to endothelium and increased oxidation [13].

The overall role of HDL, synthesized in both enterocytes and the liver, is to obtain cholesterol from peripheral tissues and other lipoproteins and transport it to other cells, other lipoproteins (using cholesteryl ester transfer protein (CETP)) and the liver. Efflux of FC from cells [14] is mediated by adenosine triphosphate-binding cassette transporter A1 (ABCA1), which combines with apoA-I to produce nascent HDL. FC in nascent HDL is then esterified by the Lecithin-Cholesterol Acyl Transferase (LCAT), producing mature HDL [15, 16]. HDL exerts various anti-atherogenic properties, including reverse transport of cholesterol from cells of the arterial wall to the liver [17, 18], inhibition of LDL oxidation by HDL-bound paraoxonase-1 [19, 20], regulation of coagulation and fibrinolysis and inhibition of platelet activation [21], neutralization of endotoxin or lipopolysaccharide [22], inhibition of the chemotaxis of monocytes and the adhesion of leukocytes to the endothelium [21] and promotion of endothelial progenitor cell-mediated endothelial repair [23].

Lipoprotein(a) (Lp(a)) is LDL that contains apolipoprotein(a), characterized by 5 cysteine-rich regions called kringles. One of these regions is homologous with plasminogen and is thought to competitively inhibit fibrinolysis and thus predispose to thrombus [24, 25]. Because Lp(a) has LDL as its component, oxidized Lp(a) is avidly taken up by the scavenger receptor pathway and promotes cholesterol delivery into the artery wall [24], inducing atherosclerosis.

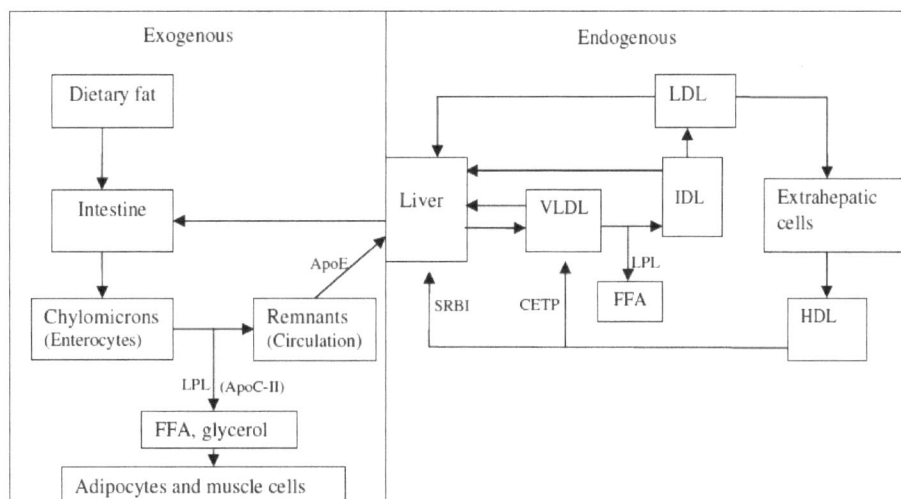

Figure 1: Summary of exogenous and endogenous lipid metabolism. FFA: free fatty acid; LDL: low-density lipoprotein; IDL: intermediate-density lipoprotein; HDL: high-density lipoprotein; LCAT: lecithin-cholesterol acyl transferase; LPL: lipoprotein lipase; ApoC-II: apolipoprotein C-II; SRBI: scavenger receptor class B type I; CETP: cholesteryl ester transfer protein

5.1.2. Prevalence of Dyslipidemia and Related Risk Factors

Lipids and lipoproteins abnormalities are major metabolic disorders, commonly including elevated levels of TC, LDL-C, Lp(a) and TG and reduced levels of HDL-C. In patients with type 2 diabetes, elevated TG and reduced HDL-C [26-28] are most common lipid profiles. These abnormalities can be present alone or in combination with other metabolic disorders. The prevalence of dyslipidemia varies depending on the population studied, geographic location, socioeconomic development and the definition used [29-46]. Caucasians generally have higher mean TC concentrations than do populations of Asian or African origin [47, 48]. In general populations, the highest prevalence of hypercholesterolemia (TC ≥ 6.5 mmol/l) has been seen in Malta (up to 50% in women) and the lowest in China (2.7% in men) according to the report of the World Health Organization (WHO) Inter-Health Programme [31]. The prevalence of dyslipidemia may have changed recently in Asia and Africa because of the changes in dietary factors and lifestyles as a consequence of economic development.

There is a large body of evidence showing that diabetes is associated with a high prevalence of dyslipidemia [49-64]. In the Framingham Heart Study [49], the prevalence of low HDL-C (21% *vs.* 12% in men and 25% *vs.* 10% in women, respectively) and high TG levels (19% *vs.* 9% in men and 17% *vs.* 8% in women, respectively) in people with diabetes was almost twice as high as the prevalence in non-diabetic individuals. By contrast, TC and LDL-C levels did not differ from those of non-diabetic counterparts. A similar pattern of lipid profiles was observed in the UK Prospective Diabetes Study (UKPDS) [51]. In this study, the plasma TG levels were substantially increased whereas HDL-C levels were markedly reduced in both men and women with diabetes compared with the non-diabetic controls. Higher prevalence has been reported in other studies. Data from a primary care-based 7692 patients with type 2 diabetes in the United States showed nearly half of the patients had low HDL-C [65]. The figure was even worse in an urban Indian cohort of 5088 type 2 diabetes patients, with more than half having low HDL-C (52.3%) or high TG (57.9%) [55]. In addition to the traditional lipid measurement, increased levels of apoB were also seen in patients with diabetes compared with non-diabetic individuals [66]. Increasing evidence has suggested that dyslipidemia is present not only in diabetic but also in prediabetic subjects. The relationship between lipid and glucose levels has been investigated in both European [67] and Asian populations [68] who did not have a prior history of diabetes. Within each glucose category, FPG levels were correlated with increasing levels of TGs, TC, TC to HDL ratio and non-HDL-C and inversely associated with HDL-C. The association of lipids with 2hPG followed a similar pattern as that for the FPG [67, 68]. When assessing the risk of cardiovascular disease, the association of the dyslipidemia with intermediate hyperglycemia needs to be considered.

There are several factors that contribute to the development of dyslipidemia [69], including genetic factors [70] and acquired factors [71-73] such as overweight and obesity [74-76], physical inactivity [77, 78], cigarette smoking [65, 79-88], high fat intake [89-91], very high carbohydrate diets (> 60 percent of total energy) [92] and certain drugs [93-97] (such as beta-blockers, anabolic steroids, progestational agents, *et al.,*). Excess alcohol intake is also documented as a risk factor [81, 83, 85] despite that moderate alcohol consumption may have a beneficial effect on improving HDL-C concentrations [98, 99]. In addition, glycemic control is an important determinant of dyslipidemia in patients with diabetes [56, 65, 100, 101]. Among these acquired factors, overweight, obesity and physical inactivity appear to be most important [74-78]. They are also the most important lifestyle variables that decrease insulin action and increase the risk of diabetes.

5.1.3. Dyslipidemia in Individuals with Hyperglycemia: The Role in the Progress of Atherosclerosis

Diabetic dyslipidemia is associated with specific abnormalities in lipoprotein metabolism and abnormalities in insulin action. The most fundamental defect in these patients is resistance to cellular actions of insulin, particularly resistance to insulin-stimulated glucose uptake [102, 103]. In both fasting and postprandial states, deficient action of insulin on adipocytes results in reduced suppression of lipolysis of stored TG, increasing the release of FFA. Higher uptake of FFAs in the liver results in an increased hepatic production of VLDL [104, 105]. The reduced action of insulin also impairs LPL action, resulting in impaired clearance of VLDL from the circulation. The final result is an elevation of circulating TG concentration.

A low level of HDL-C is closely linked to the overproduction of TG-rich lipoproteins such as VLDL and chylomicrons [106, 107]. In the presence of hypertriglyceridemia, and insulin resistance, the metabolic activity of the TG-rich lipoproteins is enhanced that over-exchange their core lipid with both HDL and LDL, a process facilitated by CETP [108]. This results in TG enrichment of HDL and LDL. Although the mechanisms are not entirely clear, available data suggest that the TG-enrichment of HDL particles leads to particle instability and degradation and enhances catabolism of HDL [109]. ApoA-I may dissociate from TG-enriched HDL and is then cleared rapidly from plasma, further reducing the availability of HDL for reverse cholesterol transport. It is also possible that insulin resistance and low HDL-C levels may have a common mediator such as tumor necrosis factor-α that is found to down-regulate the apoA-I gene expression and can lower serum HDL-C levels [110]. On the other hand, TG-enriched LDL particles due to the hypertriglyceridemia and increased CETP activity undergo lipolysis and thus convert into small dense LDL [28].

Diabetic dyslipidemia is a major predisposing factor to the development of atherosclerosis [111]. Small dense LDL particles penetrate the endothelial barrier 1.7 times more easily than do larger LDL particles, and they remain longer in the subendothelial matrix [112]. Moreover, small dense LDL particles are more easily modified by oxidation and, particularly in type 2 diabetes, by glycation, and are more atherogenic [113]. Oxidative modification of LDL particles results in rapid uptake by macrophages, with subsequent formation of foam cells [114]. LDL particles can promote inflammatory and immune changes *via* cytokine released from macrophages [115]. Foam cells can rupture and release oxidized LDL particles, intracellular enzymes and oxygen-free radicals that can further damage the vessel wall. The increased synthesis of VLDL particles are taken up by receptors located on macrophages, thus promoting the accumulation of lipids within macrophages and contributing to the formation of foam cells in vessel walls as well. Furthermore, hypertriglyceridemia is associated with prothrombotic and inflammatory changes that may contribute to the increased risk of cardiovascular disease (CVD) [116]. HDL from patients with type 2 diabetes may have substantially impaired endothelial-protective effects compared with HDL from healthy subjects [117]. In addition, low HDL may disturb reverse cholesterol transport, a process by which excess amounts of cholesterol located in cells and atherosclerotic plaques are removed [118].

5.2. ETHNIC VARIATION IN LIPIDS PROFILES IN RELATION TO GLUCOSE INTOLERANCE

It has been shown that the prevalence of lipid and/or glucose abnormality differs between ethnic groups. Elevated TG and reduced HDL-C, as the components of the metabolic syndrome and atherogenic dyslipidemia, was seen more common in Asian Indians than in the whites [119-122], Chinese [119, 120, 123-125], Japanese [124, 125] or Africans [122]. In a nationally representative sample of seven ethnic groups in the UK [126], the prevalence of low HDL-C was highest in south Asian groups such as Bangladeshi, Indian and Pakistani, followed by Chinese, Irish and those from the general population living in private households. In contrast, the lowest prevalence was seen in black Caribbean. Similar finding was reported in another study where the comparison was made between non-South-Asians and South Asians [127]. In addition, African Americans have been reported to have less adverse lipid profiles than Whites or Hispanics despite the presence of diabetes [50, 128, 129]. The causes of ethnic difference in levels of CVD risk factor are complex and may include genetic, environmental, dietary and cultural factors [126]. Lipid profiles were also investigated among the DECODE and the DECODA participants controlling for glucose tolerance status. Data from 31 DECODE and DECODA study cohorts of 12 countries, consisting of 24, 760 men and 27, 595 women (aged 25-74 years) showed that compared with central and northern Europeans, multivariable adjusted odds ratios (95% confidence intervals) for having low HDL-C were 4.74 (4.19-5.37), 5.05 (3.88-6.56), 3.07 (2.15-4.40), and 2.37 (1.67-3.35) in Asian Indian men, but 0.12 (0.09-0.16), 0.07 (0.04-0.13), 0.11 (0.07-0.20), and 0.16 (0.08-0.32) in Chinese men who had normoglycemia, prediabetes, undiagnosed and diagnosed diabetes, respectively. Similar results were obtained for women. The prevalence of low HDL-C remained higher in Asian Indians (62.8% of the nondiabetic and 67.4% of the diabetic) than in Europeans (20.3 and 37.3%), Japanese (25.7 and 34.1%), or Chinese in Qingdao, China (15.7 and 17.0%), even in individuals with LDL-C of less than 3 mmol/l (Table 2) [130]. These findings suggest that ethnic-specific strategies and guidelines on risk assessment and prevention of cardiovascular disease are required.

Table 2: Proportions (%) of individuals according to lipid levels stratified by diabetic status in each ethnic group

	LDL-C < 3 mmol/liter				LDL-C ≥ 3 mmol/liter			
	Normal HDL-C and normal TG	Low HDL-C[a] alone	High TG[b] alone	Both	Normal HDL-C and normal TG	Low HDL-C[a] alone	High TG[b] alone	Both
Nondiabetic population								
Hong Kong Chinese	29.3	9.9	1.6	4.2	32.1	12.9	3.7	6.2
Qingdao Chinese	31.0	5.4	8.3	1.9	40.5	2.4	9.8	0.7
Asian Indian	23.2	33.6	3.2	11.0	9.2	10.7	2.8	6.4
Mauritian Indian	23.9	15.8	5.0	4.7	23.2	14.7	5.7	7.0
Japanese	25.2	6.4	3.4	3.5	38.2	13.0	5.0	5.3
C&N European	13.3	2.3	2.0	1.6	48.6	9.7	12.6	10.0
Southern European	14.2	4.3	1.1	2.1	45.5	15.1	7.8	10.0
Diabetic population								
Hong Kong Chinese	12.4	9.6	1.4	11.0	22.6	18.1	7.6	17.2
Qingdao Chinese	21.1	3.5	11.1	3.1	37.9	2.7	19.1	1.5
Asian Indian	12.8	17.4	6.0	21.4	8.1	12.4	7.2	14.7
Mauritian Indian	12.4	8.6	6.4	10.2	21.2	15.5	10.2	15.5
Japanese	14.3	6.0	7.1	5.1	34.3	11.6	12.2	9.4
C&N European	10.5	2.8	4.9	6.4	30.4	9.3	16.4	19.4
Southern European	7.5	3.3	6.0	10.2	24.4	11.2	12.8	14.8

Data are expressed as percentage. [a] Less than 1.03 mmol/l in men and <1.29mmol/l in women. [b] ≥1.70 mmol/l. This table was adapted from [130].

5.3. LIPIDS AND CARDIOVASCULAR DISEASE IN RELATION TO GLYCEMIC LEVELS

In the past decades, genetic, histopathologic and epidemiological studies have established the primary role of lipids and lipoproteins in the development of CVD, either in general population or in patients with diabetes. It is well-established that TC, LDL-C, low HDL-C and calculated indices such as TC/HDL-C or non-HDL-C are predictors of cardiovascular events. Whether fasting TG is an independent predictor of CVD, however, remains unsettled.

5.3.1. Lipids and Cardiovascular Risk in General Populations

The link between levels of TC and the risk of CHD has been well established. There is a strong and graded positive association between TC as well as LDL-C and the risk of CHD [131, 132]. Data from the Multiple Risk Factor Intervention Trial (MRFIT) study [133] demonstrate a curvilinear relation between TC level and CHD mortality. Clinical trials using lipid-modifying drugs have unequivocally demonstrated that lowering LDL-C yields significant reductions in both morbidity and mortality from CHD in people with or without established CHD [134, 135], supporting that the reduction of LDL-C should be of prime concern in both primary and secondary prevention of atherosclerotic disease.

The role of HDL-C as an independent and powerful inverse predictor of CHD has been well established [126, 136-148]. An analysis of data from the Framingham study, the Coronary Primary Prevention Trial (CPPT), and the MRFIT study indicates that the risk for CHD decreases by 2%-3% for each 0.03 mmol/l increase in HDL-C, after controlling for other risk factors [149]. In the Lipid Research Clinics Prevalence Mortality Follow-up Study (LRCF), the same increment (0.03 mmol/l) in HDL-C was associated with a significant CVD mortality decrement of 3.7% in men and 4.7% in women [149]. Although the benefits of raising HDL-C levels remain to be confirmed in randomized clinical trials, it appears in a most recent report that the modest improvement in HDL-C levels (per 0.13 mmol/l) is associated with a 21% reduction in cardiovascular risk independent of the effect on other lipid measures [150].

The association between hypertriglyceridemia and risk of CVD is not as strong as it is for TC and HDL-C. High TG is consistently shown to be a significant CVD risk factor in most of the univariate analyses [147, 151-164] and in some of the multivariate models including HDL-C [151, 154, 156, 157, 161-164] but not in others [147, 152-155, 158, 160-166]. In many early prospective studies, the predictive value of fasting TG tended to diminish or even disappear when other lipid or non-lipid risk factors were considered. This failure may result from the large number of intercorrelated variables associated with elevated TG. Renewed interest in the importance of elevated TG has been, however, stimulated by the publication of meta-analyses that found that raised TG is in fact an independent risk factor for CHD [167, 168]. A number of epidemiological studies published in the past few years [147, 153, 154, 160] have also supported the role of TG as an independent risk factor. Recently, the use of TC/HDL-C [142, 146] and non-HDL-C [138] for CVD risk assessment has increased. The Framingham Heart Study and the Quebec Cardiovascular Study have demonstrated that TC/HDL-C appears to predict CHD events better than any single lipid parameter [169, 170]. Non-HDL-C is also shown to be a better predictor of CVD mortality than LDL-C [138, 146, 171, 172] because it includes all atherogenic lipoprotein particles.

In addition, apoB and apoB/apoA-I are useful indicators of risk of atherosclerosis. Data from the Health Professionals Follow-up Study, a nested case-control study with a 6-years follow up of 18, 225 male participants, showed that apoB is more predictive of the development of CHD than non-HDL-C [147]. The finding from the INTERHEART study, another case-control study with 21, 465 participants from 262 centres in 52 countries, strengthened the predictive ability of apoB/apoA1 for Myocardial Infarction (MI) [173]. This has been supported by recent reports from prospective studies, such as Apolipoprotein Mortality Risk study [166], the European Prospective Investigation of Cancer-Norfolk study [174], Uppsala Longitudinal Study of Adult Men [175] and the MONItoring of trends and determinants in Cardiovascular disease Augsburg/KOoperative Gesundheitsforschung in der Region Augsburg [176]. In a most recent report from the Third National Health and Nutrition Examination Survey mortality study, the predictive ability of apoB to detect CHD death was better than any of the routine clinical lipid measurement and as powerful as apoB/apoA-I [177]. Whereas, standardized apoB measures are not widely available and apoB is not included in the current recommendations for assessing cardiovascular risk.

5.3.2. Lipids and Cardiovascular Risk in Individuals with Hyperglycemia

It is well known that the risk of morbidity and mortality from CVD is increased by two- to four-fold in diabetic patients compared with the general population [49, 178, 179]. A number of studies have determined the association of dyslipidemia with cardiovascular risk in people with hyperglycemia, and most of them were conducted in patients with diabetes. The majority of these studies have shown that dyslipidemia increased cardiovascular risk in patients with diabetes, with only a few exceptions [180, 181]. Cross-sectional studies have found positive associations of atherosclerotic vascular disease with TC [58, 182], LDL-C [58, 62, 183], non-HDL-C [58], TG [182, 184, 185], apoB [182] and Lp(a) [186-188], but inverse associations with HDL-C [58, 65, 182, 183, 185, 188] and apoA-I [182, 189].

Prospective data have provided with strong evidence. The UKPDS study [190] has demonstrated that high LDL-C and low HDL-C are potentially modifiable risk factors for Coronary Artery Disease (CAD) in patients with type 2 diabetes. TG, however, was not independently associated with CAD risk in this study, possibly because of its close inverse relationship with HDL-C. Results from the MRFIT [191], in which 356499 nondiabetic and 5163 diabetic men without CHD at baseline were followed for 12 years, indicated that serum cholesterol is an independent predictor of CHD mortality in men with diabetes. Rosengren *et al.,* [192] showed similar results in a prospective study of 6897 middle aged diabetic men. Patients with TC > 7.3 mmol/l had a significantly higher incidence of CHD during the 7-years follow-up than those with TC ≤ 5.5 mmol/l (28.3% *vs.* 5.4%, p<0.05). Long term follow-up of the London cohort of the WHO Multinational Study of Vascular Disease in Diabetics, consisting of 254 type 2 diabetic patients, has showed that TC was associated with increased incidence of MI [193] and overall cardiovascular mortality [194]. The role of TC in predicting CHD was also confirmed in another study among female patients with diabetes [171].

In general, the lipid profile in patients with type 2 diabetes is most commonly characterized by hypertriglyceridemia and reduced HDL-C. Most of the studies consistently addressed the role of HDL-C in predicting CVD in patients with hyperglycemia. In the Honolulu Heart Program [195], both HDL-C and TC were significant predictors of incident CHD in men with diabetes (diagnosis based on use of oral hypoglycemic agent) or abnormal glucose tolerance (1-h glucose ≥ 12.5 mmol/l after 50 g oral glucose challenge), independent of age, Body Mass Index (BMI), Systolic Blood Pressure (SBP), smoking and alcohol consumption. In the Helsinki Heart Study, both low HDL-C and high LDL-C were independently related to CHD incidence in 135 diabetic patients during a 5-years follow-up [196]. Laakso *et al.,* [145] gave further evidence in a Finnish cohort that low HDL-C and HDL_2 cholesterol are powerful risk indicators of CHD events in 313 diabetic patients during a 7-years follow-up.

In spite of the fact that the role of TG in predicting cardiovascular events remains controversial in the general population, the evidence in diabetic populations is better established [145, 190, 196-204]. In the WHO multinational study, ischemic heart disease was more strongly associated with TG than with TC concentrations, particularly in obese diabetic patients [203]. During an 11-year follow-up of 943 patients with either IGT or diabetes in the Paris Prospective Study, TG was the only lipid variable significantly associated with coronary deaths in multivariate regression analysis [202]. In the Schwabing Study of 542 diabetic patients, TG was shown to be a significant predictor of 5-years incidence of major macrovascular complications such as cardiovascular death, gangrene or MI [197]. Data from a Finnish study [145] showed that both high total and VLDL-TG were predictive of CHD events in 313 diabetic patients who were followed up for 7 years. In another Finnish study, LDL-TG but not total TG was found to be associated with cardiovascular death [198]. This may be due to the impact of LDL particles enriched with TG on atherogenesis. The role of TG was also confirmed separately in women patients with type 2 diabetes enrolled in the Nurses' Health Study [171]. In addition, data from diabetic patients of races other than Caucasian confirmed the predictive value of TG. Chan and colleagues [200], following 517 Chinese patients with newly diagnosed type 2 diabetes for 4.6 years, found that TG was significantly associated with cardiovascular mortality in these patients. These epidemiological findings have been supported by randomized clinical trials in which reduction of TG was related to decreased risk of CVD in patients with low HDL-C [205, 206].

In the Hoorn Study [199], high TG was shown to be a risk factor for CVD in subjects with diabetes or prediabetes, but only in those with high non-HDL-C. This finding, together with other emerging evidence, implies that non-HDL-C may be a useful marker for CVD not only in diabetic patients [171, 207, 208] but also in the general population [138, 147, 172, 209]. In the Strong Heart study, a 9-years follow-up study of 2108 American-Indian patients with diabetes but free of CVD at baseline, non-HDL-C (highest *vs.* lowest tertile) was strongly associated with incidence of overall CVD in both male (HR 2.23 [1.41-3.43]) and female (1.80 [1.32-2.46]) patients [207]. The finding was further confirmed in diabetic men in the Health

Professionals' Follow-up Study [208]. However, among diabetic women in the Nurses' Health Study [171], non-HDL-C predicted CHD risk only among those with elevated TG levels, implying that non-HDL-C may provide little additional information over that of the TG in predicting future CHD.

Recently, the utility of TC/HDL-C as a CVD predictor is increasing in diabetic population and has been evaluated in several studies. TC/HDL-C was as a good CVD risk predictor as non-HDL-C in the Strong Heart Study [207] and shown to be the best predictor in diabetic men in the Health Professionals' Follow-up Study [208], but was not a predictor in diabetic women in the Nurses' Health Study [171].

Previous studies have shown that patients with diabetes have elevated apoB [66, 210], apoC-III/C-II, apoE and decreased concentrations of apoA-I [210]. In two prospective studies, apoB seems to be a potent predictor of CVD in both diabetic men [208] and women [171]. Nevertheless, evidence is still limited concerning the role of apoB in predicting CVD risk in diabetic patients.

Although the role of lipid parameters in predicting cardiovascular risk has, as above summarized, been well addressed in either general or diabetic populations, it is still unclear that whether dyslipidemia predicts CVD/CHD events in people with prediabetes (*i.e.*, IGT and IFG), who are already exposed to a cluster of risk factors. Recently the DECODE study examined the impact of dyslipidemia on CVD mortality in relation to FPG and 2hPG levels in individuals without a prior history of diabetes. Data from 14 European population-based prospective studies of 9132 men and 8631 women aged 25-89 years showed that low HDL-C and high TC/HDL-C increase CVD mortality in either diabetic or non-diabetic individuals defined based on the fasting glucose criteria, but not the 2-h criteria. TG is a significant CVD risk predictor only in the presence of combined hyperglycemia or diabetes [211]. The difference between fasting and post-load hyperglycemia with regard to the lipid-CVD relation may suggest a different pathophysiology underlying these two prediabetic status.

5.4. MANAGEMENT OF DYSLIPIDEMIA IN INDIVIDUALS WITH HYPERGLYCEMIA

Epidemiological investigations of human populations have revealed a robust relationship between lipids and CVD risk. Furthermore, the benefit of lipid-modifying strategy on cardiovascular events has been demonstrated from a large number of randomized clinical trials [134, 135], especially from those using 3-hydroxy-3-methyl-glutaryl-CoA (HMG-CoA) reductase inhibitors (*i.e.*, statins) [212-218]. Intensive control of dyslipidemia has been greatly emphasized in the prevention and management of CVD. Current guidelines from the National Cholesterol Education Program Adult Treatment Panel III (ATP III) [219], the European Society of Cardiology [220] and the American Diabetes Association [221] consistently recommend that LDL-C should be the primary target of therapy not only in patients with CHD or diabetes but also in persons with increased cardiovascular risk. In addition, non-HDL-C is set by ATP III as a secondary target of therapy and HDL-C and TG as potential target.

Guidelines for treatment of dyslipidemia have been made targeting at lowering the LDL-C levels, but the elevated LDL-C is not the sole abnormal lipid profile that defines the vascular risk. Therapies which aim to raise HDL-C attract less attention currently in spite of the unfavorable CVD effect of the low HDL-C. A most recent study showed that Extended-Release Niacin (ERN) therapy could not only increase plasma HDL-C levels but also substantially improve endothelial-protective properties of HDL in diabetic patients [117]. Moreover, ERN therapy in combination with a statin induces regression of carotid intima-media thickness in patients with CHD or CHD equivalent including diabetes, peripheral vascular disease, or cerebrovascular disease [222]. The current evidence implies that pharmacological HDL-raising therapies may restore the vascular function and needs to be further examined.

REFERENCES

[1]   Breckenridge WC, Little JA, Steiner G, Chow A, Poapst M. Hypertriglyceridemia associated with deficiency of apolipoprotein C-II. N Engl J Med 1978; 298: 1265-73.
[2]   Mahley RW, Ji ZS. Remnant lipoprotein metabolism: key pathways involving cell-surface heparan sulfate proteoglycans and apolipoprotein E. J Lipid Res 1999; 40: 1-16.

[3]   Eisenberg S. High density lipoprotein metabolism. J Lipid Res 1984; 25: 1017-58.

[4]   Poapst M, Reardon M, Steiner G. Relative contribution of triglyceride-rich lipoprotein particle size and number to plasma triglyceride concentration. Arteriosclerosis 1985; 5: 381-90.

[5]   Steiner G, Schwartz L, Shumak S, Poapst M. The association of increased levels of intermediate-density lipoproteins with smoking and with coronary artery disease. Circulation 1987; 75: 124-30.

[6]   Attie AD, Pittman RC, Steinberg D. Hepatic catabolism of low density lipoprotein: mechanisms and metabolic consequences. Hepatology 1982; 2: 269-81.

[7]   Spady DK, Dietschy JM. Dietary saturated triacylglycerols suppress hepatic low density lipoprotein receptor activity in the hamster. Proc Natl Acad Sci USA 1985; 82: 4526-30.

[8]   Fox JC, McGill HC, Jr., Carey KD, Getz GS. *In vivo* regulation of hepatic LDL receptor mRNA in the baboon. Differential effects of saturated and unsaturated fat. J Biol Chem 1987; 262: 7014-20.

[9]   Austin MA, King MC, Vranizan KM, Newman B, Krauss RM. Inheritance of low-density lipoprotein subclass patterns: results of complex segregation analysis. Am J Hum Genet 1988; 43: 838-46.

[10]   Barakat HA, Carpenter JW, McLendon VD, *et al.* Influence of obesity, impaired glucose tolerance, and NIDDM on LDL structure and composition. Possible link between hyperinsulinemia and atherosclerosis. Diabetes 1990; 39: 1527-33.

[11]   Austin MA, Breslow JL, Hennekens CH, Buring JE, Willett WC, Krauss RM. Low-density lipoprotein subclass patterns and risk of myocardial infarction. JAMA 1988; 260: 1917-21.

[12]   Aguilera CM, Gil-Campos M, Canete R, Gil A. Alterations in plasma and tissue lipids associated with obesity and metabolic syndrome. Clin Sci (Lond) 2008; 114: 183-93.

[13]   Nigon F, Lesnik P, Rouis M, Chapman MJ. Discrete subspecies of human low density lipoproteins are heterogeneous in their interaction with the cellular LDL receptor. J Lipid Res 1991; 32: 1741-53.

[14]   Johnson WJ, Bamberger MJ, Latta RA, Rapp PE, Phillips MC, Rothblat GH. The bidirectional flux of cholesterol between cells and lipoproteins. Effects of phospholipid depletion of high density lipoprotein. J Biol Chem 1986; 261: 5766-76.

[15]   Rye KA, Clay MA, Barter PJ. Remodelling of high density lipoproteins by plasma factors. Atherosclerosis 1999; 145: 227-38.

[16]   Santamarina-Fojo S, Lambert G, Hoeg JM, Brewer HB, Jr. Lecithin-cholesterol acyltransferase: role in lipoprotein metabolism, reverse cholesterol transport and atherosclerosis. Curr Opin Lipidol 2000; 11: 267-75.

[17]   Miller NE, La Ville A, Crook D. Direct evidence that reverse cholesterol transport is mediated by high-density lipoprotein in rabbit. Nature 1985; 314: 109-11.

[18]   Tall AR. An overview of reverse cholesterol transport. Eur Heart J 1998; 19 (Suppl A): A31-5.

[19]   Mackness MI, Arrol S, Abbott C, Durrington PN. Protection of low-density lipoprotein against oxidative modification by high-density lipoprotein associated paraoxonase. Atherosclerosis 1993; 104: 129-35.

[20]   Mackness MI, Mackness B, Durrington PN, Connelly PW, Hegele RA. Paraoxonase: biochemistry, genetics and relationship to plasma lipoproteins. Curr Opin Lipidol 1996; 7: 69-76.

[21]   Nofer JR, Kehrel B, Fobker M, Levkau B, Assmann G, von Eckardstein A. HDL and arteriosclerosis: beyond reverse cholesterol transport. Atherosclerosis 2002; 161: 1-16.

[22]   Huuskonen J, Olkkonen VM, Jauhiainen M, Ehnholm C. The impact of phospholipid transfer protein (PLTP) on HDL metabolism. Atherosclerosis 2001; 155: 269-81.

[23]   Sumi M, Sata M, Miura S, *et al.* Reconstituted high-density lipoprotein stimulates differentiation of endothelial progenitor cells and enhances ischemia-induced angiogenesis. Arterioscler Thromb Vasc Biol 2007; 27: 813-8.

[24]   Jialal I. Evolving lipoprotein risk factors: lipoprotein(a) and oxidized low-density lipoprotein. Clin Chem 1998; 44: 1827-32.

[25]   Maher VM, Brown BG. Lipoprotein (a) and coronary heart disease. Curr Opin Lipidol 1995; 6: 229-35.

[26]   Goldberg IJ. Clinical review 124: Diabetic dyslipidemia: causes and consequences. J Clin Endocrinol Metab 2001; 86: 965-71.

[27]   Krauss RM. Lipids and lipoproteins in patients with type 2 diabetes. Diabetes Care 2004; 27: 1496-504.

[28]   Kendall DM. The dyslipidemia of diabetes mellitus: giving triglycerides and high-density lipoprotein cholesterol a higher priority? Endocrinol Metab Clin North Am 2005; 34: 27-48.

[29]   Wood PD, Stern MP, Silvers A, Reaven GM, von der Groeben J. Prevalence of plasma lipoprotein abnormalities in a free-living population of the Central Valley, California. Circulation 1972; 45: 114-26.

[30]   Onat A, Surdum-Avci G, Senocak M, Ornek E, Gozukara Y. Plasma lipids and their interrelationship in Turkish adults. J Epidemiol Community Health 1992; 46: 470-6.

[31] Berrios X, Koponen T, Huiguang T, Khaltaev N, Puska P, Nissinen A. Distribution and prevalence of major risk factors of noncommunicable diseases in selected countries: the WHO Inter-Health Programme. Bull World Health Organ 1997; 75: 99-108.

[32] Ezenwaka CE, Premanand N, Orrett FA. Studies on plasma lipids in industrial workers in central Trinidad and Tobago. J Natl Med Assoc 2000; 92: 375-81.

[33] Foucan L, Kangambega P, Koumavi Ekouevi D, Rozet J, Bangou-Bredent J. Lipid profile in an adult population in Guadeloupe. Diabetes Metab 2000; 26: 473-80.

[34] Hanh TTM, Komatsu T, Hung NT, *et al.* Nutritional status of middle-aged Vietnamese in Ho Chi Minh City. J Am Coll Nutr 2001; 20: 616-22.

[35] Zaman MM, Yoshiike N, Rouf MA, *et al.* Cardiovascular risk factors: distribution and prevalence in a rural population of Bangladesh. J Cardiovasc Risk 2001; 8: 103-8.

[36] Li Z, Yang R, Xu G, Xia T. Serum lipid concentrations and prevalence of dyslipidemia in a large professional population in Beijing. Clin Chem 2005; 51: 144-50.

[37] Pang RW, Tam S, Janus ED, *et al.* Plasma lipid, lipoprotein and apolipoprotein levels in a random population sample of 2875 Hong Kong Chinese adults and their implications (NCEP ATP-III, 2001 guidelines) on cardiovascular risk assessment. Atherosclerosis 2006; 184: 438-45.

[38] Zhao WH, Zhang J, Zhai Y, *et al.* Blood lipid profile and prevalence of dyslipidemia in Chinese adults. Biomed Environ Sci 2007; 20: 329-35.

[39] Erem C, Hacihasanoglu A, Deger O, Kocak M, Topbas M. Prevalence of dyslipidemia and associated risk factors among Turkish adults: Trabzon lipid study. Endocrine 2008; 34: 36-51.

[40] Azizi F, Rahmani M, Ghanbarian A, *et al.* Serum lipid levels in an Iranian adults population: Tehran Lipid and Glucose Study. Eur J Epidemiol 2003; 18: 311-9.

[41] Pongchaiyakul C, Hongsprabhas P, Pisprasert V. Rural-urban difference in lipid levels and prevalence of dyslipidemia: a population-based study in Khon Kaen province, Thailand. J Med Assoc Thai 2006; 89: 1835-44.

[42] Mann JI, Lewis B, Shepherd J, *et al.* Blood lipid concentrations and other cardiovascular risk factors: distribution, prevalence, and detection in Britain. Br Med J (Clin Res Ed) 1988; 296: 1702-6.

[43] Hertz RP, Unger AN, Ferrario CM. Diabetes, hypertension, and dyslipidemia in Mexican Americans and non-Hispanic whites. Am J Prev Med 2006; 30: 103-10.

[44] Tekes-Manova D, Israeli E, Shochat T, *et al.* The prevalence of reversible cardiovascular risk factors in Israelis aged 25-55 years. Isr Med Assoc J 2006; 8: 527-31.

[45] Steinhagen-Thiessen E, Bramlage P, Losch C, *et al.* Dyslipidemia in primary care--prevalence, recognition, treatment and control: data from the German Metabolic and Cardiovascular Risk Project (GEMCAS). Cardiovasc Diabetol 2008; 7: 31.

[46] Florez H, Silva E, Fernandez V, *et al.* Prevalence and risk factors associated with the metabolic syndrome and dyslipidemia in White, Black, Amerindian and Mixed Hispanics in Zulia State, Venezuela. Diabetes Res Clin Pract 2005; 69: 63-77.

[47] Fuentes R, Uusitalo T, Puska P, Tuomilehto J, Nissinen A. Blood cholesterol level and prevalence of hypercholesterolemia in developing countries: a review of population-based studies carried out from 1979 to 2002. Eur J Cardiovasc Prev Rehabil 2003; 10: 411-9.

[48] Tolonen H, Keil U, Ferrario M, Evans A. Prevalence, awareness and treatment of hypercholesterolemia in 32 populations: results from the WHO MONICA Project. Int J Epidemiol 2005; 34: 181-92.

[49] Kannel WB. Lipids, diabetes, and coronary heart disease: insights from the Framingham Study. Am Heart J 1985; 110: 1100-7.

[50] Cowie CC, Howard BV, Harris MI. Serum lipoproteins in African Americans and whites with non-insulin-dependent diabetes in the US population. Circulation 1994; 90: 1185-93.

[51] Manley SE. U.K. Prospective Diabetes Study Investigators. U.K. Prospective Diabetes Study 27. Plasma lipids and lipoproteins at diagnosis of NIDDM by age and sex. Diabetes Care 1997; 20: 1683-7.

[52] Jacobs MJ, Kleisli T, Pio JR, *et al.* Prevalence and control of dyslipidemia among persons with diabetes in the United States. Diabetes Res Clin Pract 2005; 70: 263-9.

[53] Bruckert E, Baccara-Dinet M, Eschwege E. Low HDL-cholesterol is common in European Type 2 diabetic patients receiving treatment for dyslipidemia: data from a pan-European survey. Diabet Med 2007; 24: 388-91.

[54] Okafor CI, Fasanmade OA, Oke DA. Pattern of dyslipidemia among Nigerians with type 2 diabetes mellitus. Niger J Clin Pract 2008; 11: 25-31.

[55] Surana SP, Shah DB, Gala K, *et al.* Prevalence of metabolic syndrome in an urban Indian diabetic population using the NCEP ATP III guidelines. J Assoc Physicians India 2008; 56: 865-8.

[56] Ahmed N, Khan J, Siddiqui TS. Frequency of dyslipidemia in type 2 diabetes mellitus in patients of Hazara division. J Ayub Med Coll Abbottabad 2008; 20: 51-4.

[57] Abdel-Aal NM, Ahmad AT, Froelicher ES, Batieha AM, Hamza MM, Ajlouni KM. Prevalence of dyslipidemia in patients with type 2 diabetes in Jordan. Saudi Med J 2008; 29: 1423-8.

[58] Jurado J, Ybarra J, Solanas P, *et al.* Prevalence of cardiovascular disease and risk factors in a type 2 diabetic population of the North Catalonia diabetes study. J Am Acad Nurse Pract 2009; 21: 140-8.

[59] Papazafiropoulou A, Sotiropoulos A, Skliros E, *et al.* Familial history of diabetes and clinical characteristics in Greek subjects with type 2 diabetes. BMC Endocr Disord 2009; 9: 12.

[60] Roberto Robles N, Barroso S, Marcos G, Sanchez Munoz-Torrero JF. (Lipid control in diabetic patients in Extremadura (Spain)). Endocrinol Nutr 2009; 56: 112-7.

[61] Seyum B, Mebrahtu G, Usman A, *et al.* Profile of patients with diabetes in Eritrea: results of first phase registry analyses. Acta Diabetol 2010; 47: 23-7.

[62] Agarwal AK, Singla S, Singla R, Lal A, Wardhan H, Yadav R. Prevalence of coronary risk factors in type 2 diabetics without manifestations of overt coronary heart disease. J Assoc Physicians India 2009; 57: 135-42.

[63] Temelkova-Kurktschiev TS, Kurktschiev DP, Vladimirova-Kitova LG, Vaklinova I, Todorova BR. Prevalence and type of dyslipidemia in a population at risk for cardiovascular death in Bulgaria. Folia Med (Plovdiv) 2009; 51: 26-32.

[64] Zhang X, Sun Z, Zhang D, *et al.* Prevalence and association with diabetes and obesity of lipid phenotypes among the hypertensive Chinese rural adults. Heart Lung 2009; 38: 17-24.

[65] Grant RW, Meigs JB. Prevalence and treatment of low HDL cholesterol among primary care patients with type 2 diabetes: an unmet challenge for cardiovascular risk reduction. Diabetes Care 2007; 30: 479-84.

[66] Bangou-Bredent J, Szmidt-Adjide V, Kangambega-Nouvier P, *et al.* Cardiovascular risk factors associated with diabetes in an Indian community of Guadeloupe. A case control study. Diabetes Metab 1999; 25: 393-8.

[67] Zhang L, Qiao Q, Tuomilehto J, *et al.* Blood lipid levels in relation to glucose status in European men and women without a prior history of diabetes: the DECODE Study. Diabetes Res Clin Pract 2008; 82: 364-77.

[68] Zhang L, Qiao Q, Tuomilehto J, *et al.* Blood lipid levels in relation to glucose status in seven populations of Asian origin without a prior history of diabetes: the DECODA study. Diabetes Metab Res Rev 2009; 25: 549-57.

[69] Grundy SM, Becker D, Clark LT, *et al.* Expert panel on detection E, and treatment of high blood cholesterol in adults. Executive Summary of The Third Report of The National Cholesterol Education Program (NCEP) Expert Panel on Detection, Evaluation, And Treatment of High Blood Cholesterol In Adults (Adult Treatment Panel III). JAMA 2001; 285: 2486-97.

[70] Cohen JC, Wang Z, Grundy SM, Stoesz MR, Guerra R. Variation at the hepatic lipase and apolipoprotein AI/CIII/AIV loci is a major cause of genetically determined variation in plasma HDL cholesterol levels. J Clin Invest 1994; 94: 2377-84.

[71] Chait A, Brunzell JD. Acquired hyperlipidemia (secondary dyslipoproteinemias). Endocrinol Metab Clin North Am 1990; 19: 259-78.

[72] Devroey D, De Swaef N, Coigniez P, Vandevoorde J, Kartounian J, Betz W. Correlations between lipid levels and age, gender, glycemia, obesity, diabetes, and smoking. Endocr Res 2004; 30: 83-93.

[73] Ruixing Y, Jinzhen W, Yaoheng H, *et al.* Associations of diet and lifestyle with hyperlipidemia for middle-aged and elderly persons among the Guangxi Bai Ku Yao and Han populations. J Am Diet Assoc 2008; 108: 970-6.

[74] Denke MA, Sempos CT, Grundy SM. Excess body weight. An underrecognized contributor to high blood cholesterol levels in white American men. Arch Intern Med 1993; 153: 1093-103.

[75] Denke MA, Sempos CT, Grundy SM. Excess body weight. An under-recognized contributor to dyslipidemia in white American women. Arch Intern Med 1994; 154: 401-10.

[76] Brown CD, Higgins M, Donato KA, *et al.* Body mass index and the prevalence of hypertension and dyslipidemia. Obes Res 2000; 8: 605-19.

[77] Berg A, Halle M, Franz I, Keul J. Physical activity and lipoprotein metabolism: epidemiological evidence and clinical trials. Eur J Med Res 1997; 2: 259-64.

[78] Hardman AE. Physical activity, obesity and blood lipids. Int J Obes Relat Metab Disord 1999; 23 (Suppl 3): S64-71.

[79] Criqui MH, Wallace RB, Heiss G, Mishkel M, Schonfeld G, Jones GT. Cigarette smoking and plasma high-density lipoprotein cholesterol. The Lipid Research Clinics Program Prevalence Study. Circulation 1980; 62: IV70-6.

[80] Cade J, Margetts B. Cigarette smoking and serum lipid and lipoprotein concentrations. BMJ 1989; 298: 1312.

[81]   Umeda T, Kono S, Sakurai Y, *et al.* Relationship of cigarette smoking, alcohol use, recreational exercise and obesity with serum lipid atherogenicity: a study of self-defense officials in Japan. J Epidemiol 1998; 8: 227-34.

[82]   Fisher SD, Zareba W, Moss AJ, *et al.* Effect of smoking on lipid and thrombogenic factors two months after acute myocardial infarction. Am J Cardiol 2000; 86: 813-8.

[83]   Wu DM, Pai L, Sun PK, Hsu LL, Sun CA. Joint effects of alcohol consumption and cigarette smoking on atherogenic lipid and lipoprotein profiles: results from a study of Chinese male population in Taiwan. Eur J Epidemiol 2001; 17: 629-35.

[84]   Maeda K, Noguchi Y, Fukui T. The effects of cessation from cigarette smoking on the lipid and lipoprotein profiles: a meta-analysis. Prev Med 2003; 37: 283-90.

[85]   Mammas IN, Bertsias GK, Linardakis M, Tzanakis NE, Labadarios DN, Kafatos AG. Cigarette smoking, alcohol consumption, and serum lipid profile among medical students in Greece. Eur J Public Health 2003; 13: 278-82.

[86]   Venkatesan A, Hemalatha A, Bobby Z, Selvaraj N, Sathiyapriya V. Effect of smoking on lipid profile and lipid peroxidation in normal subjects. Indian J Physiol Pharmacol 2006; 50: 273-8.

[87]   Batic-Mujanovic O, Beganlic A, Salihefendic N, Pranjic N, Kusljugic Z. Influence of smoking on serum lipid and lipoprotein levels among family medicine patients. Med Arh 2008; 62: 264-7.

[88]   Arslan E, Yakar T, Yavasoglu I. The effect of smoking on mean platelet volume and lipid profile in young male subjects. Anadolu Kardiyol Derg 2008; 8: 422-5.

[89]   Millen BE, Quatromoni PA, Nam BH, O'Horo CE, Polak JF, D'Agostino RB. Dietary patterns and the odds of carotid atherosclerosis in women: the Framingham Nutrition Studies. Prev Med 2002; 35: 540-7.

[90]   Hennig B, Toborek M, McClain CJ. High-energy diets, fatty acids and endothelial cell function: implications for atherosclerosis. J Am Coll Nutr 2001; 20: 97-105.

[91]   Tanasescu M, Cho E, Manson JE, Hu FB. Dietary fat and cholesterol and the risk of cardiovascular disease among women with type 2 diabetes. Am J Clin Nutr 2004; 79: 999-1005.

[92]   McNamara DJ, Howell WH. Epidemiologic data linking diet to hyperlipidemia and arteriosclerosis. Semin Liver Dis 1992; 12: 347-55.

[93]   Lehtonen A. Effect of beta blockers on blood lipid profile. Am Heart J 1985; 109: 1192-6.

[94]   Fogari R, Zoppi A, Pasotti C, Poletti L, Tettamanti F, Maiwald C. Effects of different beta-blockers on lipid metabolism in chronic therapy of hypertension. Int J Clin Pharmacol Ther Toxicol 1988; 26: 597-604.

[95]   Roberts WC. Recent studies on the effects of beta blockers on blood lipid levels. Am Heart J 1989; 117: 709-14.

[96]   Middeke M, Richter WO, Schwandt P, Beck B, Holzgreve H. Normalization of lipid metabolism after withdrawal from antihypertensive long-term therapy with beta blockers and diuretics. Arteriosclerosis 1990; 10: 145-7.

[97]   Stone NJ. Secondary causes of hyperlipidemia. Med Clin North Am 1994; 78: 117-41.

[98]   De Oliveira ESER, Foster D, McGee Harper M, *et al.* Alcohol consumption raises HDL cholesterol levels by increasing the transport rate of apolipoproteins A-I and A-II. Circulation 2000; 102: 2347-52.

[99]   Shai I, Rimm EB, Schulze MB, Rifai N, Stampfer MJ, Hu FB. Moderate alcohol intake and markers of inflammation and endothelial dysfunction among diabetic men. Diabetologia 2004; 47: 1760-7.

[100]   Ismail IS, Nazaimoon W, Mohamad W, *et al.* Ethnicity and glycemic control are major determinants of diabetic dyslipidemia in Malaysia. Diabet Med 2001; 18: 501-8.

[101]   Gatti A, Maranghi M, Bacci S, *et al.* Poor glycemic control is an independent risk factor for low HDL cholesterol in patients with type 2 diabetes. Diabetes Care 2009; 32: 1550-2.

[102]   Ginsberg HN. Insulin resistance and cardiovascular disease. J Clin Invest 2000; 106: 453-8.

[103]   Avramoglu RK, Basciano H, Adeli K. Lipid and lipoprotein dysregulation in insulin resistant states. Clin Chim Acta 2006; 368: 1-19.

[104]   Howard BV. Lipoprotein metabolism in diabetes mellitus. J Lipid Res 1987; 28: 613-28.

[105]   Lewis GF. Fatty acid regulation of very low density lipoprotein production. Curr Opin Lipidol 1997; 8: 146-53.

[106]   Bakogianni MC, Kalofoutis CA, Skenderi KI, Kalofoutis AT. Clinical evaluation of plasma high-density lipoprotein subfractions (HDL2, HDL3) in non-insulin-dependent diabetics with coronary artery disease. J Diabetes Complications 2001; 15: 265-9.

[107]   Semenkovich CF. Insulin resistance and atherosclerosis. J Clin Invest 2006; 116: 1813-22.

[108]   Hayek T, Azrolan N, Verdery RB, *et al.* Hypertriglyceridemia and cholesteryl ester transfer protein interact to dramatically alter high density lipoprotein levels, particle sizes, and metabolism. Studies in transgenic mice. J Clin Invest 1993; 92: 1143-52.

[109]   Rashid S, Watanabe T, Sakaue T, Lewis GF. Mechanisms of HDL lowering in insulin resistant, hypertriglyceridemic states: the combined effect of HDL triglyceride enrichment and elevated hepatic lipase activity. Clin Biochem 2003; 36: 421-9.

[110] Haas MJ, Horani M, Mreyoud A, Plummer B, Wong NC, Mooradian AD. Suppression of apolipoprotein AI gene expression in HepG2 cells by TNF alpha and IL-1beta. Biochim Biophys Acta 2003; 1623: 120-8.

[111] Syvanne M, Taskinen MR. Lipids and lipoproteins as coronary risk factors in non-insulin-dependent diabetes mellitus. Lancet 1997; 350 (Suppl 1): SI20-3.

[112] de Graaf J, Hak-Lemmers HL, Hectors MP, Demacker PN, Hendriks JC, Stalenhoef AF. Enhanced susceptibility to *in vitro* oxidation of the dense low density lipoprotein subfraction in healthy subjects. Arterioscler Thromb 1991; 11: 298-306.

[113] Brinton EA. Controversies in dyslipidemias: atheroprevention in diabetes and insulin resistance. Ann N Y Acad Sci 2005; 1055: 159-78.

[114] Pastromas S, Terzi AB, Tousoulis D, Koulouris S. Postprandial lipemia: an under-recognized atherogenic factor in patients with diabetes mellitus. Int J Cardiol 2008; 126: 3-12.

[115] Hammad SM, Twal WO, Barth JL, *et al.* Oxidized LDL immune complexes and oxidized LDL differentially affect the expression of genes involved with inflammation and survival in human U937 monocytic cells. Atherosclerosis 2009; 202: 394-404.

[116] Krentz AJ. Lipoprotein abnormalities and their consequences for patients with type 2 diabetes. Diabetes Obes Metab 2003; 5 (Suppl 1): S19-27.

[117] Sorrentino SA, Besler C, Rohrer L, *et al.* Endothelial-vasoprotective effects of high-density lipoprotein are impaired in patients with type 2 diabetes mellitus but are improved after extended-release niacin therapy. Circulation 2010; 121: 110-22.

[118] Gotto AM, Jr., Brinton EA. Assessing low levels of high-density lipoprotein cholesterol as a risk factor in coronary heart disease: a working group report and update. J Am Coll Cardiol 2004; 43: 717-24.

[119] Anand SS, Yusuf S, Vuksan V, *et al.* Differences in risk factors, atherosclerosis, and cardiovascular disease between ethnic groups in Canada: the Study of Health Assessment and Risk in Ethnic groups (SHARE). Lancet 2000; 356: 279-84.

[120] Razak F, Anand S, Vuksan V, *et al.* Ethnic differences in the relationships between obesity and glucose-metabolic abnormalities: a cross-sectional population-based study. Int J Obes (Lond) 2005; 29: 656-67.

[121] Chandalia M, Mohan V, Adams-Huet B, Deepa R, Abate N. Ethnic difference in sex gap in high-density lipoprotein cholesterol between Asian Indians and Whites. J Investig Med 2008; 56: 574-80.

[122] Mulukutla SR, Venkitachalam L, Marroquin OC, *et al.* Population variation in atherogenic dyslipidemia: A report from the Heart SCORE and India SCORE Studies. J Clin Lipido 2008; 2: 410-7.

[123] Tan CE, Emmanuel SC, Tan BY, Jacob E. Prevalence of diabetes and ethnic differences in cardiovascular risk factors. The 1992 Singapore National Health Survey. Diabetes Care 1999; 22: 241-7.

[124] Karthikeyan G, Teo KK, Islam S, *et al.* Lipid profile, plasma apolipoproteins, and risk of a first myocardial infarction among Asians: an analysis from the INTERHEART Study. J Am Coll Cardiol 2009; 53: 244-53.

[125] Nyamdorj R, Qiao Q, Tuomilehto J, *et al.* The DECODA Study Group. Prevalence of the metabolic syndrome in populations of Asian origin. Comparison of the IDF definition with the NCEP definition. Diabetes Res Clin Pract 2007; 76: 57-67.

[126] Zaninotto P, Mindell J, Hirani V. Prevalence of cardiovascular risk factors among ethnic groups: results from the Health Surveys for England. Atherosclerosis 2007; 195: e48-57.

[127] France MW, Kwok S, McElduff P, Seneviratne CJ. Ethnic trends in lipid tests in general practice. QJM 2003; 96: 919-23.

[128] Sharma MD, Pavlik VN. Dyslipidemia in African Americans, Hispanics and whites with type 2 diabetes mellitus and hypertension. Diabetes Obes Metab 2001; 3: 41-5.

[129] Werk EE, Jr., Gonzalez JJ, Ranney JE. Lipid level differences and hypertension effect in blacks and whites with type II diabetes. Ethn Dis 1993; 3: 242-9.

[130] Zhang L, Qiao Q, Tuomilehto J, *et al.* Distinct ethnic differences in lipid profiles across glucose categories. J Clin Endocrinol Metab 2010; 95: 1793-801.

[131] Neaton JD, Blackburn H, Jacobs D, *et al.* Serum cholesterol level and mortality findings for men screened in the Multiple Risk Factor Intervention Trial. Multiple Risk Factor Intervention Trial Research Group. Arch Intern Med 1992; 152: 1490-500.

[132] Nobili A, D'Avanzo B, Santoro L, Ventura G, Todesco P, La Vecchia C. Serum cholesterol and acute myocardial infarction: a case-control study from the GISSI-2 trial. Gruppo Italiano per lo Studio della Sopravvivenza nell'Infarto-Epidemiologia dei Fattori di Rischio dell'Infarto Miocardico Investigators. Br Heart J 1994; 71: 468-73.

[133] LaRosa JC, Hunninghake D, Bush D, *et al.* The cholesterol facts. A summary of the evidence relating dietary fats, serum cholesterol, and coronary heart disease. A joint statement by the American Heart Association and the National Heart, Lung, and Blood Institute. The Task Force on Cholesterol Issues, American Heart Association. Circulation 1990; 81: 1721-33.

[134] Mills EJ, Rachlis B, Wu P, Devereaux PJ, Arora P, Perri D. Primary prevention of cardiovascular mortality and events with statin treatments: a network meta-analysis involving more than 65, 000 patients. J Am Coll Cardiol 2008; 52: 1769-81.

[135] Thavendiranathan P, Bagai A, Brookhart MA, Choudhry NK. Primary prevention of cardiovascular diseases with statin therapy: a meta-analysis of randomized controlled trials. Arch Intern Med 2006; 166: 2307-13.

[136] Gordon T, Castelli WP, Hjortland MC, Kannel WB, Dawber TR. High density lipoprotein as a protective factor against coronary heart disease. The Framingham Study. Am J Med 1977; 62: 707-14.

[137] Rywik SL, Manolio TA, Pajak A, *et al.* Association of lipids and lipoprotein level with total mortality and mortality caused by cardiovascular and cancer diseases (Poland and United States collaborative study on cardiovascular epidemiology). Am J Cardiol 1999; 84: 540-8.

[138] Cui Y, Blumenthal RS, Flaws JA, *et al.* Non-high-density lipoprotein cholesterol level as a predictor of cardiovascular disease mortality. Arch Intern Med 2001; 161: 1413-9.

[139] Mazza A, Tikhonoff V, Schiavon L, Casiglia E. Triglycerides + high-density-lipoprotein-cholesterol dyslipidemia, a coronary risk factor in elderly women: the CArdiovascular STudy in the ELderly. Intern Med J 2005; 35: 604-10.

[140] Bass KM, Newschaffer CJ, Klag MJ, Bush TL. Plasma lipoprotein levels as predictors of cardiovascular death in women. Arch Intern Med 1993; 153: 2209-16.

[141] Qiao Q, Pitkäniemi J, Tuomilehto J, *et al.* The DECODE Study Group. Comparison of different definitions of the metabolic syndrome in relation to cardiovascular mortality in European men and women. Diabetologia 2006; 49: 2837-46.

[142] Barzi F, Patel A, Woodward M, *et al.* A comparison of lipid variables as predictors of cardiovascular disease in the Asia Pacific region. Ann Epidemiol 2005; 15: 405-13.

[143] Tanko LB, Bagger YZ, Qin G, Alexandersen P, Larsen PJ, Christiansen C. Enlarged waist combined with elevated triglycerides is a strong predictor of accelerated atherogenesis and related cardiovascular mortality in postmenopausal women. Circulation 2005; 111: 1883-90.

[144] Tunstall-Pedoe H, Woodward M, Tavendale R, A'Brook R, McCluskey MK. Comparison of the prediction by 27 different factors of coronary heart disease and death in men and women of the Scottish Heart Health Study: cohort study. BMJ 1997; 315: 722-9.

[145] Laakso M, Lehto S, Penttila I, Pyorala K. Lipids and lipoproteins predicting coronary heart disease mortality and morbidity in patients with non-insulin-dependent diabetes. Circulation 1993; 88: 1421-30.

[146] Ridker PM, Rifai N, Cook NR, Bradwin G, Buring JE. Non-HDL cholesterol, apolipoproteins A-I and B100, standard lipid measures, lipid ratios, and CRP as risk factors for cardiovascular disease in women. JAMA 2005; 294: 326-33.

[147] Pischon T, Girman CJ, Sacks FM, Rifai N, Stampfer MJ, Rimm EB. Non-high-density lipoprotein cholesterol and apolipoprotein B in the prediction of coronary heart disease in men. Circulation 2005; 112: 3375-83.

[148] Cooney MT, Dudina A, De Bacquer D, *et al.* HDL cholesterol protects against cardiovascular disease in both genders, at all ages and at all levels of risk. Atherosclerosis 2009; 206: 611-6.

[149] Gordon DJ, Probstfield JL, Garrison RJ, *et al.* High-density lipoprotein cholesterol and cardiovascular disease. Four prospective American studies. Circulation 1989; 79: 8-15.

[150] Grover SA, Kaouache M, Joseph L, Barter P, Davignon J. Evaluating the incremental benefits of raising high-density lipoprotein cholesterol levels during lipid therapy after adjustment for the reductions in other blood lipid levels. Arch Intern Med 2009; 169: 1775-80.

[151] Stampfer MJ, Krauss RM, Ma J, *et al.* A prospective study of triglyceride level, low-density lipoprotein particle diameter, and risk of myocardial infarction. JAMA 1996; 276: 882-8.

[152] Cremer P, Nagel D, Mann H, *et al.* Ten-years follow-up results from the Goettingen Risk, Incidence and Prevalence Study (GRIPS). I. Risk factors for myocardial infarction in a cohort of 5790 men. Atherosclerosis 1997; 129: 221-30.

[153] Dunder K, Lind L, Lagerqvist B, Zethelius B, Vessby B, Lithell H. Cardiovascular risk factors for stable angina pectoris *versus* unheralded myocardial infarction. Am Heart J 2004; 147: 502-8.

[154] Eberly LE, Stamler J, Neaton JD. Relation of triglyceride levels, fasting and nonfasting, to fatal and nonfatal coronary heart disease. Arch Intern Med 2003; 163: 1077-83.

[155] Hulley SB, Rosenman RH, Bawol RD, Brand RJ. Epidemiology as a guide to clinical decisions. The association between triglyceride and coronary heart disease. N Engl J Med 1980; 302: 1383-9.

[156] Iso H, Naito Y, Sato S, *et al.* Serum triglycerides and risk of coronary heart disease among Japanese men and women. Am J Epidemiol 2001; 153: 490-9.

[157] Jeppesen J, Hein HO, Suadicani P, Gyntelberg F. Low triglycerides-high high-density lipoprotein cholesterol and risk of ischemic heart disease. Arch Intern Med 2001; 161: 361-6.

[158] Pirro M, Mauriege P, Tchernof A, *et al.* Plasma free fatty acid levels and the risk of ischemic heart disease in men: prospective results from the Quebec Cardiovascular Study. Atherosclerosis 2002; 160: 377-84.

[159] Psaty BM, Anderson M, Kronmal RA, *et al.* The association between lipid levels and the risks of incident myocardial infarction, stroke, and total mortality: The Cardiovascular Health Study. J Am Geriatr Soc 2004; 52: 1639-47.

[160] Shai I, Rimm EB, Hankinson SE, *et al.* Multivariate assessment of lipid parameters as predictors of coronary heart disease among postmenopausal women: potential implications for clinical guidelines. Circulation 2004; 110: 2824-30.

[161] Sharrett AR, Ballantyne CM, Coady SA, *et al.* Coronary heart disease prediction from lipoprotein cholesterol levels, triglycerides, lipoprotein(a), apolipoproteins A-I and B, and HDL density subfractions: The Atherosclerosis Risk in Communities (ARIC) Study. Circulation 2001; 104: 1108-13.

[162] Talmud PJ, Hawe E, Miller GJ, Humphries SE. Nonfasting apolipoprotein B and triglyceride levels as a useful predictor of coronary heart disease risk in middle-aged UK men. Arterioscler Thromb Vasc Biol 2002; 22: 1918-23.

[163] Yarnell JW, Patterson CC, Sweetnam PM, *et al.* Do total and high density lipoprotein cholesterol and triglycerides act independently in the prediction of ischemic heart disease? Ten-years follow-up of Caerphilly and Speedwell Cohorts. Arterioscler Thromb Vasc Biol 2001; 21: 1340-5.

[164] Bansal S, Buring JE, Rifai N, Mora S, Sacks FM, Ridker PM. Fasting compared with nonfasting triglycerides and risk of cardiovascular events in women. JAMA 2007; 298: 309-16.

[165] Avins AL, Neuhaus JM. Do triglycerides provide meaningful information about heart disease risk? Arch Intern Med 2000; 160: 1937-44.

[166] Walldius G, Jungner I, Holme I, Aastveit AH, Kolar W, Steiner E. High apolipoprotein B, low apolipoprotein A-I, and improvement in the prediction of fatal myocardial infarction (AMORIS study): a prospective study. Lancet 2001; 358: 2026-33.

[167] Austin MA, Hokanson JE, Edwards KL. Hypertriglyceridemia as a cardiovascular risk factor. Am J Cardiol 1998; 81: 7B-12B.

[168] Assmann G, Schulte H, Funke H, von Eckardstein A. The emergence of triglycerides as a significant independent risk factor in coronary artery disease. Eur Heart J 1998; 19 (Suppl M): M8-14.

[169] Natarajan S, Glick H, Criqui M, Horowitz D, Lipsitz SR, Kinosian B. Cholesterol measures to identify and treat individuals at risk for coronary heart disease. Am J Prev Med 2003; 25: 50-7.

[170] Lemieux I, Lamarche B, Couillard C, *et al.* Total cholesterol/HDL cholesterol ratio *vs.* LDL cholesterol/HDL cholesterol ratio as indices of ischemic heart disease risk in men: the Quebec Cardiovascular Study. Arch Intern Med 2001; 161: 2685-92.

[171] Schulze MB, Shai I, Manson JE, *et al.* Joint role of non-HDL cholesterol and glycated hemoglobin in predicting future coronary heart disease events among women with type 2 diabetes. Diabetologia 2004; 47: 2129-36.

[172] Liu J, Sempos C, Donahue RP, Dorn J, Trevisan M, Grundy SM. Joint distribution of non-HDL and LDL cholesterol and coronary heart disease risk prediction among individuals with and without diabetes. Diabetes Care 2005; 28: 1916-21.

[173] McQueen MJ, Hawken S, Wang X, *et al.* Lipids, lipoproteins, and apolipoproteins as risk markers of myocardial infarction in 52 countries (the INTERHEART study): a case-control study. Lancet 2008; 372: 224-33.

[174] Vaessen SF, Schaap FG, Kuivenhoven JA, *et al.* Apolipoprotein A-V, triglycerides and risk of coronary artery disease: the prospective Epic-Norfolk Population Study. J Lipid Res 2006; 47: 2064-70.

[175] Dunder K, Lind L, Zethelius B, Berglund L, Lithell H. Evaluation of a scoring scheme, including proinsulin and the apolipoprotein B/apolipoprotein A1 ratio, for the risk of acute coronary events in middle-aged men: Uppsala Longitudinal Study of Adult Men (ULSAM). Am Heart J 2004; 148: 596-601.

[176] Meisinger C, Loewel H, Mraz W, Koenig W. Prognostic value of apolipoprotein B and A-I in the prediction of myocardial infarction in middle-aged men and women: results from the MONICA/KORA Augsburg cohort study. Eur Heart J 2005; 26: 271-8.

[177] Sierra-Johnson J, Fisher RM, Romero-Corral A, *et al.* Concentration of apolipoprotein B is comparable with the apolipoprotein B/apolipoprotein A-I ratio and better than routine clinical lipid measurements in predicting coronary heart disease mortality: findings from a multi-ethnic US population. Eur Heart J 2009; 30: 710-7.

[178] Morrish NJ, Stevens LK, Fuller JH, Keen H, Jarrett RJ. Incidence of macrovascular disease in diabetes mellitus: the London cohort of the WHO Multinational Study of Vascular Disease in Diabetics. Diabetologia 1991; 34: 584-9.

[179] Almdal T, Scharling H, Jensen JS, Vestergaard H. The independent effect of type 2 diabetes mellitus on ischemic heart disease, stroke, and death: a population-based study of 13, 000 men and women with 20 years of follow-up. Arch Intern Med 2004; 164: 1422-6.

[180] Roselli della Rovere G, Lapolla A, Sartore G, *et al.* Plasma lipoproteins, apoproteins and cardiovascular disease in type 2 diabetic patients. A nine-year follow-up study. Nutr Metab Cardiovasc Dis 2003; 13: 46-51.

[181] Vlajinac H, Ilic M, Marinkovic J. Cardiovascular risk factors and prevalence of coronary heart disease in type 2 (non-insulin-dependent) diabetes. Eur J Epidemiol 1992; 8: 783-8.

[182] Ronnemaa T, Laakso M, Kallio V, Pyorala K, Marniemi J, Puukka P. Serum lipids, lipoproteins, and apolipoproteins and the excessive occurrence of coronary heart disease in non-insulin-dependent diabetic patients. Am J Epidemiol 1989; 130: 632-45.

[183] Reckless JP, Betteridge DJ, Wu P, Payne B, Galton DJ. High-density and low-density lipoproteins and prevalence of vascular disease in diabetes mellitus. Br Med J 1978; 1: 883-6.

[184] Santen RJ, Willis PW, 3rd, Fajans SS. Atherosclerosis in diabetes mellitus. Correlations with serum lipid levels, adiposity, and serum insulin level. Arch Intern Med 1972; 130: 833-43.

[185] Gomes MB, Giannella-Neto D, Faria M, *et al.* Estimating cardiovascular risk in patients with type 2 diabetes: a national multicenter study in Brazil. Diabetol Metab Syndr 2009; 1: 22.

[186] Mohan V, Deepa R, Haranath SP, *et al.* Lipoprotein(a) is an independent risk factor for coronary artery disease in NIDDM patients in South India. Diabetes Care 1998; 21: 1819-23.

[187] Murakami K, Ishibashi S, Yoshida Y, Yamada N, Akanuma Y. Lipoprotein(a) as a coronary risk factor in Japanese patients with Type II (non-insulin-dependent) diabetes mellitus. Relation with apolipoprotein(a) phenotypes. Diabetologia 1998; 41: 1397-8.

[188] Smaoui M, Hammami S, Chaaba R, *et al.* Lipids and lipoprotein(a) concentrations in Tunisian type 2 diabetic patients; Relationship to glycemic control and coronary heart disease. J Diabetes Complications 2004; 18: 258-63.

[189] Seviour PW, Teal TK, Richmond W, Elkeles RS. Serum lipids, lipoproteins and macrovascular disease in non-insulin-dependent diabetics: a possible new approach to prevention. Diabet Med 1988; 5: 166-71.

[190] Turner RC, Millns H, Neil HA, *et al.* Risk factors for coronary artery disease in non-insulin dependent diabetes mellitus: United Kingdom Prospective Diabetes Study (UKPDS: 23). BMJ 1998; 316: 823-8.

[191] Stamler J, Vaccaro O, Neaton JD, Wentworth D. Diabetes, other risk factors, and 12-years cardiovascular mortality for men screened in the Multiple Risk Factor Intervention Trial. Diabetes Care 1993; 16: 434-44.

[192] Rosengren A, Welin L, Tsipogianni A, Wilhelmsen L. Impact of cardiovascular risk factors on coronary heart disease and mortality among middle aged diabetic men: a general population study. BMJ 1989; 299: 1127-31.

[193] Morrish NJ, Stevens LK, Fuller JH, Jarrett RJ, Keen H. Risk factors for macrovascular disease in diabetes mellitus: the London follow-up to the WHO Multinational Study of Vascular Disease in Diabetics. Diabetologia 1991; 34: 590-4.

[194] Morrish NJ, Stevens LK, Head J, Fuller JH, Jarrett RJ, Keen H. A prospective study of mortality among middle-aged diabetic patients (the London Cohort of the WHO Multinational Study of Vascular Disease in Diabetics) II: Associated risk factors. Diabetologia 1990; 33: 542-8.

[195] Laws A, Marcus EB, Grove JS, Curb JD. Lipids and lipoproteins as risk factors for coronary heart disease in men with abnormal glucose tolerance: the Honolulu Heart Program. J Intern Med 1993; 234: 471-8.

[196] Koskinen P, Manttari M, Manninen V, Huttunen JK, Heinonen OP, Frick MH. Coronary heart disease incidence in NIDDM patients in the Helsinki Heart Study. Diabetes Care 1992; 15: 820-5.

[197] Janka HU. Five-years incidence of major macrovascular complications in diabetes mellitus. Horm Metab Res Suppl 1985; 15: 15-9.

[198] Uusitupa MI, Niskanen LK, Siitonen O, Voutilainen E, Pyorala K. Ten-year cardiovascular mortality in relation to risk factors and abnormalities in lipoprotein composition in type 2 (non-insulin-dependent) diabetic and non-diabetic subjects. Diabetologia 1993; 36: 1175-84.

[199] Bos G, Dekker JM, Nijpels G, *et al.* A combination of high concentrations of serum triglyceride and non-high-density-lipoprotein-cholesterol is a risk factor for cardiovascular disease in subjects with abnormal glucose metabolism--The Hoorn Study. Diabetologia 2003; 46: 910-6.

[200] Chan WB, Tong PC, Chow CC, *et al.* Triglyceride predicts cardiovascular mortality and its relationship with glycemia and obesity in Chinese type 2 diabetic patients. Diabetes Metab Res Rev 2005; 21: 183-8.

[201] Tseng CH, Tseng CP, Chong CK, Cheng JC, Tai TY. Independent association between triglycerides and coronary artery disease in Taiwanese type 2 diabetic patients. Int J Cardiol 2006; 111: 80-5.

[202] Fontbonne A, Eschwege E, Cambien F, *et al.* Hypertriglyceridemia as a risk factor of coronary heart disease mortality in subjects with impaired glucose tolerance or diabetes. Results from the 11-years follow-up of the Paris Prospective Study. Diabetologia 1989; 32: 300-4.

[203] West KM, Ahuja MM, Bennett PH, *et al.* The role of circulating glucose and triglyceride concentrations and their interactions with other "risk factors" as determinants of arterial disease in nine diabetic population samples from the WHO multinational study. Diabetes Care 1983; 6: 361-9.

[204] Giorda CB, Avogaro A, Maggini M, *et al.* Recurrence of cardiovascular events in patients with type 2 diabetes: epidemiology and risk factors. Diabetes Care 2008; 31: 2154-9.

[205] Rubins HB, Robins SJ, Collins D, *et al.* Gemfibrozil for the secondary prevention of coronary heart disease in men with low levels of high-density lipoprotein cholesterol. Veterans Affairs High-Density Lipoprotein Cholesterol Intervention Trial Study Group. N Engl J Med 1999; 341: 410-8.

[206] Keech A, Simes RJ, Barter P, *et al.* Effects of long-term fenofibrate therapy on cardiovascular events in 9795 people with type 2 diabetes mellitus (the FIELD study): randomised controlled trial. Lancet 2005; 366: 1849-61.

[207] Lu W, Resnick HE, Jablonski KA, *et al.* Non-HDL cholesterol as a predictor of cardiovascular disease in type 2 diabetes: the strong heart study. Diabetes Care 2003; 26: 16-23.

[208] Jiang R, Schulze MB, Li T, *et al.* Non-HDL cholesterol and apolipoprotein B predict cardiovascular disease events among men with type 2 diabetes. Diabetes Care 2004; 27: 1991-7.

[209] Rallidis LS, Pitsavos C, Panagiotakos DB, Sinos L, Stefanadis C, Kremastinos DT. Non-high density lipoprotein cholesterol is the best discriminator of myocardial infarction in young individuals. Atherosclerosis 2005; 179: 305-9.

[210] Thomas GN, Jiang CQ, McGhee SM, *et al.* Association of vascular risk factors with increasing glycemia even in normoglycemic subjects in an older Chinese population: the Guangzhou Biobank Cohort Study. Metabolism 2006; 55: 1035-41.

[211] Zhang L, Qiao Q, Tuomilehto J, *et al.* The impact of dyslipidemia on cardiovascular mortality in individuals without a prior history of diabetes in the DECODE Study. Atherosclerosis 2009; 206: 298-302.

[212] Colhoun HM, Betteridge DJ, Durrington PN, *et al.* Primary prevention of cardiovascular disease with atorvastatin in type 2 diabetes in the Collaborative Atorvastatin Diabetes Study (CARDS): multicentre randomised placebo-controlled trial. Lancet 2004; 364: 685-96.

[213] Pyorala K, Ballantyne CM, Gumbiner B, *et al.* Reduction of cardiovascular events by simvastatin in nondiabetic coronary heart disease patients with and without the metabolic syndrome: subgroup analyses of the Scandinavian Simvastatin Survival Study (4S). Diabetes Care 2004; 27: 1735-40.

[214] Collins R, Armitage J, Parish S, Sleigh P, Peto R. MRC/BHF Heart Protection Study of cholesterol-lowering with simvastatin in 5963 people with diabetes: a randomised placebo-controlled trial. Lancet 2003; 361: 2005-16.

[215] Goldberg RB, Mellies MJ, Sacks FM, *et al.* Cardiovascular events and their reduction with pravastatin in diabetic and glucose-intolerant myocardial infarction survivors with average cholesterol levels: subgroup analyses in the cholesterol and recurrent events (CARE) trial. The Care Investigators. Circulation 1998; 98: 2513-9.

[216] Shepherd J, Barter P, Carmena R, *et al.* Effect of lowering LDL cholesterol substantially below currently recommended levels in patients with coronary heart disease and diabetes: the Treating to New Targets (TNT) study. Diabetes Care 2006; 29: 1220-6.

[217] Sever PS, Poulter NR, Dahlof B, *et al.* Reduction in cardiovascular events with atorvastatin in 2, 532 patients with type 2 diabetes: Anglo-Scandinavian Cardiac Outcomes Trial-lipid-lowering arm (ASCOT-LLA). Diabetes Care 2005; 28: 1151-7.

[218] Knopp RH, d'Emden M, Smilde JG, Pocock SJ. Efficacy and safety of atorvastatin in the prevention of cardiovascular end points in subjects with type 2 diabetes: the Atorvastatin Study for Prevention of Coronary Heart Disease Endpoints in non-insulin-dependent diabetes mellitus (ASPEN). Diabetes Care 2006; 29: 1478-85.

[219] Grundy SM, Becker D, Clark LT, *et al.* Adult Treatment panel III. Third Report of the National Cholesterol Education Program (NCEP) Expert Panel on Detection, Evaluation, and Treatment of High Blood Cholesterol in Adults (Adult Treatment Panel III) final report. Circulation 2002; 106: 3143-421.

[220] Graham I, Atar D, Borch-Johnsen K, *et al.* European guidelines on cardiovascular disease prevention in clinical practice: executive summary. Fourth Joint Task Force of the European Society of Cardiology and other societies on cardiovascular disease prevention in clinical practice (constituted by representatives of nine societies and by invited experts). Eur J Cardiovasc Prev Rehabil 2007; 14 (Suppl 2): E1-40.

[221] American Diabetes Association. Standards of medical care in diabetes--2009. Diabetes Care 2009; 32 (Suppl 1): S13-61.

[222] Villines TC, Stanek EJ, Devine PJ, *et al.* The ARBITER 6-HALTS Trial (Arterial Biology for the Investigation of the Treatment Effects of Reducing Cholesterol 6-HDL and LDL Treatment Strategies in Atherosclerosis) Final results and the impact of medication adherence, dose, and treatment duration. J Am Coll Cardiol 2010; 55:2721-6.

CHAPTER 6

Uric Acid, Hyperuricemia and Diabetes

Hairong Nan*

Department of Community Medicine, School of Public Health, The University of Hong Kong, Hong Kong SAR, China

Abstract: We began this chapter by summarizing the definition of hyperuricemia and its increasing prevalence in different ethnic groups that accompany the increase in obesity, diabetes and metabolic syndrome worldwide. This was followed by a discussion on complex associations between serum Uric Acid (UA) and Fasting and 2-hour Plasma Glucose (FPG and 2hPG) in both pre-diabetes and diabetic patients. The UA-glucose association was positive in the low FPG and low 2hPG distributions, but negative in the upper FPG and 2hPG distributions. In spite of inconsistent findings among studies, most prospective data found that higher levels of baseline UA predicted a future risk of developing type 2 diabetes independently. The direction of causality between value of UA and the development of type 2 diabetes is, however, uncertain. Further studies to investigate the pathophysiological mechanism underlying the relationship between glucose, UA and cardio-metabolic risk factors are gravely needed.

Keywords: Diabetes and non-diabetic hyperglycemia, serum uric acid, hyperuricemia.

Serum Uric Acid (UA) concentration as an end product of the purine metabolism in humans, is determined by an interaction of genetic and environmental factors. The UA levels are higher in humans and the Great and Lesser Apes due to parallel mutations of the uricase gene that occurred during the mid Miocene era [1]. The consequence of the mutation is that humans not only have higher UA levels than most other mammals but they can not regulate UA levels as effectively as others either [2, 3].

The uricase mutation may have conferred a survival advantage by helping to maintain Blood Pressure (BP), stimulate salt-sensitivity, and induce insulin resistance and mild obesity, thereby helping promote survival during a period of famine or stress [4]. As a consequence of westernization and during the past few decades including physical inactivity, high intake of meat and fructose, both which generate UA, humans today have higher UA levels (range 238-595 µmol/l) compared with primates that lack uricase (whose UA levels are typically in the 178-238 µmol/l range) [3].

People with elevated UA, but without the symptoms of gout, nephropathy, or kidney stones are classified as having asymptomatic hyperuricemia. If the gouty symptom does not occur, people with asymptomatic hyperuricemia are usually unaware of their condition and the possible consequences such as hypertension, diabetes, renal disease, and cardiovascular diseases. Increased urbanization, westernization, and economic development have already contributed to a worldwide substantial rise in obesity and diabetes. Interestingly, the prevalence of hyperuricemia has shown a rise in both developing and developed countries, accompanied by a rapid increased rate in obesity and diabetes [5-7].

Since hyperuricemia was first described as being associated with hyperglycemia and hypertension by Kylin in 1923 [8], there has been a heightened interest in the association between elevated UA and other metabolic abnormalities of hyperglycemia, abdominal obesity, dyslipidemia, and hypertension. Serum UA is positively associated with plasma glucose in healthy subjects [9, 10]. This association is, however, different between healthy and diabetic individuals [11-13]. It is still not clear whether elevated serum UA can be used as an early sign of the development of diabetes and other metabolic disorders. A systematic review on the prevalence of hyperuricemia and the complex association between the UA levels and glucose concentrations in diabetic and pre-diabetic ranges is conducted in the chapter.

*Address correspondence to Hairong Nan: Department of Community Medicine, School of Public Health, The University of Hong Kong, 21 Sassoon Road, Pokfulam, Hong Kong SAR, China; E-mail: hnan@hku.hk

6.1. DEFINITION AND PREVALENCE OF HYPERURICEMIA

6.1.1. Definition of Hyperuricemia

The serum UA level is determined by the balance between purine intake and UA production on the one hand and UA elimination by renal and extrarenal routes on the other. Approximately two thirds of total body urate are produced endogenously, the remaining one third is accounted for by dietary purines. However, approximately 70% of the urate produced daily is excreted by the kidneys, the rest is eliminated by the intestines. Normal serum UA levels are less than 420 µmol/l in men and 330-360 µmol/l in women [14]. UA levels are lower in premenopausal women because estrogen is uricosuric [15]. After menopause, UA levels in women are similar to men. UA levels also increase with age [16]. Furthermore, UA levels may vary in the same individual by as much as 59 to 119 µmol/l during the course of a day, due to the effects of diet and exercise.

Hyperuricemia is arbitrarily defined as a serum UA concentration in excess of urate solubility, which is about 420 µmol/l in men and 360 µmol/l in women. Hyperuricemia may occur from excessive production of urate (overproduction) or decreased elimination (underexcretion), and frequently a combination of both processes occur in the same individual. Long-term hyperuricemia is a causal factor to develop damages in joints, connective tissues and kidney.

The rise in UA concentration has historically been viewed as simply a potential risk factor for inducing gout, a clinical diagnosis of gout is, however, only the top of the iceberg. If the gouty symptom does not occur, people with asymptomatic hyperuricemia are usually unaware of their conditions. Hyperuricemia is associated with and may predispose individuals to hypertension, diabetes, renal disease and cardiovascular disease.

6.1.2. Prevalence of Hyperuricemia

The prevalence of hyperuricemia varies markedly depending on differences in races, geographic regions and survey years (Table **1**). Among twenty seven [5-7, 11, 17-39] studies that used hyperuricemia definition of > 420 µmol/l for men and of > 360 µmol/l for women, the prevalence of hyperuricemia ranged from 0.05% in Chinese women in Shandong, China in 1995-96 to 82.0% in male aborigines in Taiwan in 1993-96. The prevalence was lowest among Mainland Chinese and Indians in Amazon region in Brazil and highest among aborigines in Taiwan Mountainous area and Maori in New Zealand in both men and women (Table **1**).

Table 1: Prevalence (%) of hyperuricemia in different ethnic groups and geographic regions

Ethnicity	Survey Year	Geographic Locations	Age	Number	Prevalence (%)		References
			(years)	men/women	men	women	
Caucasian	1970	Birminham, Winfrish and Glasgow, UK	Adult	849/254	7.2	0.4 [a]	Sturge, 1977 [17]
Caucasian	1989	Southern Germany			28.6[b]	2.6 [b]	Gresser, 1990 [18]
Caucasian	1990-1992	New Zealand	≥19	139/176	9.4	10.5	Klemp, 1997 [19]
Chinese	1980	Beijing, Shanghai and Guangzhou, China	≥20	267/235	1.4	1.3	Fang, 1983 [20]
Chinese	1987-1988	Beijing urban area, China	40-58	1 062/951	15.4	11.0	Li, 1997 [21]
		Beijing rural area, China	40-58	558/949	11.3	8.4	Li, 1997 [21]
Chinese	1995-1996	Littoral area, Shandong, China	≥20	-	5.8	0.05	Jiang, 1999 [22]
Chinese	1998	Shanghai, China	≥15	913/1 124	14.2	7.1	Chen, 1998 [23]
Chinese, Han	2002	Urban of Qingdao, China	20-74	903/1 535	32.1	21.8	Nan, 2006 [24]
Chinese	2002	Urban of Shanghai, China	40-74	3 978/-	25.0	-	Villegas, 2010 [25]
Chinese	2004	5 coastal cities of Shandong,	20-80	2395/2068	18.3	8.6	Miao, 2008 [26]

		China					
Chinese	2004-2006	Hangzhou, China	Adult	1 468/906	19.1	3.4	Chen, 2007 [27]
Chinese (Han and Muslim)	2006	Beijing, China	Adult	1 217/780	13.8	6.0	Fang, 2006 [28]
Chinese, Han	1991-1992	Taiwan Kin-Hu, Kinmen	≥30	1 515/1 670	25.8	15.0	Lin, 2000 [29]
Chinese, Han	1993-1996	Taiwan	≥19	1 348/1 498	42.1	27.4	Chang, 2001 [7]
					26.1[b]	17.0[b]	Chang, 2001 [7]
Taiwanese	1993-1996	Taiwan Metropolitan cities	≥19	204/201	48.0	20.7	Chang, 2001 [7]
Taiwanese	1993-1996	Taiwan Mountainous area	≥19	206/233	82.0	64.3	Chang, 2001 [7]
Taiwan aborigines	1990	Taiwan Mountainous area	≥18	145/197	53.8	30.7	Chou, 1998 [30]
Taiwan aborigines	1994-1999	Taiwan	12-15	476/464	50.4	37.7	Ko, 2002 [31]
Chinese and Taiwan aborigines	1999-2000	Taiwan	≥65	1 225/1 167	46.0	26.0	Lee, 2005 [32]
Thai	1999-2000	Bangkok, Thailand	≥15	376/1 005	18.4	7.8	Lohsoonthorn, 2006 [33]
Melanesian	1980	Fiji	≥20	643/697	26.7	27.1	Tuomilehto, 1988 [11]
Asian Indian	1980	Fiji	≥20	598/700	21.7	10.9	Tuomilehto, 1988 [11]
Maori	1963	New Zealand	≥15	388/378	49.0	42.0	Brauer, 1978 [34]
Maori	1990-1992	New Zealand	≥19	130/212	27.1	26.6	Klemp, 1997 [19]
Micronesian-Polynesian	1978	Urban area in Nauru	≥20	217/238	63.6	60.0	Zimmet, 1978 [35]
Malayo-Polynesian	1992	Rural area in Java		Total: 4 683	24.3	12.2	Darmawan, 1992 [5]
African descent	1994	Seychelles	25-64	482/529	35.2	8.7	Conen, 2004 [6]
Arab	1998-1999	Saudi Arabia	≥14	250/237	8.0	8.9	Al-Arfaj, 2001 [36]
Parkateje Indian	1997	Amazon region, Brazil	≥20	56/34	5.6	-	Tavares, 2003 [37]
Japanese	2000	Okinawa, Japan	18-89	2 927/1 562	32.6	9.0	Nagahama, 2004 [38]
White and African-American	1987-1989	4 communities, US	45-64	Total: 14 481	11.2[c]		Schmidt, 1996 [39]

[a] Hyperuricemia defined as UA >420 µmol/l for women; [b] Hyperuricemia defined as UA ≥458 µmol/l for men and ≥393 µmol/l for women; [c] Hyperuricemia defined as UA ≥480 µmol/l; the rest using uric acid >420 µmol/l for men and >360 µmol/l for women.

Early evidence suggests that the Maori people of New Zealand were virtually untroubled by gout or obesity at a time when these disorders were rife in the best fed and hardest drinking sections of the Northern European population [40]. During the past decades, with the introduction of a Western culture and diet, there has been a significant change. By the mid 20th Century with an apparent decline of gout in Europe and North America, hyperuricemia and gout appeared on a large scale in Maori and in other indigenous inhabitants of the Pacific islands. Half the Polynesian population of New Zealand, Rarotonga, Puka Puka, and the Tokelau Islands had hyperuricemia by accepted European and North American standards, the associated gout rate reached 10.2% in Maori males aged 20 and over [40]. Studies of indigenous Pacific populations have also documented that the serum UA is higher in Maori in New Zealand [19, 34], Filipinos in Hawaii and Alaska [41], Chamorros and Carolinians in the Marianas Islands [42].

Recently, accompanying the increase in obesity, diabetes and metabolic syndrome worldwide hyperuricemia has been shown to increase in different areas of the world [43]. Trend studies in Caucasian [18] and Han Chinese in Taiwan [7, 29] showed the prevalence of hyperuricemia has increased over past decades. A German study [18] showed that the UA levels had increased in both genders over secular periods, from 1962 to 1971, 1984 and 1989. The prevalence of hyperuricemia reached 2.6% for women and 28.6% for men in southern Germany in 1989. Earlier studies among immigrants have shown that the serum UA concentrations were higher among Chinese immigrants in Malaya and western Canada compared with their relatives who lived in Taiwan [44]; the urban African black populations have higher serum UA levels than their counterparts living in the rural community [45]. These studies suggested that the elevation in serum UA was associated with the degree of urbanization and economic development.

Serum UA levels tend to be higher in certain populations (*e.g.,* Pacific Islanders and Taiwan aborigines in high Mountainous area), with certain phenotypes (obesity, metabolic syndrome) and with special diets (meat eaters) [19, 34, 46]. Australian indigenous [47] and Taiwanese aborigines have higher UA levels than Caucasian and Chinese population in the same residential areas [7]. Taiwanese aborigines are genetically related to the Malayo-Polynesians [7], have different genetic background compare with Han Chinese population in Taiwan, most of the Han Chinese came from southern mainland China some 400 years ago and some of whom arrived from the central and northern mainland China 60 years ago [30, 48].

6.2. HYPERURICEMIA AND DIABETES

6.2.1. Diabetes, Hyperglycemia and Insulin Resistance

Type 2 diabetes results from the body's ineffective use of insulin and is characterized by insulin resistance and relative insulin deficiency, either of which may be present at the time that diabetes becomes clinically manifested [49, 50]. Type 2 diabetes comprises 90% of people with diabetes around the world, and is largely the result of excess body weight and physical inactivity. In 1985, only 30 million people worldwide were estimated to have diabetes. In 2000, the figure rose to over 150 million. In 2011, an estimated 366 million adults were affected worldwide according to the *Diabetes Atlas* of the International Diabetes Federation and this will have risen to 552 million by 2030 [51]. Approximately 85% to 95% of affected people have type 2 diabetes in developed countries, and account for an even higher percentage in developing countries.

The Bruneck Study, based on a random sample of the general population (n = 888, age 40-79), reported that the prevalence of insulin resistance is 62.8% in subjects with hyperuricemia [52]. It has been reported that the degree of insulin resistance (measured in everyday practice by the homeostasis model assessment index and the quantitative insulin sensitivity check index) [53] may be directly related to serum UA levels [10, 54]. The increased purine biosynthesis and turnover, with consequent increases in serum UA concentrations caused by the increased activity of the hexose monophosphate shunt, may link to insulin resistance and/or hyperinsulinemia [10]. Especially, the impairment of the glycolytic pathway can increase the flux of glucose-6-phosphate through the hexose monophosphate shunt, resulting in the accumulation of ribose-5-phosphate and other intermediates, which are major substrates for UA production [55, 56]. On the other hand, there is evidence that UA may not only be a consequence of insulin resistance, but it may actually promote or worsen insulin resistance. A recent study [57] showed that UA plays an important role in the pathogenesis of the metabolic syndrome, probably due to its ability to inhibit endothelial function through inhibiting nitric oxide bioavailability [58]. Since insulin needs nitric oxide to stimulate glucose uptake, the investigators hypothesized that hyperuricemia may have a key role in the pathogenesis of insulin resistance [57].

In addition, drugs that improve insulin sensitivity, such as metformin [59], troglitazone [60], sibutramine [61, 62], and orlistat [59, 63] have also been reported to be able to lower UA levels. Furthermore, insulin receptors were found in different tubular segments of human kidney [64]. Insulin can enhance renal proximal tubular UA reabsorption in humans due to an active transport mechanism closely linked to the tubular reabsorption of sodium [65-67]. The possible mechanisms linking hyperinsulinemia (a consequence of insulin resistance) with hyperuricemia include the direct stimulations of tubular ion (UA-Na) exchange or the acceleration of cellular metabolism in spite of the site of the tubular effects of insulin [68].

6.2.2. UA Concentration in Relation to Pre-Diabetes and Type 2 Diabetes

6.2.2.1. Cross-Sectional Studies

A few cross-sectional studies have shown that diabetic patients have the low UA levels [11, 69, 70]; the UA concentration was significantly elevated in people with impaired glucose tolerance [11], impaired fasting glucose and newly diagnosed diabetes in white populations [71, 72]. A study among Chinese in Taiwan [73] revealed that among non-diabetic subjects, FPG increased with increasing UA levels in women, but not in men.

The association of serum UA with glucose levels was also extensively investigated in two consecutive population-based cross-sectional studies in mainland China in 2002 and 2006 [74, 75]. The studies further showed that the UA-glucose association was positive in the low FPG and low 2hPG distributions, but negative in the upper FPG and 2hPG distributions in both men and women as shown in the Table **2** and Figs. **1-2** [75]. Multivariate adjustment for various potential confounders did not alter the UA-glucose association substantially although the regression coefficients were reduced in some of the models as shown in the Table **2**. Additional adjustment for seafood consumption, systolic (or diastolic) BP, HDL-C, ApoB or ApoB to ApoA ratio, and menopause status did not change the observed associations either. Only a few studies have investigated the relationship between 2hPG and UA due to the fact that 2h OGTT have not been widely applied. Another population-based cross-sectional study that has examined the UA-2hPG association revealed that serum UA was strongly correlated with 2hPG in non-diabetic Mauritian men (r=0.15) and women (r=0.22) (p<0.001 for both) [76]. Since the results from the cross-sectional studies probably reflected the biochemical interaction between glucose, insulin and purine metabolism, with increased excretions of UA during hyperglycemia and glycosuria [10, 65, 72], the association detected need to be further examined in prospective studies.

Findings from a recent medical screening program in Taiwan including 484 568 men and women 20 years and older showed that the relationship between glucose and UA levels was in opposite direction in nondiabetics and diabetics; increased in UA levels in the former and decreased in the latter [89]. Similar findings have been reported in Taiwanese nondiabetic patients that serum UA levels increased with blood glucose levels [73]. The threshold for this uricosuric effect of glycosuria occurred when FPG level was reportedly at 10 mmol/l or hemoglobin HbA1c level was at 7% in the Third National Health and Nutrition Examination Survey of US populations [90].

Studies have revealed that insulin can enhance renal proximal tubular UA reabsorption in humans, linking to the tubular reabsorption of sodium [65-67]. In addition, insulin resistance increases serum UA through the hexose monophosphate shunt connecting with UA production [10, 55]. Thus, high insulin levels can lead to hyperuricemia. The high baseline fasting insulin levels may explain the high baseline UA levels in individuals with diabetes at follow-up, but can not explain the decrease in UA levels after the onset of diabetes. The reduction in UA levels after the onset of diabetes may be a consequence of the excess excretion of UA due to the hyperosmotic effect caused by high blood glucose concentration and glycosuria [72]. To summarize, the high serum UA in pre-diabetic individuals is a net result of increased UA reabsorption due to insulin resistance while the low serum UA in diabetic patients is attributed to the uricosuria due to osmotic diuresis.

Table 2: Standardized linear regression coefficient for serum uric acid concentration (μmol/l) in relation to fasting plasma glucose (FPG) or 2h plasma glucose (2hPG) concentration (mmol/l) [a]

Adjustment for	Men		Women		Men		Women	
	FPG<7.0	FPG≥7.0	FPG<7.0	FPG≥7.0	2hPG<10.0	2hPG≥10.0	2hPG<10.0	2hPG≥10.0
Number	1357	133	2152	173	1119	136	1639	207
Model 1: Age+Resident area +Alcohol drinking	0.11 [‡]	-0.21 *	0.09 [‡]	-0.31 [‡]	0.16 [‡]	-0.24 [†]	0.09 [‡]	-0.17 *
Model 2: 1+ Triglycerides	0.04	-0.23 [†]	0.07 [†]	-0.29 [‡]	0.11 [‡]	-0.25 [†]	0.06 *	-0.17 *
Model 3: 1+ Body mass index	0.07 [†]	-0.18 *	0.07 [†]	-0.27 [‡]	0.12 [‡]	-0.22 *	0.06 *	-0.16 *
Model 4: 1+ Fasting insulin [b]	0.10 *	-0.20	0.07 *	-0.17	0.15 [‡]	-0.25 *	0.13 [‡]	-0.13
Model 5: 1+Body mass index +Triglycerides	0.02	-0.20 *	0.06 [†]	-0.27 [†]	0.09 [†]	-0.25 [†]	0.04	-0.16 *
Model 6: 5+ Creatinine + C-reactive protein	0.01	-0.13	0.05 *	-0.21 [†]	0.09 [†]	-0.17 *	0.07 [†]	-0.12
Model 7: 6+others [c]	0.01	-0.13	0.06 [†]	-0.21 [†]	0.02	-0.20 *	0.01	-0.12

* p<0.05, [†] p<0.01, [‡] p<0.001. [a] the models were made separately for FPG <7.0 and ≥7.0 mmol/l, or 2hPG <10.0 and ≥10.0 in individuals without prior history of diabetes and gout. [b] N=976 and 79, for FPG<7.0 and FPG ≥7.0 in men, and 1433 and 96 in women; N=809 and 92 for 2hPG <10.0 and 2hPG≥10.0 in men, and 1079 and 138 in women. [c] previous history of hypertension, cardiovascular disease, dyslipidemia and kidney diseases. This table was adapted from [75].

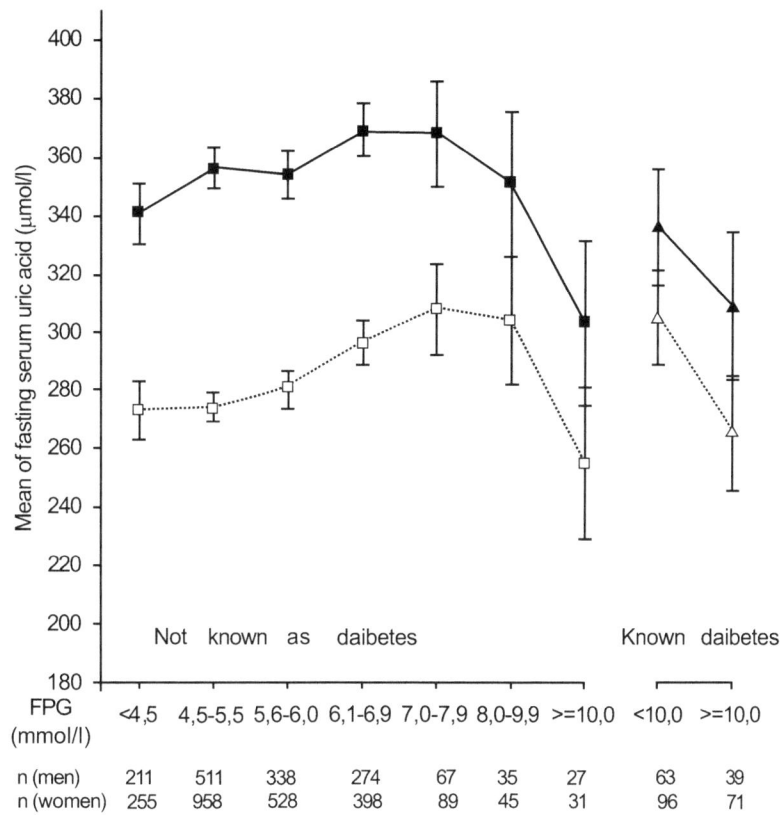

FPG (mmol/l)	<4,5	4,5-5,5	5,6-6,0	6,1-6,9	7,0-7,9	8,0-9,9	>=10,0	<10,0	>=10,0
n (men)	211	511	338	274	67	35	27	63	39
n (women)	255	958	528	398	89	45	31	96	71

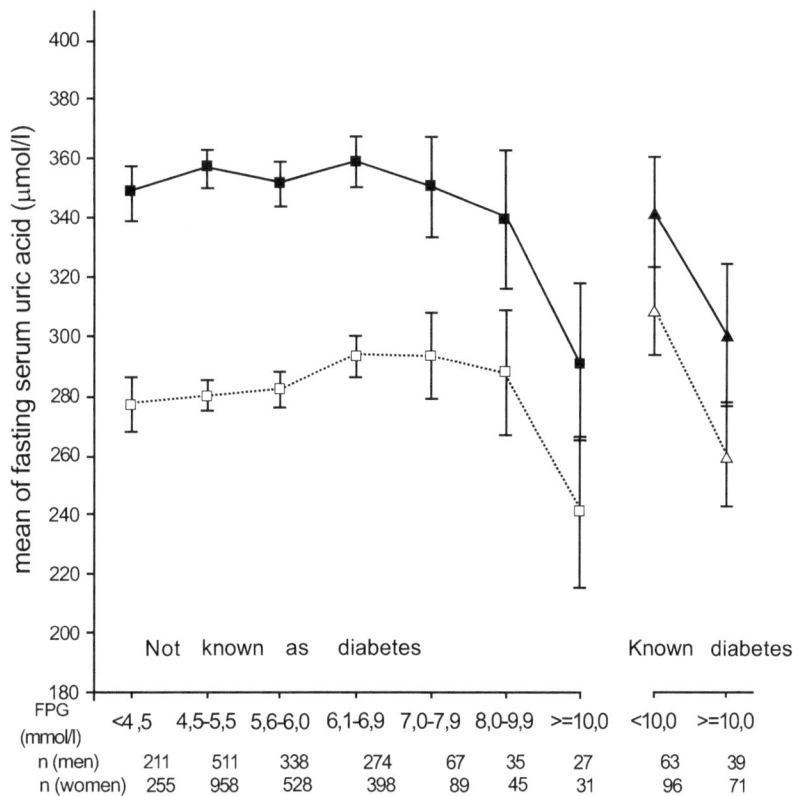

FPG (mmol/l)	<4,5	4,5-5,5	5,6-6,0	6,1-6,9	7,0-7,9	8,0-9,9	>=10,0	<10,0	>=10,0
n (men)	211	511	338	274	67	35	27	63	39
n (women)	255	958	528	398	89	45	31	96	71

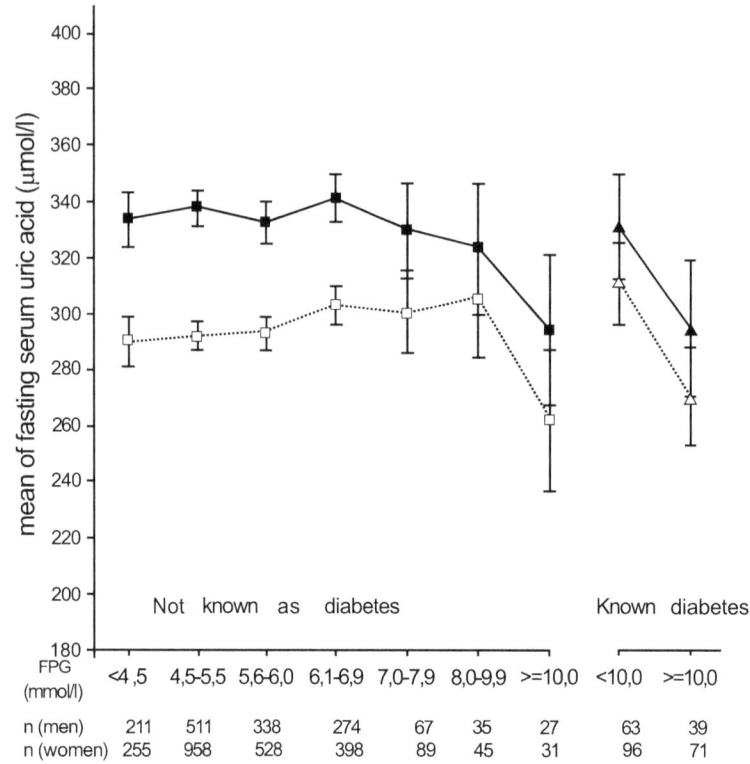

Figure 1: Mean serum uric acid (μ mol/l) (line) and their 95% confidence intervals (bar) in men (solid line) and women (dashed line) according to fasting plasma glucose categories, after adjustment for age, residential areas and alcohol consumption **(A)**; additional adjustment for body mass index and triglycerides **(B)**; and further adjustment for creatinine, C-reactive protein, previous history of hypertension, cardiovascular disease, and dislipidemia **(C)**. This figure was adapted from [75].

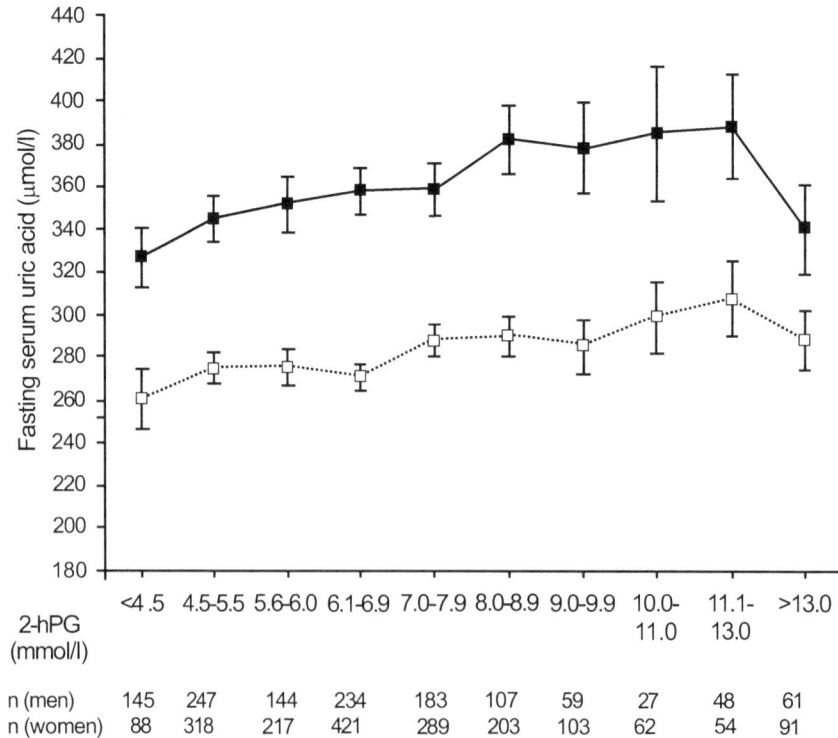

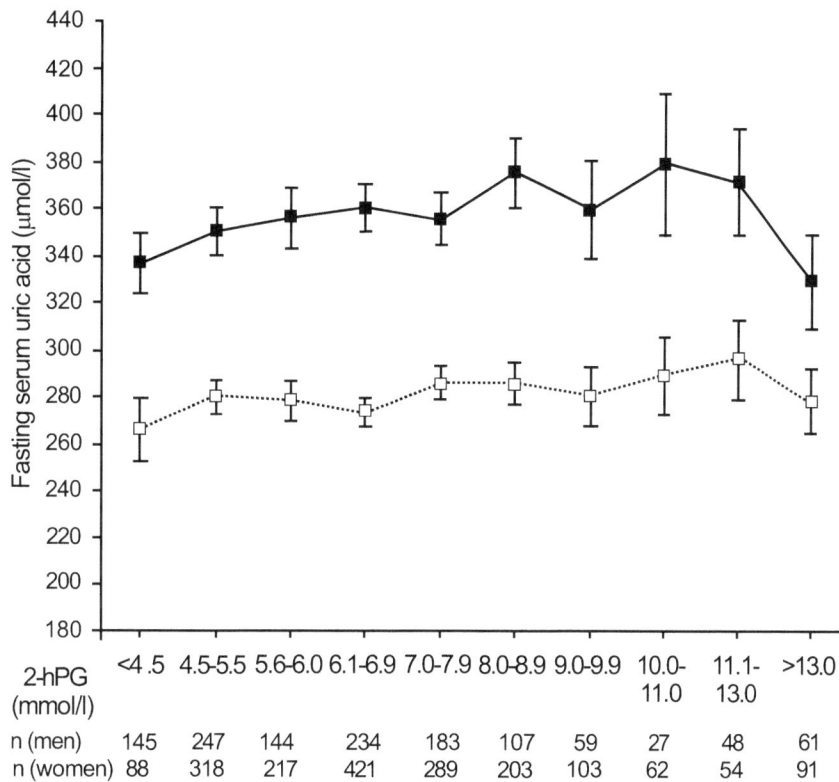

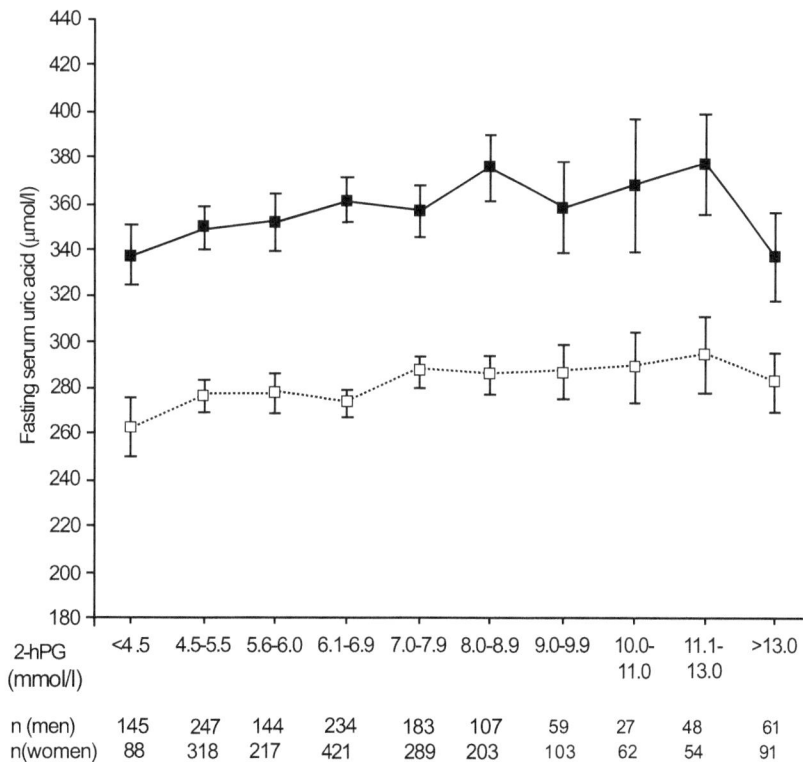

Figure 2: Mean serum uric acid (μmol/l) (line) and their 95% confidence intervals (bar) in men (solid line) and women (dashed line) according to 2h post-load plasma glucose categories, after adjustment for age and residential areas **(A)**; additional adjustment for body mass index and triglycerides **(B)**; and further adjustment for creatinine, previous history of hypertension, cardiovascular disease, and dislipidemia **(C)**. This figure was adapted from [75].

Table 3: Elevated serum uric acid as a predictor for the development of new cases of type 2 diabetes

Study	Study Region	Baseline Study Year	Population, Age (y)	Ethnicity	Follow-up Years	Hazard Ratio (95% CI)	Covariate
Israeli Heart Disease Study [77]	Israel	1963	10 000 Men, age ≥40	Asian, African and European immigrants, and Israeli	5	1.14 per 1 mg/dl	Age, BMI, SBP, total cholesterol, hemoglobin, education, and birthplace.
Rancho Bernardo Study [78]	United States	1984-1987	566 (41% men)	Caucasian	13	1.65 (1.25-2.18) per 1 mg/dl	Age, sex, BMI, diuretic use, and estimated glomerular filtration rate.
Monica Augsburg Cohort Study [79]	Augsburg, Germany	1984-1995	3 052 Men and 3 114 Women, age 35-74	Caucasian	3-15	Men 1.1 (0.9-1.4), women 2.2 (1.6-3.0) per 1mmol/l	Age, BMI, SBP, HDL-C, smoking and alcohol drinking status, family history of DM, physical activity, and cohort.
Hyperuricemic Chinese Study [80]	Taiwan	1991-1992	391 Men and 250 Women, age ≥30	Chinese	7	Men 0.76 (0.51-1.22), Women 1.44 (1.13-2.25) per 1 mg/dl	Age, FPG, BMI, SBP (DBP), menopause status (women), HDL-C, serum creatinine, triglyceride, total cholesterol, and fasting serum insulin.
Mauritius national Surveys [81]	Mauritius	1987, 1992-1998	1 941 men and 2 318 women, age 25-74	Indian and African	5-11	Men 1.19 (1.07, .34), Women 1.05 (0.95, 1.16) per 1 S.D.	Cohort, BMI, FPG, triglycerides, serum creatinine, alcohol consumption, history of hypertension, family history of diabetes, fasting serum insulin, and ethnicity.
Swedish Study [82]	Gothenburg, Sweden	1967	766 Men, mean age 54	Caucasian	13.5	Q5 *vs.* Q1 5.8(2.2-16.0)	Age, BMI (WHR), SBP (DBP), FPG, triglycerides, GOT(GPT), and Bilirubin.
British Regional Heart Study [83]	Great Britain	1977-1980	7 735 Men, age 40-59	Caucasian	12.8	Q5 *vs.* Q1 1.5 (0.9-2.5)	Age, BMI, SBP, HDL-C, smoking and alcohol drinking status, prevalent CHD, heart rate, and physical activity.
Japanese office worker Study [13]	Osaka, Japan	1981-1991	6 356 Men, age 35-60	Japanese	9	Q5 *vs.* Q1 1.24 (0.9-1.7)	Age, BMI, daily alcohol consumption, smoking habits (current, past-, non-smokers), leisure-time physical activity (regular physical activity <= once per week), the duration of the walk to work, FPG, and a parental history of Type 2 diabetes.
Japanese office worker Study [12]	Japan	1994	2 310 Men, age 39-59	Japanese	6	Q5 *vs.* Q1 1.78 (1.11-2.85)	Age, BMI, family history of diabetes, cigarette smoking, alcohol intake, regular physical exercise, mean BP, FPG, triglycerides, total

								cholesterol, and HDL-C.
Community Cardiovascular Cohort Study [84]	Taiwan	1990	1 392 Men and 1 566 Women, age ≥35	Chinese	9		Q5 *vs.* Q1 1.40 (1.02-1.92) for total population	Age, sex, BMI, SBP (DBP), FPG, triglycerides, HDL-C, alcohol intake, marital status, education level, occupation, and family history of diabetes.
Multiple Risk Factor Intervention Trial [85]	United States	1973-1976	11 351 Men	US populations	6		Q5 *vs.* Q1 1.70 (1.38-2.11)	Age, family history of diabetes, smoking status, BMI, hypertension, FPG, physical activity, and gout status annual during follow-up.
Rotterdam Study [86]	Netherlands	1990-1993	4 536 Men and women, age ≥55		10.1		Quartile 4 *vs.* Quartile 1 1.68 (1.22-2.30)	Age, sex, BMI, waist circumference, SBP. DBP, and HDL-C
Finnish Diabetes Prevention Study [87]	Finland	1999	522 impaired glucose tolerance	Finnish	4.1		Tertile 3 *vs.* Tertile 1 1.87 (1.07-3.26)	Age, sex, group, BP medication, and baseline creatinine, SBP, triglycerides, BMI, levels of daily energy intake, intakes of poly-, monounsaturated, and saturated fat and fiber, and leisure-time physical activity and their changes during the follow-up.
Framingham Heart Study [88]	United States	Original cohort: 1948-	4883 (45% men)	US populations			1.20 (1.11-1.28) per 1 mg/dl	Age, sex, BMI, alcohol consumption, smoking, physical activity, hypertension, blood glucose level (casual glucose for original cohort, fasting glucose for offspring cohort), blood cholesterol level, creatinine level, and serum triglyceride level.
		Offspring cohort: 1971-	4292 (48% men)	US populations			1.15 (1.06-1.23) per 1 mg/dl	

6.2.2.2. Prospective Studies

Based on a 5-years follow-up of a population-based study in Mauritius, it has been previous reported that the relationship of UA with risk of diabetes is direct and graded [91]. Recently based on data collected over a maximum of 11 years of follow-up of the same study population, the UA-diabetes relationship was further investigated [81]. Among 1941 men and 2318 non-pregnant women aged 25-74 years and free of diabetes at baseline examination, a total of 337 (17.4%) men (252 Indians and 85 Africans) and 379 (16.4%) women (257 Indians and 122 Africans) developed diabetes at the end of the 11-years follow-up. The interesting findings were that baseline UA levels were significant higher in individuals who developed diabetes (423 µmol/l in men and 311 µmol/l in women) than in those who retained free of diabetes at the end of the follow-up (384 µmol/l in men and 292 µmol/l in women) [81]. Considering the difference between cohorts both chronologically and methodologically, Z scores of blood UA were calculated and compared between baseline and follow-up examinations. The UA levels (Z-scores) fell significantly from baseline to follow-up in men (from 0.35 to 0.02) and pre-menopausal women (from 0.04 to -0.21) who developed diabetes (p < 0.001 for both), but not in the post-menopausal women (from 0.38 to 0.45). Multivariate adjusted hazard ratios (95% CIs) for the incidence of diabetes corresponding to a one SD increase in UA at baseline in

Mauritius Indians, Mauritius Africans and both combined were 1.14 (1.01-1.30), 1.37(1.11-1.68) and 1.19 (1.07-1.34) in men, and 1.07 (0.95-1.22), 1.01 (0.84-1.22) and 1.05 (0.95-1.16) in women, respectively, after adjusting for FPG, BMI, triglycerides, fasting insulin, serum creatinine, alcohol consumption, history of hypertension, family history of diabetes, and cohort [81]. Replacing BMI, history of hypertension, triglycerides, fasting insulin, and FPG with waist circumference, systolic or diastolic BP, HDL-C or total cholesterol, HOMA-IR, and 2hPG, did not change the results substantially. Adjustment for the baseline smoking status did not alter the relationships observed between UA and diabetes either. The prediction was not significant for either pre-menopausal or post-menopausal women [81]. Aging and sex hormones may contribute to the gender difference, but the mechanism is uncertain. In addition, the difference in smoking and diet between men and women may be involved, since smoking and drinking alcohol were more popular in men than in women in Mauritius. This needs to be further investigated.

In the literature only a few studies have investigated the relationship between fasting serum UA and the development of type 2 diabetes, and most of these studies were conducted in male population alone (Table **3**) [12, 78-80, 83, 86]. Recently, a community-based prospective cohort study of Chinese participants (age range, 35-97 years) over a median follow-up of 9.0 years in Chin-Shan town, Taiwan [84] found that high baseline UA levels predicted future type 2 diabetes development in both men and women. Another prospective data from two generations of the Framingham Heart Study found that higher levels of baseline UA were associated with an increased future risk of developing type 2 diabetes in a graded manner, independent of other known risk factors [88].

More earlier in a 13-years follow-up of Rancho Bernardo Study of 566 middle-class old Caucasians, each 1 mg/dl increment in UA levels independently predicted incident type 2 diabetes among participants who had impaired fasting glucose (odds ratio 1.75, 95% CI 1.1-2.9, P = 0.02) [78]. The baseline serum UA level has also been found to independently predict the 2hPG levels during 13.5 years follow-up in a Swedish male population, with a low regression coefficient of 0.01 (p = 0.026) [82]. In the Finnish Diabetes Prevention Study [87], baseline UA levels were associated with the changes in insulin levels after adjustment for changes in UA during follow-up in a model including age, sex, randomization group, BP medication, and baseline creatinine, systolic BP, triglycerides, BMI, levels of daily energy intake, intakes of poly-, monounsaturated, and saturated fat and fiber, and leisure time physical activity and their changes during the follow-up (p = 0.001). The changes in UA levels were also associated with changes in FPG and 2hPG and 2h insulin concentrations during the follow-up after adjustment for baseline UA [87]. The researchers concluded that baseline UA and its changes predicted a 2-fold increase in the likelihood of developing type 2 diabetes in this lifestyle intervention study among high-risk middle-aged Finns with impaired glucose tolerance [87].

In addition to its interaction with insulin resistance, UA may play a direct role in the pathogenesis of diabetes by the possible inhibition of endothelial function [57], inhibition of nitric oxide bioavailability [58] and stimulation of vascular smooth muscle cell proliferation [92]. Furthermore, deficiency of endothelial-derived nitric oxide is believed to be the primary defect that links insulin resistance and cellular disturbances in glucose and lipid metabolism [93]. The underlying mechanism of UA in the process of deterioration of glucose metabolism is still not clear, and needs to be further investigated.

6.3. EFFECT OF UA LOWERING THERAPY ON INTERVENTION

The urate-lowering therapy allopurinol, a xanthine oxidase inhibitor, has been the mainstay of prophylactic treatment for gout and conditions associated with hyperuricemia for many years [43]. It is the treatment of choice for urate overproducers, tophaceous gout, nephrolithiasis or urate nephropathy, and in patients with renal insufficiency [94].

In a short-term, crossover designed clinical trial of adolescents with newly diagnosed hypertension, treatment with allopurinol resulted in reduction of BP [95]. The results represent a new potential therapeutic approach, although not a fully developed therapeutic strategy due to potential adverse effects. Recently, in a double-blinded randomized controlled trial on 40 patients with type 2 diabetes mellitus and diabetic nephropathy (proteinuria, at least 500 mg/24 h and a serum creatinine level less than 3 mg/dl), allopurinol (100 mg/dl) was compared with placebo [96]. Administration of antihypertensive and renoprotective drugs (angiotensin-converting enzyme inhibitors and angiotensin receptor blockers) continued for both groups, without changes in dosage. Low-dose allopurinol can ameliorate severity of proteinuria in diabetic patients with nephropathy after 4 months by decreasing the UA levels [96].

In another randomized, controlled trial of 74 adult men who were administered 200 g fructose daily for 2 weeks with or without allopurinol, the ingestion of fructose resulted in significant increase in fasting insulin and HOMA indices, an increase by 25% and 33% for metabolic syndrome regarding to the NCEP-ATP Ш definition and IDF definition respectively, but the plasma glucose level did not change [97]. The most encouraging findings were, a) allopurinol lowered the serum UA level ($P<0.0001$) and prevented the increase in 24-h ambulatory diastolic BP and daytime systolic BP and diastolic BP; b) allopurinol treatment lowered low-density lipoprotein cholesterol as compared to control ($P<0.02$) although did not reduce HOMA or fasting plasma triglyceride levels; c) also prevented the increase in newly diagnosed metabolic syndrome (0-2%, $P=0.009$) [97].

These preliminary findings require confirmation in larger randomized, controlled clinical trails. Febuxostat is a novel potent selective inhibitor of xanthine oxidase that appears to be well tolerated in all groups of patients, including those who are sensitive to allopurinol [98]. Allopurinol and other agents of febuxostat, or pegylated, would be potential candidate drugs for intervention, but the safety and cost-effectiveness of these medications in pre-diabetes or diabetes individuals first need to be studied. Insulin resistance is well known perpetuating factor once obesity and intracellular lipid accumulation manifest [99]. Thus, lowering UA might be expected to provide some benefits once insulin resistance and diabetes develop but may not be able to fully reverse these conditions; if UA can be identified as true remediable risk factors, then a new chapter in the prevention of obesity, diabetes and metabolic syndrome will unfold [100].

6.4. CONCLUSIONS

The UA levels increase in pre-diabetes and undiagnosed diabetes but gradually decline in known diabetes with increasing degree of hyperglycemia. Individuals with higher levels of baseline UA are at a risk of development type 2 diabetes independent of other known risk factors. Although current evidence from both cross-sectional and prospective data provide support for the independent association between UA levels and the risk of developing diabetes, the direction of causality between hyperuricemia and deterioration of glucose metabolism remains to be clarified by future studies. In particular, to investigate the pathophysiological mechanism underlying the relationship between glucose, insulin resistance, UA and cardio-metabolic risk factors would be valuable to clarify whether UA is an early marker of hyperglycemia, a risk factor for diabetes or an underlying cause of diabetes. Well designed randomized controlled trial on intervention may help to understand the formation of these metabolic disorders.

REFERENCES

[1]   Wu XW, Muzny DM, Lee CC, *et al.* Two independent mutational events in the loss of urate oxidase during hominoid evolution. J Mol Evol 1992; 34: 78-84.

[2]   Johnson RJ, Rideout BA. Uric acid and diet--insights into the epidemic of cardiovascular disease. N Engl J Med 2004; 350: 1071-3.

[3]   Johnson RJ, Titte S, Cade JR, *et al.* Uric acid, evolution and primitive cultures. Semin Nephrol 2005; 25: 3-8.

[4]   Johnson RJ, Gaucher EA, Sautin YY, *et al.* The planetary biology of ascorbate and uric acid and their relationship with the epidemic of obesity and cardiovascular disease. Med Hypotheses 2008; 71: 22-31.

[5]   Darmawan J, Valkenburg HA, Muirden KD, *et al.* The epidemiology of gout and hyperuricemia in a rural population of Java. J Rheumatol 1992; 19: 1595-9.

[6]   Conen D, Wietlisbach V, Bovet P, *et al.* Prevalence of hyperuricemia and relation of serum uric acid with cardiovascular risk factors in a developing country. BMC Public Health 2004; 4: 9.

[7]   Chang HY, Pan WH, Yeh WT, *et al.* Hyperuricemia and gout in Taiwan: results from the Nutritional and Health Survey in Taiwan (1993-96). J Rheumatol 2001; 28: 1640-6.

[8]   Kylin E. Studies of the hypertension-hyperglycemia hyperuricemia syndrome (Studien ueber das hypertonie-hypergly-kämie-hyperurikämiesyndrom). Zentral-blatt fuer Innere Medizin 1923; 44: 105-27.

[9]   Facchini F, Chen YD, Hollenbeck CB, *et al*. Relationship between resistance to insulin-mediated glucose uptake, urinary uric acid clearance, and plasma uric acid concentration. JAMA 1991; 266: 3008-11.

[10]   Modan M, Halkin H, Karasik A, *et al*. Elevated serum uric acid-a facet of hyperinsulinemia. Diabetologia 1987; 30: 713-8.

[11]   Tuomilehto J, Zimmet P, Wolf E, *et al*. Plasma uric acid level and its association with diabetes mellitus and some biological parameters in a biracial population of Fiji. Am J Epidemiol 1988; 127: 321-36.

[12]   Nakanishi N, Okamoto M, Yoshida H, *et al*. Serum uric acid and risk for development of hypertension and impaired fasting glucose or Type II diabetes in Japanese male office workers. Eur J Epidemiol 2003; 18: 523-30.

[13]   Taniguchi Y, Hayashi T, Tsumura K, *et al*. Serum uric acid and the risk for hypertension and Type 2 diabetes in Japanese men: The Osaka Health Survey. J Hypertens 2001; 19: 1209-15.

[14]   Johnson RJ, Kivlighn SD, Kim YG, *et al*. Reappraisal of the pathogenesis and consequences of hyperuricemia in hypertension, cardiovascular disease and renal disease. Am J Kidney Dis 1999; 33: 225-34.

[15]   Nicholls A, Snaith M, Scott J. Effect of estrogen therapy on plasma and urinary levels of uric acid. Br Med J 1973; 1: 449-51.

[16]   Glynn RJ, Campion EW, Silbert JE. Trends in serum uric acid levels 1961-1980. Arthritis Rheum 1983; 26: 87-93.

[17]   Sturge RA, Scott JT, Kennedy AC, *et al*. Serum uric acid in England and Scotland. Ann Rheum Dis 1977; 36: 420-7.

[18]   Gresser U, Gathof B, Zollner N. Uric acid levels in southern Germany in 1989. A comparison with studies from 1962, 1971, and 1984. Klin Wochenschr 1990; 68: 1222-8.

[19]   Klemp P, Stansfield SA, Castle B, *et al*. Gout is on the increase in New Zealand. Ann Rheum Dis 1997; 56: 22-6.

[20]   Fang Q, Chen HZ, Yu ZFe. Survey of uric acid among healthy Chinese and its relation to blood lipids (Chinese). Zhonghua Nei Ke Za Zhi 1983; 22: 434-8.

[21]   Li Y, Stamler J, Xiao Z, *et al*. Serum uric acid and its correlate in Chinese adult population, urban and rural, of Beijing. The PRC-USA Collaborative Study in Cardiovascular and Cardiopulmonary Epidemiology. Int J Epidemiol 1997; 26: 288-96.

[22]   Jiang FB, Zhang YS, Xu XF, *et al*. Epidemiological survey of gout and hyperuricemia in littoral of shandong province (Chinese). Zhong Guo Gong Gong Wei Sheng 1999; 15: 205-6.

[23]   Chen S, Du H, Wang Y, *et al*. The epidemiology study of hyperuricemia and gout in a community population of Huangpu District in Shanghai. Chin Med J (Engl) 1998; 111: 228-30.

[24]   Nan H, Qiao Q, Dong Y, *et al*. The prevalence of hyperuricemia in a population of the coastal city of Qingdao, China. J Rheumatol 2006; 33: 1346-50.

[25]   Villegas R, Xiang YB, Cai Q, *et al*. Prevalence and determinants of hyperuricemia in middle-aged, urban Chinese men. Metab Syndr Relat Disord 2010; 8: 263-70.

[26]   Miao Z, Li C, Chen Y, *et al*. Dietary and lifestyle changes associated with high prevalence of hyperuricemia and gout in the Shandong coastal cities of Eastern China. J Rheumatol 2008; 35: 1859-64.

[27]   Chen LY, Zhu WH, Chen ZW, *et al*. Relationship between hyperuricemia and metabolic syndrome. J Zhejiang Univ Sci B 2007; 8: 593-8.

[28]   Fang WG, Zeng XJ, Li MT, *et al*. (Decision-making about gout by physicians of China and influencing factors thereof). Zhonghua yi xue za zhi 2006; 86: 1901-5.

[29]   Lin KC, Lin HY, Chou P. Community based epidemiological study on hyperuricemia and gout in Kin-Hu, Kinmen. J Rheumatol 2000; 27: 1045-50.

[30]   Chou CT, Lai JS. The epidemiology of hyperuricemia and gout in Taiwan aborigines. Br J Rheumatol 1998; 37: 258-62.

[31]   Ko YC, Wang TN, Tsai LY, *et al*. High prevalence of hyperuricemia in adolescent Taiwan aborigines. J Rheumatol 2002; 29: 837-42.

[32]   Lee MS, Lin SC, Chang HY, *et al*. High prevalence of hyperuricemia in elderly Taiwanese. Asia Pac J Clin Nutr 2005; 14: 285-92.

[33]   Lohsoonthorn V, Dhanamun B, Williams MA. Prevalence of hyperuricemia and its relationship with metabolic syndrome in thai adults receiving annual health exams. Arch Med Res 2006; 37: 883-9.

[34]   Brauer GW, Prior IA. A prospective study of gout in New Zealand Maoris. Ann Rheum Dis 1978; 37: 466-72.

[35]   Zimmet PZ, Whitehouse S, Jackson L, *et al*. High prevalence of hyperuricemia and gout in an urbanised Micronesian population. Br Med J 1978; 1: 1237-9.

[36]   Al-Arfaj AS. Hyperuricemia in Saudi Arabia. Rheumatol Int. 2001; 20: 61-4.

[37]   Tavares EF, Vieira-Filho JP, Andriolo A, *et al.* Metabolic profile and cardiovascular risk patterns of an Indian tribe living in the Amazon Region of Brazil. Hum Biol 2003; 75: 31-46.

[38]   Nagahama K, Inoue T, Iseki K, *et al.* Hyperuricemia as a predictor of hypertension in a screened cohort in Okinawa, Japan. Hypertens Res 2004; 27: 835-41.

[39]   Schmidt MI, Watson RL, Duncan BB, *et al.* Clustering of dyslipidemia, hyperuricemia, diabetes, and hypertension and its association with fasting insulin and central and overall obesity in a general population. Atherosclerosis Risk in Communities Study Investigators. Metabolism 1996; 45: 699-706.

[40]   Rose BS. Gout in the Maoris. Semin Arthritis Rheum 1975; 5: 121-45.

[41]   Healey LA, Caner JE, Basset DR, *et al.* Serum uric acid and obesity in Hawaiians. JAMA 1966; 196: 364-5.

[42]   Burch TA, O'Brien WM, Need R, *et al.* Hyperuricemia and gout in the Mariana Islands. Ann Rheum Dis 1966; 25: 114-6.

[43]   Wortmann RL. Gout and hyperuricemia. Curr Opin Rheumatol 2002; 14: 281-6.

[44]   Ford DK, Demos AM. Serum uric acid levels of healthy caucasian, chinese and haida indian males in british columbia. Can Med Assoc J 1964; 90: 1295-7.

[45]   Beighton P, Solomon L, Soskolne CL, *et al.* Serum uric acid concentrations in an urbanized South African Negro population. Ann Rheum Dis 1974; 33: 442-5.

[46]   Chang SJ, Ko YC, Wang TN, *et al.* High prevalence of gout and related risk factors in Taiwan's Aborigines. J Rheumatol 1997; 24: 1364-9.

[47]   Emmerson BT, Douglas W, Doherty RL, *et al.* Serum urate concentrations in the Australian aboriginal. Ann Rheum Dis 1969; 28: 150-6.

[48]   Chungtei C. Hyperuricemia and gout among Taiwan aborigines and Taiwanese prevalence and risk factors. Chin Med J (Engl) 2003; 116: 965-7.

[49]   Reaven GM, Bernstein R, Davis B, *et al.* Nonketotic diabetes mellitus: insulin deficiency or insulin resistance? Am J Med 1976; 60: 80-8.

[50]   Tuomilehto J, Lindstrom J, Eriksson JG, *et al.* Prevention of type 2 diabetes mellitus by changes in lifestyle among subjects with impaired glucose tolerance. N Engl J Med 2001; 344: 1343-50.

[51]   Whiting DR, Guariguata L, Weil C, Shaw J. IDF diabetes atlas: global estimates of the prevalence of diabetes for 2011 and 2030. Diabetes Res Clin Pract 2011; 94: 311-21.

[52]   Bonora E, Kiechl S, Willeit J, *et al.* Prevalence of insulin resistance in metabolic disorders: the Bruneck Study. Diabetes 1998; 47: 1643-9.

[53]   Pacini G, Mari A. Methods for clinical assessment of insulin sensitivity and beta-cell function. Best Pract Res Clin Endocrinol Metab 2003; 17: 305-22.

[54]   Vuorinen-Markkola H, Yki-Jarvinen H. Hyperuricemia and insulin resistance. J Clin Endocrinol Metab 1994; 78: 25-9.

[55]   Fox IH. Metabolic basis for disorders of purine nucleotide degradation. Metabolism 1981; 30: 616-34.

[56]   Fox IH, John D, DeBruyne S, *et al.* Hyperuricemia and hypertriglyceridemia: metabolic basis for the association. Metabolism 1985; 34: 741-6.

[57]   Nakagawa T, Hu H, Zharikov S, *et al.* A causal role for uric acid in fructose-induced metabolic syndrome. Am J Physiol Renal Physiol 2006; 290: 625-31.

[58]   Baldus S, Koster R, Chumley P, *et al.* Oxypurinol improves coronary and peripheral endothelial function in patients with coronary artery disease. Free Radic Biol Med 2005; 39: 1184-90.

[59]   Gokcel A, Gumurdulu Y, Karakose H, *et al.* Evaluation of the safety and efficacy of sibutramine, orlistat and metformin in the treatment of obesity. Diabetes Obes Metab 2002; 4: 49-55.

[60]   Tsunoda S, Kamide K, Minami J, *et al.* Decreases in serum uric acid by amelioration of insulin resistance in overweight hypertensive patients: effect of a low-energy diet and an insulin-sensitizing agent. Am J Hypertens 2002; 15: 697-701.

[61]   Tambascia MA, Geloneze B, Repetto EM, *et al.* Sibutramine enhances insulin sensitivity ameliorating metabolic parameters in a double-blind, randomized, placebo-controlled trial. Diabetes Obes Metab 2003; 5: 338-44.

[62]   Filippatos TD, Kiortsis DN, Liberopoulos EN, *et al.* A review of the metabolic effects of sibutramine. Curr Med Res Opin 2005; 21: 457-68.

[63]   Kiortsis DN, Filippatos TD, Elisaf MS. The effects of orlistat on metabolic parameters and other cardiovascular risk factors. Diabetes Metab 2005; 31: 15-22.

[64]   Nakamura R, Emmanouel DS, Katz AI. Insulin binding sites in various segments of the rabbit nephron. J Clin Invest 1983; 72: 388-92.

[65] Muscelli E, Natali A, Bianchi S, *et al.* Effect of insulin on renal sodium and uric acid handling in essential hypertension. Am J Hypertens 1996; 9: 746-52.

[66] Quinones Galvan A, Natali A, Baldi S, *et al.* Effect of insulin on uric acid excretion in humans. Am J Physiol 1995; 268: E1-5.

[67] Cappuccio FP, Strazzullo P, Farinaro E, *et al.* Uric acid metabolism and tubular sodium handling. Results from a population-based study. JAMA 1993; 270: 354-9.

[68] Mandel LJ. Primary active sodium transport, oxygen consumption, and ATP: coupling and regulation. Kidney Int 1986; 29: 3-9.

[69] Herman JB, Medalie JH, Goldbourt U. Diabetes, prediabetes and uricemia. Diabetologia 1976; 12: 47-52.

[70] Yano K, Hoads G, Kagan A. Epidemiology of serum urate levels among 8000 Japanese-American men in Hawaii. J Chronic Dis 1977; 30: 171-84.

[71] Whitehead TP, Jungner I, Robinson D, *et al.* Serum urate, serum glucose and diabetes. Ann Clin Biochem 1992; 29: 159-61.

[72] Cook DG, Shaper AG, Thelle DS, *et al.* Serum uric acid, serum glucose and diabetes: relationships in a population study. Postgrad Med J 1986; 62: 1001-6.

[73] Chou P, Lin KC, Lin HY, *et al.* Gender differences in the relationships of serum uric acid with fasting serum insulin and plasma glucose in patients without diabetes. J Rheumatol 2001; 28: 571-6.

[74] Nan H, Dong Y, Gao W, *et al.* Diabetes associated with a low serum uric acid level in a general Chinese population. Diabetes Res Clin Pract 2007; 76: 68-74.

[75] Nan H, Pang Z, Wang S, *et al.* Serum uric acid, plasma glucose and diabetes. Diab Vasc Dis Res 2010; 7: 40-6.

[76] Hodge AM, Boyko EJ, de Courten M, *et al.* Leptin and other components of the Metabolic Syndrome in Mauritius--a factor analysis. Int J Obes Relat Metab Disord 2001; 25: 126-31.

[77] Medalie JH, Papier CM, Goldbourt U, *et al.* Major factors in the development of diabetes mellitus in 10, 000 men. Arch Intern Med 1975; 135: 811-7.

[78] Kramer CK, von Muhlen D, Jassal SK, *et al.* Serum uric acid levels improve prediction of incident type 2 diabetes in individuals with impaired fasting glucose: the Rancho Bernardo Study. Diabetes Care 2009; 32: 1272-3.

[79] Meisinger C, Thorand B, Schneider A, *et al.* Sex differences in risk factors for incident type 2 diabetes mellitus: the MONICA Augsburg cohort study. Arch Intern Med 2002; 162: 82-9.

[80] Lin KC, Tsai ST, Lin HY, *et al.* Different progressions of hyperglycemia and diabetes among hyperuricemic men and women in the kinmen study. J Rheumatol 2004; 31: 1159-65.

[81] Nan H, Qiao Q, Soderberg S, *et al.* Serum uric acid and incident diabetes in Mauritian Indian and Creole populations. Diabetes Res Clin Pract 2008; 80: 321-7.

[82] Ohlson LO, Larsson B, Bjorntorp P, *et al.* Risk factors for type 2 (non-insulin-dependent) diabetes mellitus. Thirteen and one-half years of follow-up of the participants in a study of Swedish men born in 1913. Diabetologia 1988; 31: 798-805.

[83] Perry IJ, Wannamethee SG, Walker MK, *et al.* Prospective study of risk factors for development of non-insulin dependent diabetes in middle aged British men. BMJ 1995; 310: 560-4.

[84] Chien KL, Chen MF, Hsu HC, *et al.* Plasma uric acid and the risk of type 2 diabetes in a Chinese community. Clin Chem 2008; 54: 310-6.

[85] Choi HK, De Vera MA, Krishnan E. Gout and the risk of type 2 diabetes among men with a high cardiovascular risk profile. Rheumatology (Oxford) 2008; 47: 1567-70.

[86] Dehghan A, van Hoek M, Sijbrands EJ, *et al.* High serum uric acid as a novel risk factor for type 2 diabetes. Diabetes Care 2008; 31: 361-2.

[87] Niskanen L, Laaksonen DE, Lindstrom J, *et al.* Serum uric acid as a harbinger of metabolic outcome in subjects with impaired glucose tolerance: the Finnish Diabetes Prevention Study. Diabetes Care 2006; 29: 709-11.

[88] Bhole V, Choi JWJ, Woo Kim S, *et al.* Serum Uric Acid Levels and the Risk of Type 2 Diabetes: A Prospective Study. Am J Med 2010; 123: 957-61.

[89] Wen CP, David Cheng TY, Chan HT, *et al.* Is high serum uric acid a risk marker or a target for treatment? Examination of its independent effect in a large cohort with low cardiovascular risk. Am J Kidney Dis 2010; 56: 273-88.

[90] Choi HK, Ford ES. Hemoglobin HbA1c, fasting glucose, serum C-peptide and insulin resistance in relation to serum uric acid levels-the Third National Health and Nutrition Examination Survey. Rheumatology (Oxford) 2008; 47: 713-7.

[91]   Boyko EJ, de Courten M, Zimmet PZ, *et al.* Features of the metabolic syndrome predict higher risk of diabetes and impaired glucose tolerance: a prospective study in Mauritius. Diabetes Care 2000; 23: 1242-8.

[92]   Price KL, Sautin YY, Long DA, *et al.* Human vascular smooth muscle cells express a urate transporter. J Am Soc Nephrol 2006; 17: 1791-5.

[93]   Cersosimo E, DeFronzo RA. Insulin resistance and endothelial dysfunction: the road map to cardiovascular diseases. Diabetes Metab Res Rev 2006; 22: 423-36.

[94]   Teng GG, Nair R, Saag KG. Pathophysiology, clinical presentation and treatment of gout. Drugs 2006; 66: 1547-63.

[95]   Feig DI, Soletsky B, Johnson RJ. Effect of allopurinol on blood pressure of adolescents with newly diagnosed essential hypertension: a randomized trial. JAMA 2008; 300: 924-32.

[96]   Momeni A, Shahidi S, Seirafian S, *et al.* Effect of allopurinol in decreasing proteinuria in type 2 diabetic patients. Iran J Kidney Dis 2010; 4: 128-32.

[97]   Perez-Pozo SE, Schold J, Nakagawa T, *et al.* Excessive fructose intake induces the features of metabolic syndrome in healthy adult men: role of uric acid in the hypertensive response. Int J Obes (Lond) 2010; 34: 454-61.

[98]   Bruce SP. Febuxostat: a selective xanthine oxidase inhibitor for the treatment of hyperuricemia and gout. Ann Pharmacother 2006; 40: 2187-94.

[99]   Zammit VA, Waterman IJ, Topping D, *et al.* Insulin stimulation of hepatic triacylglycerol secretion and the etiology of insulin resistance. J Nutr 2001; 131: 2074-7.

[100] Johnson RJ, Perez-Pozo SE, Sautin YY, *et al.* Hypothesis: could excessive fructose intake and uric acid cause type 2 diabetes? Endocr Rev 2009; 30: 96-116.

CHAPTER 7

Diabetes and Cancer Epidemiology

Xianghai Zhou*

Department of Endocrinology and Metabolism, Peking University People's Hospital, Beijing, China and Department of Public Health, Hjelt Institute, University of Helsinki, Helsinki, Finland

Abstract: It has been proposed that diabetes was associated with an increased risk of cancer mortality and morbidity. Complex mechanisms are involved in the association between diabetes and cancer. Metformin has been suggested to reduce the risk of cancer incidence (Hazard ratio 0.63 (95% CI 0.53-0.75)) or cancer mortality (Hazard ratio 0.43 (95% CI 0.23-0.80)), but insulin or sulfonylurea is suspected to increase the risk of cancer incidence (Hazard ratio 1.36 (95% CI 1.19-1.54)) or cancer mortality (Hazard ratio 1.30 (95% CI 1.10-1.60)). Evidences on these issues are reviewed and summarized in this chapter.

Keywords: Diabetes, anti-diabetic drugs, cancer motality and morbidity.

It is well known that diabetes is associated with increased cardiovascular mortality and morbidity, but whether diabetes increases cancer risk is less known. Studies on the association of diabetes with cancer have produced inconsistent results, and the issue needs to be further investigated by taking into account the differences in study design, age, obesity, lifestyle and glucose lowering drugs.

7.1. DIABETES AND CANCER MORTALITY AND MORBIDITY

Diabetes was associated with increased risk of certain types of cancers. Patients with clinically diagnosed diabetes has been reported to have increased mortality from cancer of colon and pancreas in both men and women, and from cancer of liver and bladder in men and breast in women in an American cohort of voluntary participants aged 30 years or older [1]. Fasting serum glucose level of ≥7.8 mmol/l (140 mg/dl) was associated with higher risk of death from cancer of the esophagus, liver, pancreas and colon/rectum in men and of the liver and cervix in women as compared with fasting serum glucose level of <5.0 mmol/l (90 mg/dl) in a Korean cohort who received health insurance and had biennial medical evaluations [2]. Fasting serum glucose level of ≥7.8 mmol/l (140 mg/dl) was also associated with higher risk of incident cancer of the liver and pancreas in men and of the pancreas in women [2]. Data analysis based on the Diabetes Epidemiology: Collaborative analysis of Diagnostic criteria in Europe (DECODE) Study showed that risk of death from cancer of all-types increased with deterioration in glucose tolerance status and with increments in linear form of either fasting plasma glucose or 2-h plasma glucose levels as well. Compared with individuals with normal glucose tolerance, the hazard ratio was higher for death from cancers in stomach, colon-rectum and liver in men with prediabetes and diabetes, and for deaths from cancers in liver and pancreas in women with previously diagnosed diabetes (Table **1**) [3]. Several meta-analyses have been made based on either cross-sectional or cohort studies to estimate the overall risk of site-specific cancers in relation to diabetes diagnosed by self-report, medical record or OGTT (Table **2**). The results of these studies showed that diabetes was associated with increased risk of cancer of pancreas [4], liver [5], colon-rectum [6], bladder [7], breast [8], endometrium [9], non-Hodgkin's lymphoma [10] but decreased risk of cancer of prostate [11]. The association was stronger for cancers of liver, pancreas and endometrium than for others.

* Address correspondence to Xianghai Zhou: Department of Endocrinology and Metabolism, Peking University People's Hospital, 11 Xizhimen South Street, 100044, Beijing, China and Department of Public Health, Hjelt Institute, University of Helsinki, PL41, Mannerheimintie 172, 00014, Helsinki, Finland. E-mail: xianghaizhou@yahoo.com.cn

Table 1: Multivariable-adjusted hazard ratio of site-specific cancer mortality in relation to glucose tolerance status in men and women in the DECODE study [1]

Types of Cancer	Normal Glucose	Prediabetes	Undiagnosed Diabetes	Known Diabetes	All Diabetes
Men					
Stomach or colon-rectum	1.0	1.46 (1.09, 1.94)	1.69 (1.03, 2.76)	2.07 (1.21, 3.51)	1.84 (1.25, 2.71)
Liver	1.0	2.32 (1.25, 4.33)	3.61 (1.42, 9.19)	7.50 (3.21, 17.54)	5.16 (2.56, 10.41)
Pancreas	1.0	0.88 (0.56, 1.41)	1.52 (0.74, 3.12)	1.92 (0.85, 4.33)	1.67 (0.94, 2.97)
Women					
Stomach or colon-rectum	1.0	1.52 (1.00, 2.31)	0.49 (0.15, 1.59)	0.46 (0.11, 1.93)	0.48 (0.19, 1.21)
Liver	1.0	1.58 (0.49, 5.09)	3.67 (0.89, 15.12)	10.87 (3.16, 37.39)	6.37 (2.18, 18.62)
Pancreas	1.0	1.08 (0.63, 1.85)	1.71 (0.74, 3.94)	3.13 (1.21, 8.08)	2.13 (1.09, 4.16)

Table 2: Published review articles that have made overall estimates of Odds Ratio (OR) or Relative Risk (RR) of site-specific cancers in diabetic patients as compared with non-diabetic individuals based on meta-analyses.

Study	Cancer Site	Outcome Measures	Study Design	Number of Studies Included	OR or RR (95% CI)
Huxley R et al., 2005 [4]	Pancreas	Prevalence	case-control	17	1.94 (1.53, 2.46)
		Incidence& mortality	cohort	19	1.73 (1.59, 1.88)
			pooled analysis	36	1.82 (1.66, 1.99)
El-Serag HB et al., 2006 [5]	Liver	Prevalence	case-control	13	2.5 (1.5, 3.1)
		Incidence& mortality	cohort	12	2.5 (1.9, 3.2)
			pooled analysis	25	2.5 (1.8, 2.9)
Larsson SC et al., 2005 [6]	Colon-rectum	Prevalence	case-control	6	1.36 (1.23, 1.50)
		Incidence	cohort	9	1.29 (1.16, 1.43)
		Mortality	cohort	6	1.26 (1.05, 1.50)
			pooled analysis	15	1.30 (1.20, 1.40)
Larsson SC et al., 2006 [7]	Bladder	Prevalence	case-control	7	1.37 (1.04, 1.80)
		Incidence& mortality	cohort	3	1.43 (1.18, 1.74)
		Incidence& mortality	cohort with diabetes	6	1.01 (0.90, 1.12)
			Pooled analysis	16	1.24 (1.08, 1.42)
Larsson SC et al., 2007 [8]	Breast	Prevalence	case-control	5	1.18 (1.05, 1.32)
		Incidence	cohort	15	1.20 (1.11, 1.30)
		Mortality	cohort	5	1.24 (0.95, 1.62)
			pooled analysis	20	1.20 (1.12, 1.28)
Friberg E et al., 2007 [9]	Endometrium	Prevalence	case-control	13	2.22 (1.80, 2.74)
		Incidence	cohort	3	1.62 (1.21, 2.16)
			pooled analysis	16	2.10 (1.75, 2.53)
Mitri J et al., 2008 [10]	Non-Hodgkin's lymphoma	Prevalence	case-control	11	1.12 (0.95, 1.31)
		Incidence	cohort	5	1.41 (1.07, 1.88)
			pooled analysis	16	1.19 (1.04, 1.35)
Kasper JS et al., 2006 [11]	Prostate	Prevalence	case-control	7	0.89 (0.72, 1.11)
		Incidence& mortality	cohort	12	0.81 (0.71, 0.92)
			pooled analysis	19	0.84 (0.76, 0.93)

Many factors rather than diabetes can contribute to the death of patients with cancer such as old age, late diagnosis, cancer therapies, tumor differentiation, concurrence of certain diseases and psychological factors. To avoid the confounding effect of these factors, we conducted a meta-analysis separately for cancer mortality, and incident non-fatal cancers that were first diagnosed after the baseline examination for diabetes. Cohort studies that have estimated relative risk of all-cancer incidence [2, 12-14] or all-cancer mortality [2, 3, 15-18] that were due to diabetes, were reviewed and summarized in Figs. **1-2**. Compared with non-diabetes, diabetes was associated with increased risk of both cancer incidence and cancer mortality, with an overall relative risk (95% CI) 1.21 (1.11, 1.32) for cancer incidence (Fig. **1**) and 1.40 (1.24, 1.57) for cancer mortality (Fig. **2**).

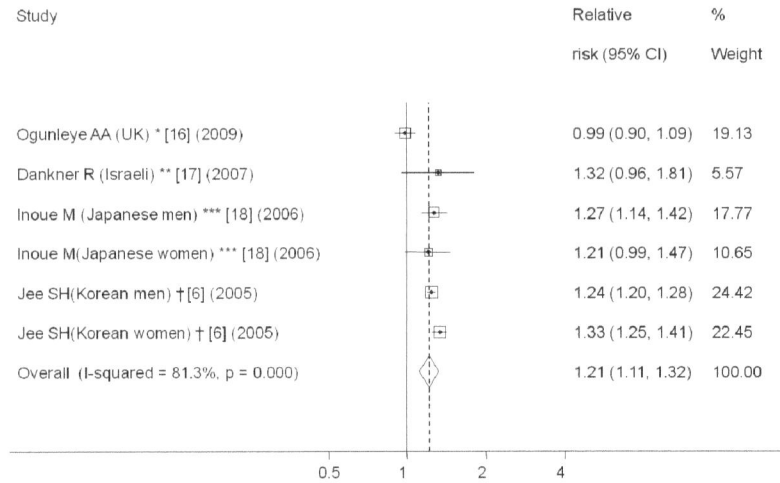

Figure 1: Multivariate adjusted relative risk (square, proportional to the percentage of weight of each study from random effects analysis) and 95% confidence interval (bars) for each study and for all studies combined for incidence of cancer of all-types in relation to diabetes status; * registered diabetes; ** OGTT diagnosed diabetes; *** self-reported diabetes; † fasting glucose ≥7.0 mmol/l or medication.

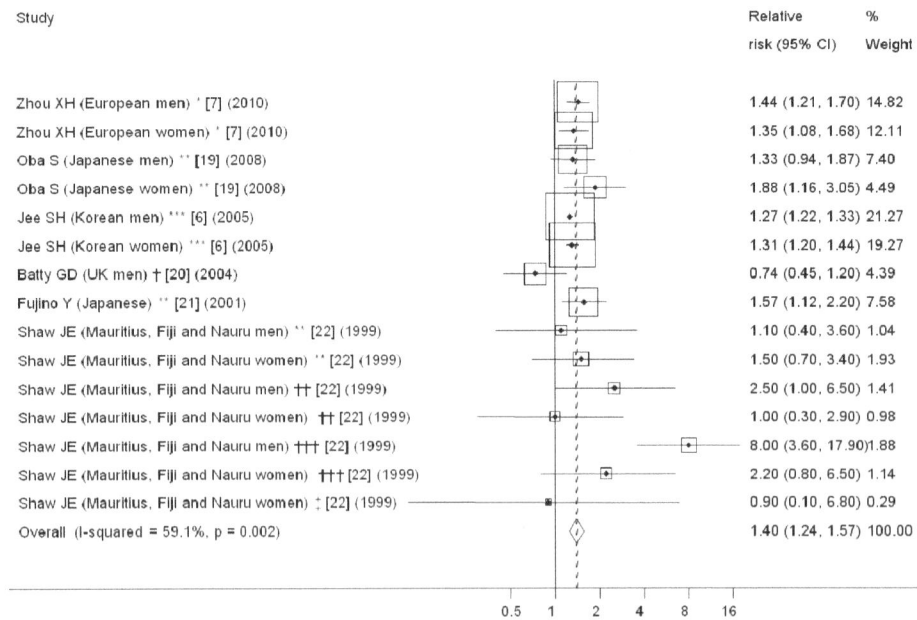

Figure 2: Multivariate adjusted relative risk (square, proportional to the percentage of weight of each study from random effects analysis) and 95% confidence interval (bars) for each study and for all studies combined for mortality from cancer of all-types in relation to diabetes status; * newly diagnosed and known diabetes; ** self-reported diabetes;

*** fasting glucose ≥7.0 mmol/l or medication; † 2h glucose ≥11.1 mmol/l or self-reported; †† fasting glucose ≥7.0mmol/l and 2h glucose ≥11.1mmol/l; ††† fasting glucose < 7.0mmol/l and 2h glucose ≥ 11.1mmol/l; ‡ fasting plasma glucose ≥ 7.0 mmol/l and 2h plasma glucose < 11.1mmol/l.

7.2. THE MECHANISM OF THE ASSOCIATION BETWEEN CANCER AND DIABETES

Several mechanisms may be involved in the relationship between glucose intolerance and the risk of cancer. Oxidative stress and accumulated advanced glycation end products induced by hyperglycemia at the cellular level may play important roles in cancer development and progression [19]. Hyperinsulinemia and increased level of bioavailable Insulin-Like Growth Factor I (IGF-I) related to insulin resistance [20] may promote cancer cell proliferation [21] and may also be related to worse cancer outcome [21]. Treatment choice for cancer patients who have diabetes may be limited by the presence of hyperglycemia and co-existing diabetes complications [22], which may also lead to the worse cancer survival in patients with diabetes.

7.3. THE ASSOCIATION BETWEEN GLUCOSE-LOWERING THERAPY AND THE RISK OF CANCER

7.3.1. Metformin and the Risk of Cancer

Metformin is a widely used glucose-lowering agent. It is speculated that metformin may reduce the risk of cancer because metformin targets at the enzyme AMP activated protein kinase (AMPK). A protein kinase named LKB1 is a tumor suppressor and is known to be an upstream regulator of AMPK [23]. A case control study in Scotland showed that metformin was associated with a reduced risk of cancer in patients with type 2 diabetes, with odds ratios (95% confidence interval) of 0.83 (0.65, 1.06), 0.86 (0.68, 1.10) and 0.57 (0.43, 0.75), respectively, corresponding to metformin of 14-672 gram, 673-964 gram and more than 964 gram dispensed between 1993-2001. Another cohort study in Scotland showed that metformin use was associated with a reduced risk of cancer by 37% in type 2 diabetes after adjusting for sex, age, BMI, HbA1c, deprivation, smoking, and other drug use [24]. In a prospective cohort study in the Netherlands, metformin use was reported to be associated with a reduced risk of cancer mortality [25]. A dose response analysis was also shown that the risk of cancer mortality decreased by 42% for every 1g per day increase in the metformin dose in that study [25]. In a randomized, double-blind, controled clinical trial (A Diabetes Outcome Progression Trial, ADOPT), 4351 patients with type 2 diabetes were randomized to glucose lowering monotherapy of metformin, rosiglitazone and glibenclamide. Cancer was reported as adverse events in 50 patients on metformin and in 55 on glibenclamide. The reduction in risk of cancer related to the metformin use was not significant as compared with glibenclamide (Hazard ratio (95% CI) was 0.78 (0.53, 1.14)) [26].

7.3.2. Sulfonylurea, Insulin and Insulin Analogues and the Risk of Cancer

As mentioned above, hyperinsulinemia might promote carcinogenesis [21]. Sulfonylurea is a kind of glucose-lowering agent that stimulates endogenous insulin secretion. It was hypothesized that patient with type 2 diabetes exposed to sulfonylurea and exogenous insulin may have an increased risk of cancer mortality as compared with those exposed to metformin [27]. A population-based cohort study in Canada reported that as compared with metformin monotherapy users, cancer mortality risk increased by 30% for sulfonylurea monotherapy users and 90% for insulin user after adjusting for age, sex and chronic disease score [27]. In a subsequent analysis of the data, cancer mortality risk was increased with increasing insulin dispensations per year [28]. In this Canadian study, potential confounders such as smoking status and glucose levels were, however, not taken into account [27, 28]. In another cohort study conducted in the Netherlands, 1353 patients with type 2 diabetes were followed up for 9.6 years. Neither sulfonylurea use nor insulin use was significantly associated with cancer mortality after adjusting for confounding factors such as smoking status and hemoglobin HbA1c levels [25]. In a retrospective cohort study in UK, sulfonylurea monotherapy and insulin-based regimens was associated with an increased risk of incident solid tumors as compared with metformin monotherapy [29]. It is unclear whether this increased risk of cancer was due to the effect of insulin or sulfonylurea use or the protective effect of metformin use.

A study *in vitro* showed that insulin analogues had different IGF-1 receptor affinity and mitogenic potency from that of human insulin [30]. Evidences from epidemiological studies didn't, however, find that insulin analogues had greater risk of incident cancer compared with human insulin [29, 31-34]. But, a nested case-control study in Italy recently showed that at high doses (≥ 0.3 IU/kg/day during the follow-up), the insulin analogue glargine was associated with increased cancer incidence [35]. The study suggested that dosage of insulin and its analogues should be considered when explore the possible association between insulin and its analogues with cancer.

7.3.3. Thiazolidinediones (TZD) and the Risk of Cancer

Studies on the TZD use and risk of cancer are still limited. TZD use was not associated with increased risk of colon/rectal cancer [36, 37], prostate cancer [36, 37] and breast cancer [37] in a retrospective cohort study [36] and in a nested case-control study [37], but associated with a reduced risk of lung cancer in a cohort study [36]. Clinical trials have shown that the use of pioglitazone, one kind of TZD, was associated with a reduced risk of breast cancer as compared with placebo [38], but that of rosiglitazone, another kind of TZD, did not alter the cancer risk, as compared with metformin use [39].

In summary, diabetes was associated with an increased risk of certain types of cancers such as cancers in liver, pancreas, colon/rectum and breast. Diabetes was associated with a reduced risk of prostate cancer. Metformin use was associated with a reduced risk of cancer as compared with sulfonylurea use and insulin use. It is recently recommended to screen for cancers among patients with diabetes but cancer risk should not be considered as a major factor in choosing therapies for diabetic patients without high risk of cancer [40].

REFERENCES

[1]   Coughlin SS, Calle EE, Teras LR, Petrelli J, Thun MJ. Diabetes mellitus as a predictor of cancer mortality in a large cohort of US adults. Am J Epidemiol 2004; 159: 1160-1167.

[2]   Jee SH, Ohrr H, Sull JW, Yun JE, Ji M, Samet JM. Fasting serum glucose level and cancer risk in Korean men and women. JAMA 2005; 293: 194-202.

[3]   Zhou XH, Qiao Q, Zethelius B, *et al.* Diabetes, prediabetes and cancer mortality. Diabetologia 2010; 53: 1867-1876.

[4]   Huxley R, Ansary-Moghaddam A, Berrington de Gonzalez A, Barzi F, Woodward M .Type-II diabetes and pancreatic cancer: a meta-analysis of 36 studies. Br J Cancer 2005; 92: 2076-2083.

[5]   El-Serag HB, Hampel H, Javadi F. The association between diabetes and hepatocellular carcinoma: a systematic review of epidemiologic evidence. Clin Gastroenterol Hepatol 2006; 4: 369-380.

[6]   Larsson SC, Orsini N, Wolk A. Diabetes mellitus and risk of colorectal cancer: a meta-analysis. J Natl Cancer Inst 2005;97: 1679-1687.

[7]   Larsson SC, Orsini N, Brismar K, Wolk A. Diabetes mellitus and risk of bladder cancer: a meta-analysis. Diabetologia 2006; 49: 2819-2823.

[8]   Larsson SC, Mantzoros CS, Wolk A. Diabetes mellitus and risk of breast cancer: a meta-analysis. Int J Cancer 2007;121: 856-862.

[9]   Friberg E, Orsini N, Mantzoros CS, Wolk A. Diabetes mellitus and risk of endometrial cancer: a meta-analysis. Diabetologia 2007; 50: 1365-1374.

[10]   Mitri J, Castillo J, Pittas AG. Diabetes and risk of Non-Hodgkin's lymphoma: a meta-analysis of observational studies. Diabetes Care 2008; 31: 2391-2397.

[11]   Kasper JS, Giovannucci E. A meta-analysis of diabetes mellitus and the risk of prostate cancer. Cancer Epidemiol Biomarkers Prev 2006; 15: 2056-2062.

[12]   Ogunleye AA, Ogston SA, Morris AD, Evans JM. A cohort study of the risk of cancer associated with type 2 diabetes. Br J Cancer 2009;101: 1199-1201.

[13]   Dankner R, Chetrit A, Segal P. Glucose tolerance status and 20 years cancer incidence. Isr Med Assoc J 2007;9: 592-596.

[14]   Inoue M, Iwasaki M, Otani T, Sasazuki S, Noda M, Tsugane S. Diabetes mellitus and the risk of cancer: results from a large-scale population-based cohort study in Japan. Arch Intern Med 2006;166: 1871-1877.

[15]   Oba S, Nagata C, Nakamura K, Takatsuka N, Shimizu H. Self-reported diabetes mellitus and risk of mortality from all causes, cardiovascular disease, and cancer in Takayama: a population-based prospective cohort study in Japan. J Epidemiol 2008; 18: 197-203.

[16]   Batty GD, Shipley MJ, Marmot M, Smith GD. Diabetes status and post-load plasma glucose concentration in relation to site-specific cancer mortality: findings from the original Whitehall study. Cancer Causes Control 2004;15: 873-881.

[17]   Fujino Y, Mizoue T, Tokui N, Yoshimura T. Prospective study of diabetes mellitus and liver cancer in Japan. Diabetes Metab Res Rev 2001;17: 374-379.

[18]   Shaw JE, Hodge AM, de Courten M, Chitson P, Zimmet PZ. Isolated post-challenge hyperglycemia confirmed as a risk factor for mortality. Diabetologia 1999; 42: 1050-1054.

[19]   Abe R, Yamagishi S. AGE-RAGE system and carcinogenesis. Curr Pharm Des 2008; 14: 940-945.

[20]   Rajpathak SN, Gunter MJ, Wylie-Rosett J, *et al.* The role of insulin-like growth factor-I and its binding proteins in glucose homeostasis and type 2 diabetes. Diabetes Metab Res Rev 2009; 25: 3-12.

[21]   Pollak M. Insulin and insulin-like growth factor signalling in neoplasia. Nat Rev Cancer 2008; 8: 915-928.

[22]   Richardson LC, Pollack LA. Therapy insight: Influence of type 2 diabetes on the development, treatment and outcomes of cancer. Nat Clin Pract Oncol 2005; 2: 48-53.

[23]   Evans JM, Donnelly LA, Emslie-Smith AM, Alessi DR, Morris AD. Metformin and reduced risk of cancer in diabetic patients. BMJ 2005; 330: 1304-1305.

[24]   Libby G, Donnelly LA, Donnan PT, Alessi DR, Morris AD, Evans JM. New users of metformin are at low risk of incident cancer: a cohort study among people with type 2 diabetes. Diabetes Care 2009; 32: 1620-1625.

[25]   Landman GW, Kleefstra N, van Hateren KJ, Groenier KH, Gans RO, Bilo HJ. Metformin associated with lower cancer mortality in type 2 diabetes: ZODIAC-16. Diabetes Care 2010; 33: 322-326.

[26]   Home PD, Kahn SE, Jones NP, Noronha D, Beck-Nielsen H, Viberti G. Experience of malignancies with oral glucose-lowering drugs in the randomised controlled ADOPT (A Diabetes Outcome Progression Trial) and RECORD (Rosiglitazone Evaluated for Cardiovascular Outcomes and Regulation of Glycemia in Diabetes) clinical trials. Diabetologia 2010; 53: 1838-1845.

[27]   Bowker SL, Majumdar SR, Veugelers P, Johnson JA. Increased cancer-related mortality for patients with type 2 diabetes who use sulfonylureas or insulin. Diabetes Care 2006; 29: 254-258.

[28]   Bowker SL, Yasui Y, Veugelers P, Johnson JA. Glucose-lowering agents and cancer mortality rates in type 2 diabetes: assessing effects of time-varying exposure. Diabetologia 2010; 53: 1631-1637.

[29]   Currie CJ, Poole CD, Gale EA. The influence of glucose-lowering therapies on cancer risk in type 2 diabetes. Diabetologia 2009; 52: 1766-1777.

[30]   Kurtzhals P, Schaffer L, Sorensen A, *et al.* Correlations of receptor binding and metabolic and mitogenic potencies of insulin analogs designed for clinical use. Diabetes 2000; 49: 999-1005.

[31]   Colhoun HM. Use of insulin glargine and cancer incidence in Scotland: a study from the Scottish Diabetes Research Network Epidemiology Group. Diabetologia 2009; 52: 1755-1765.

[32]   Hemkens LG, Grouven U, Bender R, *et al.* Risk of malignancies in patients with diabetes treated with human insulin or insulin analogues: a cohort study. Diabetologia 2009; 52: 1732-1744.

[33]   Jonasson JM, Ljung R, Talback M, Haglund B, Gudbjornsdottir S, Steineck G. Insulin glargine use and short-term incidence of malignancies-a population-based follow-up study in Sweden. Diabetologia 2009; 52: 1745-1754.

[34]   Rosenstock J, Fonseca V, McGill JB, *et al.* Similar risk of malignancy with insulin glargine and neutral protamine Hagedorn (NPH) insulin in patients with type 2 diabetes: findings from a 5 years randomised, open-label study. Diabetologia 2009; 52: 1971-1973.

[35]   Mannucci E, Monami M, Balzi D, *et al.* Doses of insulin and its analogues and cancer occurrence in insulin-treated type 2 diabetic patients. Diabetes Care 2010; 33: 1997-2003.

[36]   Govindarajan R, Ratnasinghe L, Simmons DL, *et al.* Thiazolidinediones and the risk of lung, prostate, and colon cancer in patients with diabetes. J Clin Oncol 2007; 25: 1476-1481.

[37]   Koro C, Barrett S, Qizilbash N. Cancer risks in thiazolidinedione users compared to other anti-diabetic agents. Pharmacoepidemiol Drug Saf 2007; 16: 485-492.

[38]   Dormandy JA, Charbonnel B, Eckland DJ, *et al.* Secondary prevention of macrovascular events in patients with type 2 diabetes in the PROactive Study (PROspective pioglitAzone Clinical Trial In macroVascular Events): a randomised controlled trial. Lancet 2005; 366: 1279-1289.

[39]   Home PD, Kahn SE, Jones NP, Noronha D, Beck-Nielsen H, Viberti G. Experience of malignancies with oral glucose-lowering drugs in the randomised controlled ADOPT (A Diabetes Outcome Progression Trial) and

RECORD (Rosiglitazone Evaluated for Cardiovascular Outcomes and Regulation of Glycemia in Diabetes) clinical trials. Diabetologia 2010;53: 1838-1845.

[40]   Giovannucci E, Harlan DM, Archer MC, *et al.* Diabetes and cancer: a consensus report. Diabetes Care 2010; 33: 1674-1685.

Epidemiology of Type 2 Diabetes, 2012, 105-140

CHAPTER 8

Cardiovascular Diseases and Diabetes

Feng Ning[1,*], Lei Zhang[1,2,3,4] and Qing Qiao[1,2]

[1]*Department of Public Health, Hjelt Institute, University of Helsinki, Helsinki, Finland;* [2]*Department of Chronic Disease Prevention, National Institute for Health and Welfare, Helsinki, Finland;* [3]*Qingdao Endocrine & Diabetes Hospital, Qingdao, China and* [4]*Department of Internal Medicine, Weifang Medical University, Weifang, China*

Abstract: Both micro-vascular and macro-vascular complications increase premature deaths in patients with diabetes. Hypertension, Coronary Heart Disease (CHD) and ischemic stroke are known to be highly prevalent among patients with diabetes. Cardiovascular Disease (CVD) accounts for 80% of deaths in people suffering from diabetes. There is strong evidence that diabetes is an independent risk factor for cardiovascular mortality. In addition, non-diabetic hyperglycemia defined as Impaired Fasting Glucose (IFG) or Impaired Glucose Tolerance (IGT) was also associated with risk of CVD in some, but not in all studies. Randomized controlled clinical trials have confirmed that intensive glucose control can reduce the risk of micro-vascular complications among patients with diabetes. However, whether intensive glycemic control is of great benefit to CVD reduction among patients with diabetes or impaired glucose tolerance is still inconclusive. The association between glycemic levels and risk of hypertension, CHD and ischemic stroke will be discussed in this chapter.

Keywords: Diabetic and non-diabetic hyperglycemia, coronary heart disease, stroke, hypertension, intensive glucose control, diabetes and antihypertensive drugs

8.1. CORONARY HEART DISEASE IN RELATION TO GLYCEMIC LEVELS

8.1.1. Diabetes and Risk of Coronary Heart Disease

Individuals with clinically diagnosed diabetes have a 2-to 4-fold higher risk for cardiovascular disease (CVD) than non-diabetic individuals [1-6]. A meta-analysis of 37 prospective studies has shown that the risk of fatal Coronary Heart Disease (CHD) was greater in patients with diabetes than in those without diabetes, with a Relative Risk (RR) of 1.99 (95% confidence interval 1.69-2.35) in men and 3.12 (2.34-4.17) in women [6]. Another meta-analysis of Emerging Risk Factors Collaboration (ERFC) study including 102 studies of 264353 participants with 11848 CHD events accumulated has shown a Hazard Ratio (HR) of 2.10 (1.85-2.39) for CHD after adjusting for age, sex and smoking in participants with *versus* those without diabetes; the HR for CHD was slightly attenuated but remained statistically significant after adjustment for other conventional risk factors (Fig. **1**) [7]. Diabetes has been considered as a CHD equivalent in a Finnish study among middle-aged men. The multivariate adjusted HR for diabetic subjects without a prior Myocardial Infarction (MI) was not significantly different from that for the non-diabetic subjects with a prior MI, suggesting diabetes conveys a high MI risk (Fig. **2**) [8]. The finding was further confirmed by another study of 6 countries from Australia, Brazil, Canada, the United States, Hungary and Poland, which showed the future CVD risk in diabetic patients without a prior CVD was as high as that in non-diabetic individuals with a prior CVD [9]. But inconsistent findings have been reported by other studies [10-13]. During a 20-year follow-up, the Nurses' Health Study including 121046 women aged 30 to 55 years with 1239 fatal CHD events, showed that the multivariate-adjusted RR for fatal CHD were 5.65(4.83-6.60) and 10.7(9.03-12.60), respectively, for diabetic women without CHD and for non-diabetic women with CHD, as compared with those without both conditions at baseline [10]. A recent meta-analysis of 13 studies comprising 45108 patients with either diabetes or prior MI, revealed that diabetic patients without a prior MI had a 43% lower risk of developing CHD events than non-diabetic patients with a prior MI [14].

*****Address correspondence to Feng Ning:** Department of Public Health, Hjelt Institute, University of Helsinki, PL41, Mannerheimintie 172, 00014, Helsinki, Finland; E-mail: feng.ning@helsinki.fi

HR (95% CI)

Adjusted for

Age and sex		2·06 (1·82–2·34)
Plus smoking status		2·10 (1·85–2·39)
Plus BMI		2·00 (1·78–2·25)
Plus systolic blood pressure		1·91 (1·70–2·14)
Plus non-HDL cholesterol		1·93 (1·71–2·16)
Plus HDL cholesterol		1·87 (1·67–2·09)
Plus log-triglyceride		1·87 (1·67–2·09)

1   2   4

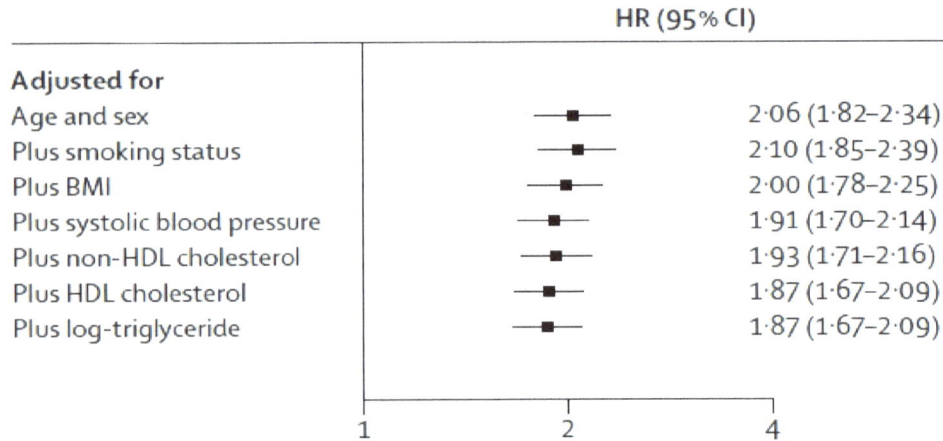

Figure 1: Hazard Ratios (HRs) for coronary heart disease in people with *versus* those without diabetes, progressively adjusted for baseline levels of conventional risk factors. BMI, body mass index. HDL, high density lipoprotein. Adapted from [7].

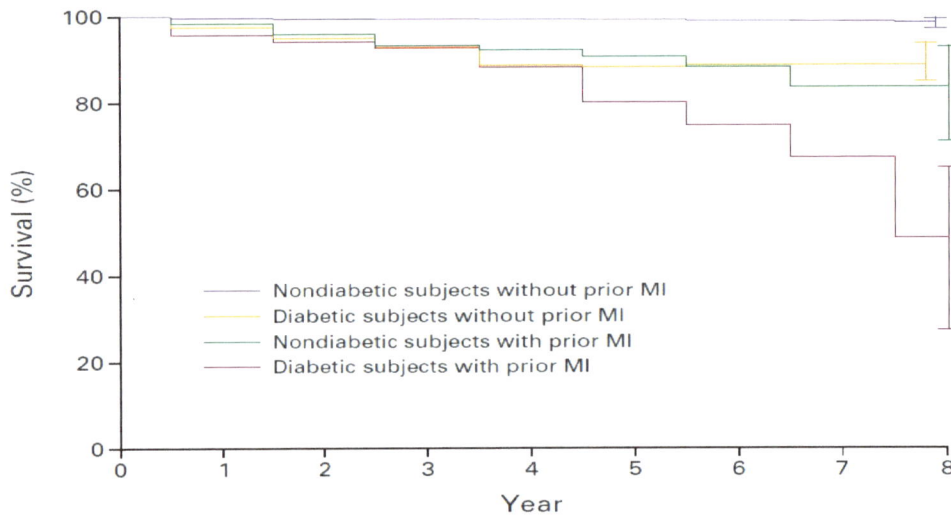

Figure 2: Kaplan-Meier estimates of the probability of death from coronary heart disease in 1059 subjects with type 2 diabetes and 1378 non-diabetic subjects with and without prior MI. MI, myocardial infarction. This figure was adapted from [8].

Numerous studies have demonstrated that the risk for CHD or CVD was also higher in subjects with newly diagnosed diabetes compared with those without diabetes [2, 15-17]. In the DECODE study (Diabetes Epidemiology: Collaborative analysis Of Diagnostic criteria in Europe), from 10 prospective cohorts including 15388 men and 7126 women aged 30 to 89 years, participants with newly diagnosed diabetes defined using fasting (FPG) and/or 2-h (2hPG) plasma glucose criteria had worse survival profiles for fatal CVD and CHD than those without diabetes during an average of 8.8-year follow-up (Fig. **3**) [4]. In the multi-ethnic Mauritius study including 9559 participants aged 20 to 82 years, the HR for CVD mortality were 2.04 (1.56-2.67) in men and 1.78 (1.29-2.46) in women who had newly diagnosed diabetes compared with individuals with normal glucose tolerance [2].

Carotid Intima-Media Thickness (CIMT) is a well-established indicator of early atherosclerosis [18-20] and is widely used as a surrogate marker of CVD [21, 22]. A meta-analysis of data from 37197 participants in 8 studies, demonstrated that each per 0.1 mm increase in CIMT was associated with a 10% increase in the risk of MI [22]. As shown in a meta-analysis including 22688 participants from 21 studies, diabetes was associated with a 13% increase in CIMT, as compared with non-diabetes (Fig. **4**) [23].

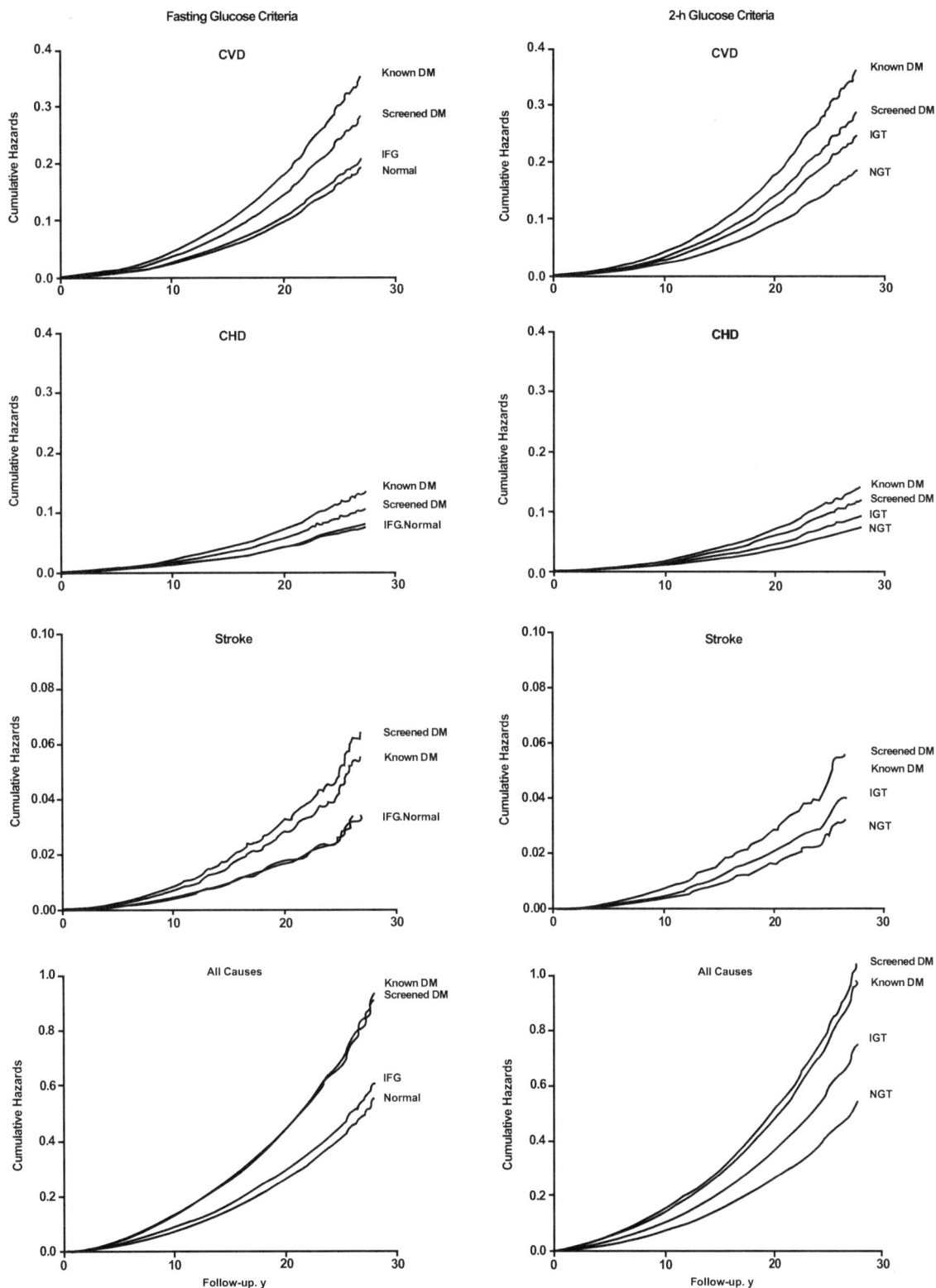

Figure 3: Cumulative hazards curves for deaths from Cardiovascular Disease (CVD), Coronary Heart Disease (CHD) and stroke, according to fasting and 2-hour glucose criteria. The cumulative hazards are estimated using Cox proportional hazards models and adjusted for age, center, sex, body mass index, blood pressure, serum cholesterol levels, and smoking status. DM, diabetes mellitus; IFG, impaired fasting glucose; IGT, impaired glucose tolerance and NGT, normal glucose tolerance. This figure was adapted from [4].

Carotid artery IMT in diabetes vs. controls

Study	Number		Mean	95% CI
		Control IMT thicker — Diabetes IMT thicker		
Folsom [13]	10 581		0.059	0.048-0.071
Hedblad [14]	5594		0.078	0.054-0.102
Wagenknecht [15]	1079		0.101	0.073-0.128
Ishizaka [16]	904		0.060	0.009-0.111
Wei [17]	867		0.057	0.033-0.080
Henry [18]	579		0.050	0.022-0.078
Taniwaki [19]	556		0.364	0.315-0.413
El-Barghouti [20]	484		0.014	-0.025-0.054
Yamasaki [21]	294		0.414	0.360-0.468
Sigurdardottir [22]	262		0.093	0.048-0.138
Mohan [23]	243		0.210	0.152-0.268
Geroulakos [26]	194		0.170	0.117-0.223
Niskanen [25]	182		0.142	0.057-0.228
Tuomilehto [27]	144		-0.080	-0.427-0.267
Temelkova-K [28]	142		0.130	0.059-0.201
Guvener [29]	122		0.180	0.116-0.244
Bonora [30]	114		0.250	0.195-0.305
Rajala [24]	111		0.090	-0.010-0.190
Puija [31]	108		0.073	0.035-0.111
Visona [32]	87		0.040	-0.010-0.089
Keven [32]	41		0.220	0.133-0.307
	22 688		0.134	0.123-0.144

-0.2 -0.1 0.0 0.1 0.2 0.3 0.4 0.5
Difference in carotid artery IMT, mm (95% CI)

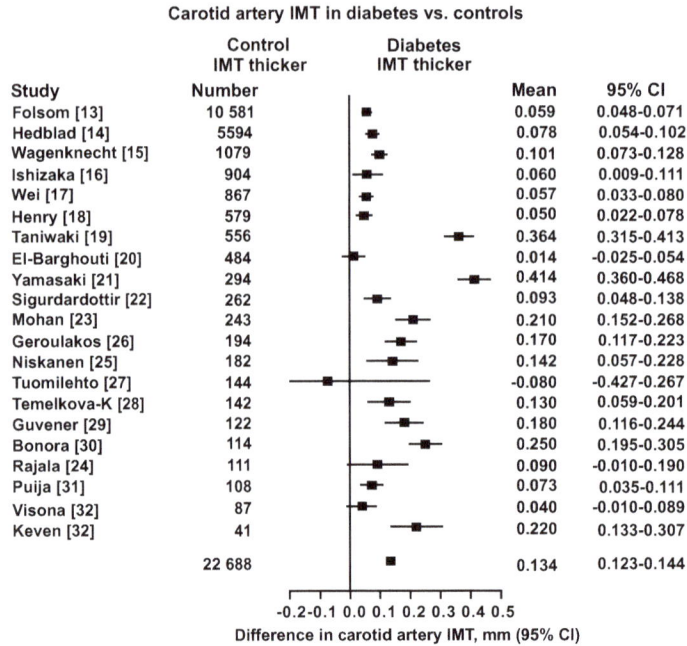

Figure 4: Mean differences in carotid artery Intima-Media Thickness (IMT) between Type 2 diabetes and control subjects. The overall difference was estimated based on the meta-analysis. This figure was adapted from [23].

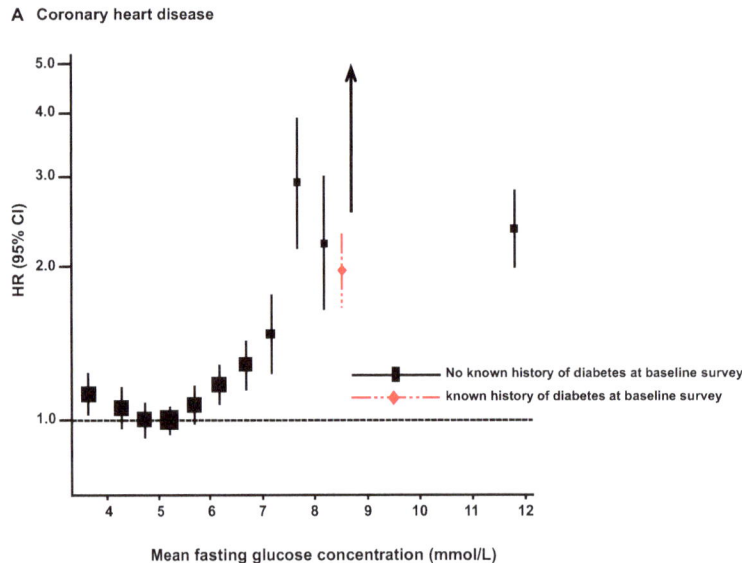

A Coronary heart disease

Figure 5: Hazard Ratios (HRs) for coronary heart disease among participants who did not have a prior history of diabetes estimated according to the baseline fasting blood glucose intervals of 0.5 mmol/l adjusted for age, smoking status, body-mass index and systolic blood pressure, and, where appropriate, stratified by sex and trial arm. HRs was plotted against mean fasting blood glucose in each group. Reference group is 5.0-5.5 mmol/l. This figure was adapted from [7].

8.1.2. CHD in Relation to Linear Forms of Glycemic Variables

The relationship between glucose levels and CVD has been extensively investigated in order to find whether there is a threshold or a change point in the glucose distribution that can be used to define diabetes according to the changes in CVD risk. In the ERFC study including 279290 participants with 14814 CHD cases accumulated, HR for CHD risk corresponding to per 1 mmol/l increase in the FPG was 1.12(1.08-1.15) within the range of FPG concentrations greater than 5.6 mmol/l (Fig. **5**) [7]. In another meta-analysis consisting of 12 studies with 45002 participants, CVD risk started to increase at the FPG cut-off value of ≥5.6 mmol/l (Fig. **6**)

[24]. In the DECODE study including 29714 subjects aged 30 to 89 years, a J-shaped relationship between FPG levels and CVD mortality was observed among Europeans who did not have a prior history of diabetes, with the lowest risk of CVD mortality observed in subjects with a FPG of 4.5-5.0 mmol/l [3] (Figs. **7-8** in the Chapter **1**). In the AusDiab (Australian Diabetes, Obesity, and Lifestyle) study based on 10026 participants aged $\geq$ 25 years, the HR for CHD corresponding to a one SD (standard deviation) (mmol/l) decrease in FPG concentrations was 4.0 (2.1-7.6) within the FPG range of < 5.1 mmol/l while to a one SD increase (mmol/l) the HR was 1.3 (1.1-1.4) in the FPG distribution of $\geq$ 5.1 mmol/l after adjustment for conventional risk factors [25]. The causes of increased CVD mortality risk associated with the low FPG level remains unclear, but the low Body Mass Index (BMI) has been considered as a potential risk factor [26, 27].

Different from the FPG-CVD relationship, a linear or graded rather than a J-shaped relationship between post-challenge glucose levels and CVD risk has been reported in many studies [3, 24, 25, 28]. This has been particularly pinpointed by the DECODE study (Figs. **7-8** in the Chapter **1**) [3] and also illustrated in the Fig. **6** based on the meta-analysis of data from 6 studies of 17081 participants [24].

These positive relationships were, however, not observed in early studies [29, 30]. Data from the International Collaborative Project, which included 11 prospective studies, failed to find a threshold or linear relationship between asymptomatic hyperglycemia and CHD mortality [29]. In a subsequent meta-analysis including 13 studies, the positive association between post-challenge glucose and CHD mortality did not reach statistical significance among half of the studies [30].

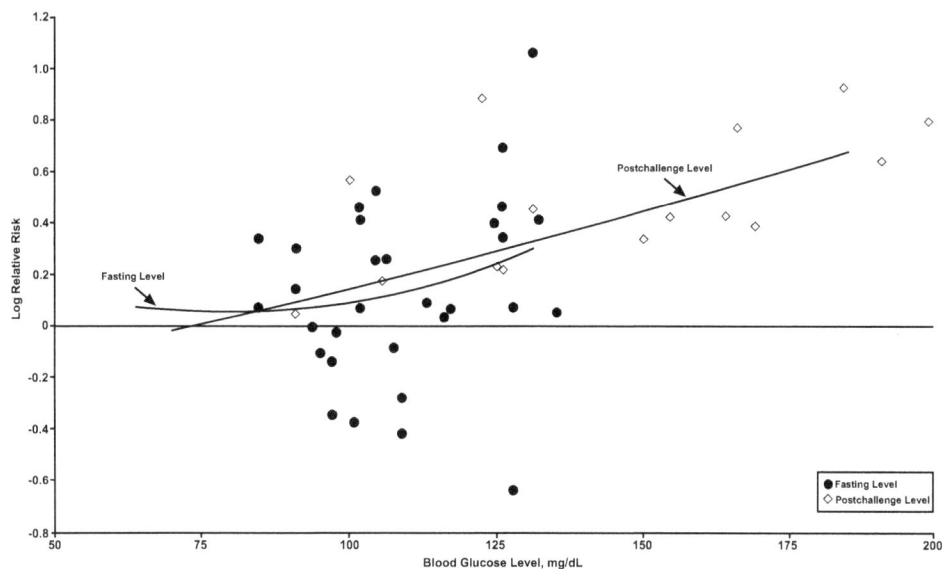

Figure 6: Dose-response relationship of cardiovascular disease with fasting and post-challenge blood glucose levels. This figure was adapted from [24].

Based on publications of prospective studies that are in English and indexed in the PubMed since 1970, we conducted an updated meta-analysis to estimate the glucose-CHD relationship. The inclusion criteria for the meta-analysis are: 1) Prospective studies with the CHD morbidity and mortality as end events; 2) Adults aged 25-89 years without diagnosed diabetes; 3) Glucose variables were estimated in their linear forms. A total of 11 studies met the inclusion criteria, with 696391 participants from eight studies providing with estimates on FPG, and 34404 participants from five studies on 2hPG. A total of 9440 CHD events for studying FPG and 4800 events for studying 2hPG were accumulated. Overall RRs for CHD were calculated by pooling study-specific estimates using a random-effects model. Variations of the effect sizes was assessed by Q statistic and I index; evidence of heterogeneity was considered if p-value less than 0.10 [31]. The overall RR per one SD increase in the FPG concentration (mmol/l or mg/dl) for CHD was 1.23(1.12-1.34) for men, 1.02(0.89-1.16) for women and 1.11(1.09-1.13) for both genders combined; the corresponding figures per one SD increase in the 2hPG concentration (mmol/l or mg/dl) were 1.19(1.14-

1.24), 1.06(0.95-1.19) and 1.17(1.13-1.21), respectively (Figs. **7** and **8**). The risk sizes for FPG were, however, heterogeneous among studies as shown by the I index and the small p value, reflecting the controversial findings among different studies for CHD-FPG relationship.

Glycated hemoglobin A1c (HbA1c) reflects the average blood glucose levels over the preceding 2-3 months. Recently, HbA1c has been adopted as a diagnostic test for diabetes by the American Diabetes Association [32]. Data from the Rancho Bernardo Study [33], the European Prospective Investigation of Cancer Study [34] and the Atherosclerosis Risk in Communities (ARIC) Study [35] have revealed that elevated HbA1c is associated with increased fatal and nonfatal CHD or CVD [36-38]. In a recent meta-analysis including 49099 participants with 1639 incident CHD cases, a 20% increase for CHD risk was seen for per 1% increase in HbA1c concentration [39].

8.1.3. CHD Risk in Relation to Impaired Fasting Glucose and Impaired Glucose Tolerance

Increasing evidence has shown that the CHD risk is higher among individuals with Impaired Fasting Glucose (IFG) and/or Impaired Glucose Tolerance (IGT) than among those with normal glucose levels. In the AusDiab study, among 10428 participants with 88 CVD deaths, IFG but not IGT were an independent risk predictor for CVD mortality after adjustment for traditional CVD risk factors as compared with normal glucose tolerance, the corresponding HRs were 2.6(1.2-5.1) and 1.2(0.7-2.2) respectively [40]. In the Framingham Heart Study including 4058 participants with 291 incident CHD cases, the multivariate adjusted OR for CHD was 1.7 (1.0 to 3.0, p = 0.048) among women with IFG defined according to the FPG of 5.6-6.9 mmol/l as compared with those with FPG<5.6 mmol/l, while the OR was 2.2 (1.1 to 4.4, p = 0.02) in women with IFG defined according to the FPG of 6.1-6.9 mmol/l as compared with those with FPG < 6.1 mmol/l [41]. Data from the multi-ethnic Mauritius study with a median of 15-year follow-up did not, however, show a significantly increased CVD mortality among individuals with IFG compared with those with normal fasting glucose with HRs of 1.24(0.82-1.87) in men and 0.66(0.32-1.38) in women [2].

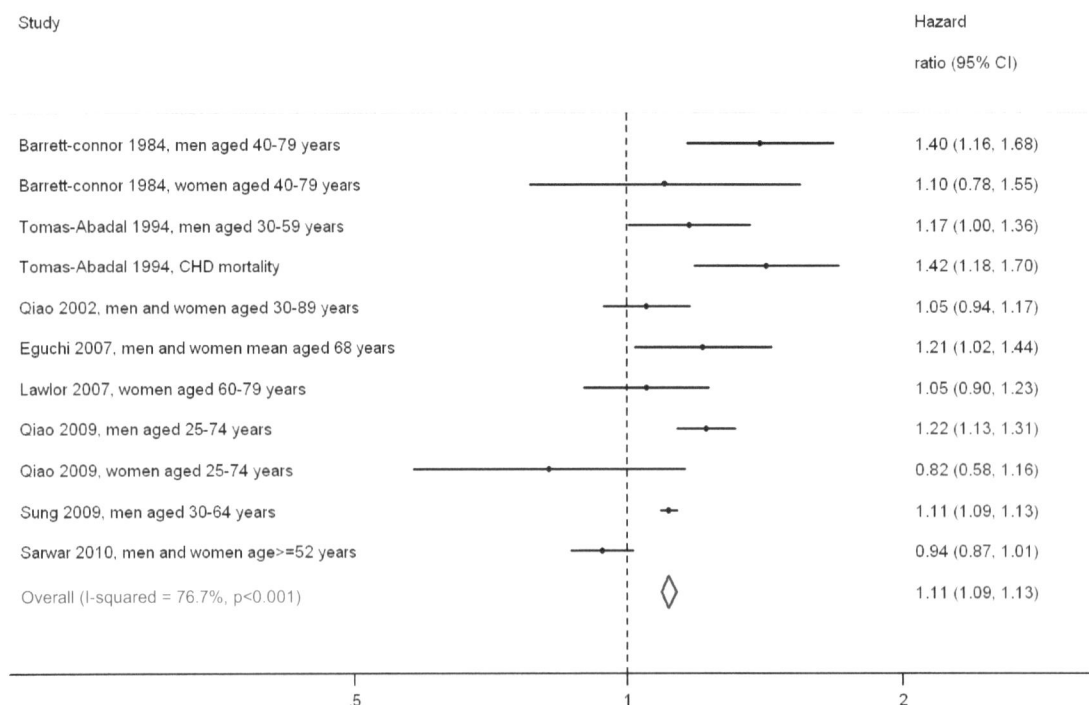

Study		Hazard ratio (95% CI)
Barrett-connor 1984, men aged 40-79 years		1.40 (1.16, 1.68)
Barrett-connor 1984, women aged 40-79 years		1.10 (0.78, 1.55)
Tomas-Abadal 1994, men aged 30-59 years		1.17 (1.00, 1.36)
Tomas-Abadal 1994, CHD mortality		1.42 (1.18, 1.70)
Qiao 2002, men and women aged 30-89 years		1.05 (0.94, 1.17)
Eguchi 2007, men and women mean aged 68 years		1.21 (1.02, 1.44)
Lawlor 2007, women aged 60-79 years		1.05 (0.90, 1.23)
Qiao 2009, men aged 25-74 years		1.22 (1.13, 1.31)
Qiao 2009, women aged 25-74 years		0.82 (0.58, 1.16)
Sung 2009, men aged 30-64 years		1.11 (1.09, 1.13)
Sarwar 2010, men and women age>=52 years		0.94 (0.87, 1.01)
Overall (I-squared = 76.7%, p<0.001)		1.11 (1.09, 1.13)

.5   1   2

Figure 7: Hazard ratio (dot) and 95% confidence interval (bar) corresponding to a one standard deviation increase in fasting plasma glucose concentration (mmol/l or mg/dl) for coronary heart disease (CHD) morbidity or mortality in participants without previously diagnosed diabetes.

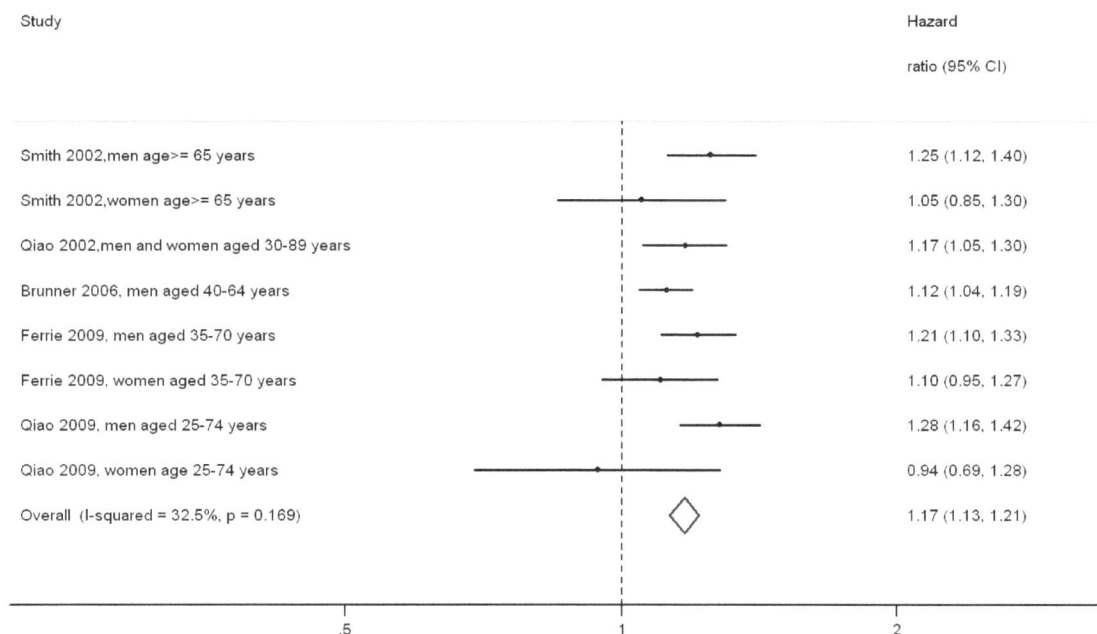

Figure 8: Hazard ratio (dot) and 95% confidence interval (bar) corresponding to a one standard deviation increase in 2-hour plasma glucose concentration (mmol/l or mg/dl) for coronary heart disease (CHD) morbidity or mortality in participants without previously diagnosed diabetes.

The Bedford Cohort Study with 10-years follow-up found that IGT carried an excess risk of CHD mortality in women but not in men [42]. In the Funagata Diabetes Study, IGT, but not IFG, increased the risk for CVD, with the corresponding Odds Ratios (ORs) of 2.22 (1.08-4.58) for IGT and 1.24 (0.64-2.38) for IFG [43]. As shown in the Fig. **3** by the DECODE study, subjects with IGT had a survival profile falling between diabetic and normal subjects according to the 2-h glucose criteria; while those with IFG had a survival profile similar to that of subjects with normoglycemia based on the fasting glucose criteria alone [4]. Based on the data analysis of a Finnish cohort study, the DECODE study group further showed that baseline IGT was an independent risk predictor for cardiovascular morbidity and mortality, and the prediction was not explained by the subsequent development of overt diabetes (Table **1**) [44].

Table 1: Ten-years incidence of Coronary Heart Disease (CHD), cardiovascular and total mortality, and the corresponding Hazard Ratios (HR), according to baseline 2-h glucose categories stratified by diabetic status at follow-up in subjects free of diabetes at baseline.

	Nondiabetic at Follow-up		Diabetic at Follow-up
Baseline 2-h glucose (mmol/l)	<6.7	6.7-9.9	<10.0
CHD incidence			
n (%)	2110 (85.9)	250 (10.2)	97 (3.9)
n (rate per 1, 000 person-years)	114 (5.3)	24 (9.7)	15 (16.1)
Age-and sex-adjusted HR (95% CI)	1	1.72 (1.11-2.69)	2.45 (1.43-4.21)
Multivariate-adjusted HR (95% CI)*	1	1.49 (0.95-2.34)	1.79 (1.02-3.16)
Cardiovascular mortality			
n (%)	2173 (85.7)	262 (10.3)	100 (3.9)
n (rate per 1, 000 person-years)	70 (3.1)	21 (7.9)	9 (8.7)
Age-and sex-adjusted HR (95% CI)	1	2.51 (1.53-4.10)	2.29 (1.14-4.60)
Multivariate-adjusted HR (95% CI)*	1	2.34 (1.42-3.85)	1.69 (0.82-3.47)
Total mortality			

n (%)	2173 (85.7)	262 (10.3)	100 (3.9)
n (rate per 1, 000 person-years)	174 (7.6)	34 (12.8)	16 (15.5)
Age-and sex-adjusted HR (95% CI)	1	1.61 (1.11-2.34)	1.71 (1.02-2.86)
Multivariate-adjusted HR (95% CI)*	1	1.65 (1.13-2.40)	1.50 (0.88-2.54)

*Adjusted for age, sex, waist-to-hip ratio, systolic blood pressure, cholesterol, high density lipoprotein cholesterol, and smoking. This table was adapted from [44].

IGT has also been found to be associated with increased IMT in some studies [45, 46], but not in others [47, 48]. In a meta-analysis including 5787 participants from 12 studies, the mean CIMT was higher in individuals with IGT than in those with normal glucose tolerance, with a mean difference of 0.03 mm (Fig. **9**) [49].

8.1.4. Comparisons of the CHD Risk in Relation to Different Glycemic Measures

It has been well documented that hyperglycemia measured by either FPG, 2hPG or HbA1c is associated with increased CHD risk [4, 15, 33, 35, 50-52], but agreement of the three is poor with regard to the classification of individuals with hyperglycemia. It is, therefore, clinically important to know whether individuals with hyperglycemia defined by different glycemic criteria have different CVD risk.

In the DECODE and the DECODA (Diabetes Epidemiology Collaborative analysis Of Diagnostic criteria in Asia) studies among 22514 Europeans and 6817 Japanese and Asian Indians, CVD mortality and all-cause mortality in relation to both FPG and 2hPG were compared (Tables **2** and **3**). Addition of the 2hPG to a model based on the FPG significantly improved the prediction of the CVD mortality; but no fundamental change was observed when FPG was fitted into the model based on the 2hPG [4, 15]. This was further supported by data from the Cardiovascular Health Study including 4014 adults, where 2hPG criteria appeared to be better than FPG criteria in predicting incident CVD among older adults [53]; and from other studies that showed the relationship between 2hPG and CVD was independent of FPG [54, 55].

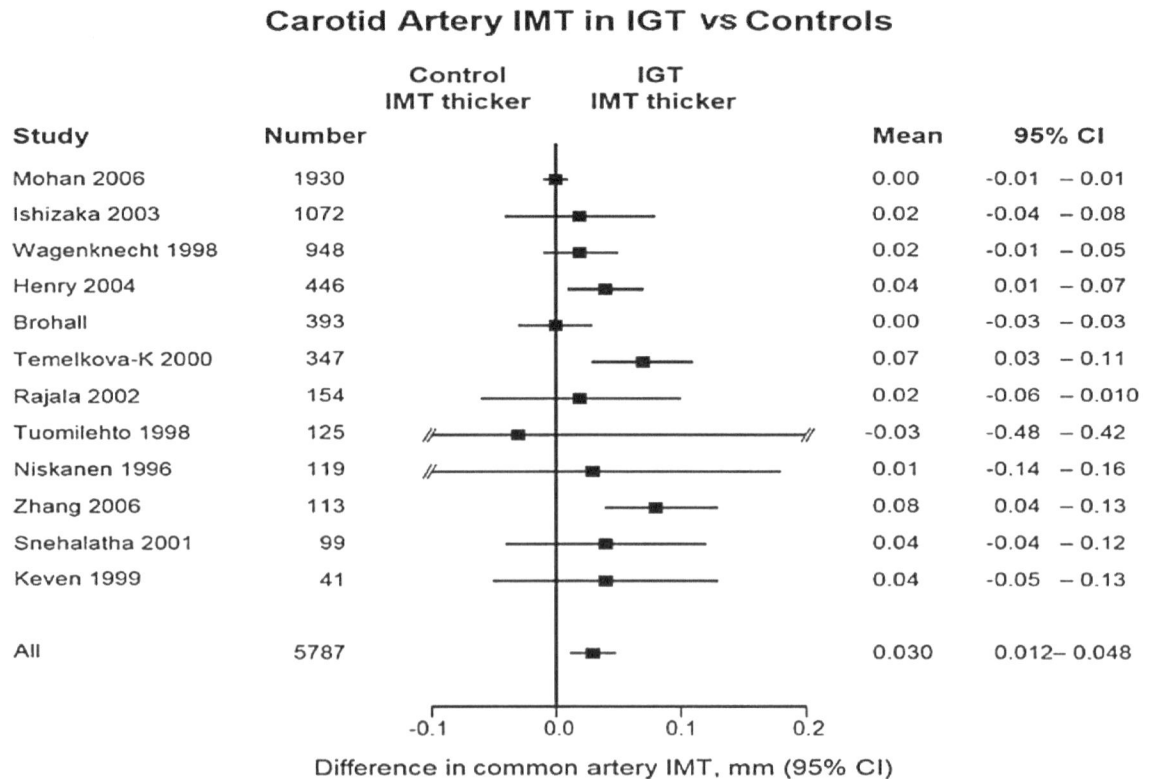

Carotid Artery IMT in IGT vs Controls

Study	Number	Control IMT thicker	IGT IMT thicker	Mean	95% CI
Mohan 2006	1930			0.00	-0.01 — 0.01
Ishizaka 2003	1072			0.02	-0.04 — 0.08
Wagenknecht 1998	948			0.02	-0.01 — 0.05
Henry 2004	446			0.04	0.01 — 0.07
Brohall	393			0.00	-0.03 — 0.03
Temelkova-K 2000	347			0.07	0.03 — 0.11
Rajala 2002	154			0.02	-0.06 — 0.010
Tuomilehto 1998	125			-0.03	-0.48 — 0.42
Niskanen 1996	119			0.01	-0.14 — 0.16
Zhang 2006	113			0.08	0.04 — 0.13
Snehalatha 2001	99			0.04	-0.04 — 0.12
Keven 1999	41			0.04	-0.05 — 0.13
All	5787			0.030	0.012– 0.048

-0.1   0.0   0.1   0.2

Difference in common artery IMT, mm (95% CI)

Figure 9: Mean difference in carotid artery Intima-Media Thickness (IMT) between groups with impaired (IGT) and normal (NGT) glucose tolerance. The overall difference was estimated based on the meta-analysis. This figure was adapted from [49].

Table 2: Hazard ratios (95% CI) for death from Cardiovascular Disease (CVD), Coronary Heart Disease (CHD), stroke and all-cause when both the fasting and the 2-h glucose classes were in the same model. Subjects not known as diabetes in the DECODE study.

	Plasma Glucose Categories (mmol/l)					
	Fasting glucose criteria [a]			2-h glucose criteria [b]		
	IFG 6.1-6.9	Diabetes ≥7.0	X^2 (p value)[c]	IGT 7.8-11.0	Diabetes ≥11.1	X^2 (p value)[d]
CVD	1.01 (0.84-1.22)	1.20 (0.88-1.64)	1.34 (>0.10)	1.32 (1.12-1.56)	1.40 (1.02-1.92)	12.09 (<0.005)
CHD	1.01 (0.77-1.31)	1.09 (0.71-1.67)	0.15 (>0.10)	1.27 (1.01-1.58)	1.56 (1.03-2.36)	6.81 (<0.05)
Stroke	1.00 (0.66-1.51)	1.64 (0.88-3.07)	2.35 (>0.10)	1.21 (0.84-1.74)	1.29 (0.66-2.54)	1.23 (>0.10)
All-cause	1.03 (0.93-1.14)	1.21 (1.01-1.44)	4.32 (>0.10)	1.37 (1.25-1.51)	1.73 (1.45-2.06)	61.35 (<0.001)

[a]Using fasting plasma glucose <6.1 mmol/l as a reference group; [b]Using 2-h post-load plasma glucose <7.8 mmol/l as a reference group; [c]Compared with the models with only the 2-h glucose criteria, 2df; [d]Compared with the models with only the fasting glucose criteria, 2df. All the models adjusted for age, sex, center, total cholesterol, body mass index, systolic blood pressure and smoking. This table was adapted from [4].

Table 3: Mortality (95% CI) per 1000 person-years, and hazard ratio (95% CI) for all-cause and cardiovascular disease (CVD) according to fasting and 2-h plasma glucose criteria.

Fasting Plasma Glucose (mmol/l)		<6.1 (n=5547)	6.1-6.9 (n=462)	≥7.0 (n=297)	p Value for Linear Trend for HR
All-cause mortality	No.	284	47	50	
	*Mortality per 1000 person-years	8.9 (8.8-8.9)	13.1 (13.0-13.2)	26.6 (26.3-26.8)	
	Model 1	1	1.19 (0.87-1.64)	1.82 (1.31-2.52)	0.001
	Model 2	1	0.94 (0.68-1.31)	0.88 (0.59-1.32)	0.81
CVD mortality	No.	127	26	29	
	Mortality per 1000 person-years	3.9 (3.9-4.0)	7.3 (7.2-7.3)	14.6 (14.5-14.8)	
	Model 1	1	1.35 (0.86-2.08)	2.01 (1.30-3.11)	0.006
	Model 2	1	1.05 (0.67-1.65)	0.88 (0.51-1.51)	0.83
2-h Plasma glucose (mmol/l)		7.8 (n=4753)	7.8-11.0 (n=1106)	≥11.1 (n=447)	p value for linear trend for HR
All-cause mortality	No.	206	87	88	
	Mortality per 1000 person-years (numbers)	8.0 (7.9-8.0)	10.5 (10.4-10.6)	28.0 (27.8-28.2)	
	Model 1	1	1.34 (1.03-1.74)	2.85 (2.16-3.75)	<0.001
	Model 3	1	1.35 (1.03-1.77)	3.03 (2.18-4.21)	<0.001
CVD mortality	No.	91	41	50	
	Mortality per 1000 person-years (numbers)	3.5 (3.5-3.6)	4.9 (4.8-4.9)	15.6 (15.5-15.8)	
	Model 1	1	1.27 (0.86-1.88)	3.21 (2.20-4.69)	<0.001
	Model 3	1	1.27 (0.86-1.88)	3.39 (2.14-5.37)	<0.001

*Mortality was age-standardized using the world standard population of subjects of 30 to 89 years of age. Model 1: adjusted for age, sex, cohort, body mass index, systolic blood pressure, total cholesterol and smoking status. Model 2: model 1 plus 2-h glucose criteria. Model 3: model 1 plus fasting glucose criteria. This table was adapted from [15].

A few studies have also compared glucose criteria with HbA1c criteria regarding to the prediction of CVD. HbA1c was found to be a better predictor of ischemic heart disease and CVD mortality than either FPG or 2hPG in some [33, 35, 52] but not in all studies [25, 56]. In the Framingham Heart Study, 2hPG appeared to be a strongest independent risk predictor among the three glycemic measures of 2hPG, FPG and HbA1c [56]. The HRs for CVD incidence were 1.42 (1.17-1.72) for one SD increase in 2hPG (mmol/l) and 0.87(0.76-1.00) in FPG (mmol/l) when the two variables were fitted in the same model; they were 1.23(1.07-1.43) for the 2hPG and 0.93(0.77-1.13) for the HbA1c when fitting the two variables simultaneously [56].

A number of studies have shown that IFG and IGT reflects different pathophysiological mechanisms of abnormal glucose homeostasis [57, 58]. The isolated IFG is associated with reduced hepatic insulin sensitivity and beta-cell dysfunction, while the isolated IGT associated with peripheral insulin resistance and defective insulin secretion. The reduced first-phase insulin release and impaired hepatic insulin sensitivity result in the fasting hyperglycemia, whereas the impaired second-phase insulin release and peripheral insulin resistance contributing to the post-challenge hyperglycemia [59, 60]. The isolated IGT are markedly more insulin resistant than the isolated IFG [59]. The difference in insulin resistance might partly explain the differences in mortality and CVD risk associated with IGT and IFG.

Both insulin resistance and endothelial dysfunction, commonly occurring with hyperglycemia, have been considered as the underlying mechanism contributing to the development of atherosclerosis [61-65]. Insulin resistance was associated with impaired nitric oxide synthase activity, a factor crucial to the normal vasodilatory response and endothelial function. Additionally, excess proinsulin has exhibited moderate but significant associations with blood pressure and total cholesterol, triglycerides, Low Density Lipoprotein-Cholesterol (LDL-C) and High Density Lipoprotein-Cholesterol (HDL-C) regardless of diabetic status [66-68]. Hyperglycemia promotes the production of reactive oxygen species and also increases the production of Advanced Glycation End-Products (AGEs), and these molecules are crucial in the pathogenesis of endothelial damage that precedes atherosclerotic changes of the vascular wall [69, 70]. In a recent experimental study, it was indicated that hyperglycemia activated the calcineurin-dependent nuclear factor of activated T cells-3 (NFATc3) signaling pathway, which upregulated the expression of osteopontin to accelerate the process of vascular diseases [71]. Despite accumulated evidence linking hyperglycemia to increased risk of micro-vascular and macro-vascular diseases [72], the molecular mechanisms underlying vascular damage need to be further investigated.

8.1.5. Normoglycemia and Risk of CVD Mortality

Recently, it has been shown that among individuals with normal fasting and 2-h plasma glucose, those with 2hPG did not return to their FPG levels during an OGTT had increased risk of type 2 diabetes [73], increased CIMT [74] and CVD mortality [75] as compared with those whose 2hPG returned to their fasting glucose levels. In the DECODE study with 23440 Europeans aged 25 to 90 years who had both normal FPG (<6.1 mmol/l) and normal 2hPG (<7.8 mmol/l) at baseline examination, the 9-year CVD mortality were higher in subjects with 2hPG > FPG than in those with 2hPG ≤ FPG in both genders (Table 4) [75]. Elevated 2hPG in the normal range increased the risk for CVD mortality independent of FPG levels. When the normal FPG was defined using strict criteria at FPG cut-off of ≤ 5.6 mmol/l, the multivariate adjusted HR for CVD mortality were 1.27(1.08-1.48) in individuals whose 2hPG > FPG than in those with 2hPG ≤ FPG [75].

Table 4: HRs (95% CIs) for death from CVD, non-CVD, and all causes for group II compared with group I*

	Model 1	Model 2	Model 3
Men			
n	12566	12566	9978
CVD	1.16 (1.01-1.34)	1.22 (1.05-1.41)	1.25 (1.05-1.50)
Non-CVD	1.01 (0.86-1.19)	1.09 (0.92-1.29)	1.09 (0.89-1.34)
All causes	1.10 (0.99-1.22)	1.16 (1.04-1.30)	1.18 (1.03-1.35)
Women			
n	10874	10874	7350
CVD	1.23 (0.91-1.65)	1.40 (1.03-1.89)	1.60 (1.03-2.48)
Non-CVD	0.92 (0.73-1.15)	0.99 (0.79-1.25)	1.05 (0.78-1.42)
All causes	1.03 (0.86-1.23)	1.13 (0.94-1.35)	1.18 (0.93-1.51)

Model 1: adjusted for age and cohort; model 2: model 1 plus fasting plasma glucose, BMI, total cholesterol, smoking and hypertension status; model 3: model 2 plus fasting insulin. *Group I, 2hPG ≤ FPG; group II, 2hPG> FPG. CVD, cardiovascular disease. This table was adapted from [75].

Both insulin resistance and reduced beta-cell function occurred during the normoglycemic stage as shown by the Québec Family Study among 643 subjects aged 18 to 71 years [76, 77]. Another cross-sectional study, with a multiethnic sample of 1020 obese youth (mean age 12.9 years) with normal FPG levels (FPG< 5.6 mmol/l), showed that insulin sensitivity decline when moving from low to high glucose levels within the normal range, independent of age, BMI, sex and ethnicity [76]. Even within normoglycemic range (FPG <5.6 mmol/l and 2hPG <7.8 mmol/l), subjects whose 2hPG did not return to FPG levels had higher CIMT and lower insulin sensitivity than subjects whose 2hPG did in a cross-sectional study [74]. However, in the Bruneck Study including subjects with normoglycemia, neither 2hPG nor FPG independently predicted the carotid atherosclerosis assessed by the IMT during a 5-years follow-up [78]. To what extent the insulin resistance contributes to the increased CVD mortality in individuals with normal glucose levels needs to be further investigated.

8.2. ISCHEMIC STROKE IN RELATION TO GLYCEMIC LEVELS

8.2.1. Diabetes and Risk of Stroke

Cerebrovascular disease, as well as CHD, is the leading causes of death and disability in diabetic patients. It is shown that participants with diabetes is two to five times more likely to develop a serious stroke compared with those without diabetes [4, 7, 79-88]. Data from 18360 Finns and Swedes aged 25 to 90 years showed the HRs for ischemic stroke incidence were 2.20(1.48-3.29) for known diabetes and 1.48(1.08-2.02) for newly diagnosed diabetes defined using the FPG criteria, and 2.26(1.51-3.38) for known diabetes and 1.60(1.18-2.16) for newly diagnosed diabetes defined using the 2hPG criteria, as compared with normal fasting or 2h glucose levels [89]. In the ERFC study including 157315 participants with 2858 stroke cases accumulated, age-, sex-and smoking-adjusted HRs were 2.59 (2.16-3.09) for ischemic stroke in subjects with diabetes compared with those without diabetes [7]. The HRs did not change substantially after additional adjustment for BMI, systolic blood pressure, HDL-C and triglycerides (Fig. **10**).

It has been noted that the effect of diabetes on the risk of CHD [6, 7, 90] and stroke [91, 92] was more pronounced in women than in men when the RR was estimated taking non-diabetic women or non-diabetic men as a reference category, respectively. The RR for fatal CHD was 3.50 (2.70-4.53) in women and 2.06 (1.81-2.34) in men with type 2 diabetes in a meta-analysis including 37 studies of 447064 individuals from Asia Pacific Cohort Studies Collaboration [6]. We have, however, shown in the DECODE study that the absolute risk of both CHD and ischemic stroke was higher for men than for women in both diabetic and non-diabetic categories; men also had higher RR than women when non-diabetic women was considered as a reference category, particularly for CHD (Table **5**) [93]. As compared with men, women had better cardiovascular risk profiles, and lower number of cardiovascular events, particularly in younger age groups [93]. It has been shown that women suffer from the stroke at a relative older age with subsequent poorer quality of life than men [94], yet the reasons for this are not well understood. Recent findings have revealed that sex steroid hormones, particularly oestrogen, may play a role in the risk of CVD either in animal models and in human studies of ischemic stroke [95, 96].

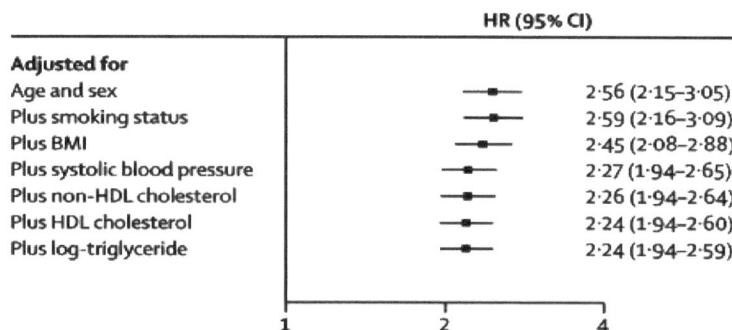

	HR (95% CI)
Adjusted for	
Age and sex	2·56 (2·15–3·05)
Plus smoking status	2·59 (2·16–3·09)
Plus BMI	2·45 (2·08–2·88)
Plus systolic blood pressure	2·27 (1·94–2·65)
Plus non-HDL cholesterol	2·26 (1·94–2·64)
Plus HDL cholesterol	2·24 (1·94–2·60)
Plus log-triglyceride	2·24 (1·94–2·59)

Figure 10: Hazard ratios (HRs) for ischemic stroke in people with *versus* those without diabetes, progressively adjusted for baseline levels of conventional risk factors. BMI, body mass index. HDL, high density lipoprotein. This figure was adapted from [7].

Table 5: Event rates per 1000 person-years and hazard ratios (HR) (95% confidence intervals) for acute coronary heart disease (CHD) and ischemic stroke events by diabetic status.

	Non-Diabetic			Diabetic		
	Age groups, yr				Age groups, yr	
	40-49	50-59	60-69	40-49	50-59	60-69
CHD						
Rates						
Women	1.09 (0.68-1.65)	2.20 (1.68-2.83)	4.61 (3.61-5.81)	5.68 (1.80-13.69)	7.50 (4.06-12.74)	12.53 (7.96-18.82)
Men	3.11 (2.31-4.10)	6.57 (5.52-7.77)	10.82 (8.97-12.95)	9.62 (4.21-19.03)	13.24 (8.59-19.55)	17.51 (11.59-25.47)
HRs						
Model 1						
Women	1	2.10 (1.26-3.49)	4.91 (2.97-8.12)	6.09 (2.08-17.82)	7.95 (3.88-16.26)	14.65 (7.87-27.28)
Men	2.90 (1.72-4.90)	6.43 (4.02-10.29)	12.34 (7.62-19.97)	10.44 (4.41-24.70)	15.98 (8.76-29.15)	22.54 (12.41-40.97)
Model 2						
Women	1	1.78 (1.06-2.97)	3.75 (2.24-6.26)	4.35 (1.48-12.80)	5.49 (2.66-11.33)	8.84 (4.68-16.72)
Men	1.94 (1.14-3.29)	4.23 (2.61-6.84)	8.40 (5.13-13.76)	5.40 (2.26-12.93)	9.54 (5.17-17.63)	13.76 (7.47-25.34
Ischemic stroke						
Rates						
Women	0.65 (0.35-1.11)	1.66 (1.22-2.22)	3.53 (2.66-4.59)	2.84 (0.48-9.38)	2.50 (0.79-6.03)	9.54 (5.65-15.17)
Men	1.06 (0.63-1.68)	2.39 (1.78-3.14)	4.18 (3.07-5.56)	4.12 (1.05-11.22)	5.18 (2.53-9.50)	11.91 (7.17-18.68)
HRs						
Model 1						
Women	1	2.62 (1.38-4.97)	5.71 (3.01-10.81)	5.08 (1.14-22.72)	4.23 (1.36-13.12)	17.78 (8.26-38.30)
Men	1.63 (0.77-3.43)	3.86 (2.05-7.26)	7.15 (3.73-13.69)	7.87 (2.22-27.93)	10.60 (4.46-25.20)	27.22 (12.76-58.10)
Model 2						
Women	1	2.48 (1.30-4.73)	5.17 (2.69-9.94)	4.14 (0.92-18.66)	3.32 (1.06-10.43)	13.91 (6.31-30.66)
Men	1.26 (0.59-2.70)	2.83 (1.48-5.42)	5.11 (2.62-9.97)	4.91 (1.36-17.74)	6.75 (2.79-16.32)	18.06 (8.29-39.37)

Model 1, adjusted for study; Model 2, adjusted for study, body mass index, hypertension, total cholesterol, high density lipoprotein-cholesterol and smoking. This table was adapted from [93].

8.2.2. Stoke in Relation to Glycemic Variables

A number of studies have demonstrated that hyperglycemia was associated with increased risk of stroke [35, 83, 97-100] but not all studies agreed on this [101, 102]. Recently, a systematic review of epidemiological studies and surveys from 52 countries showed that 13% deaths from stroke attributable to higher-than-optimum FPG [100]. In the Goettingen Risk Incidence and Prevalence Study with 5790 men aged 40.0-59.9 years followed for 10 years, RR for stroke incidence was 1.6 (1.1-2.2) in individuals with FPG > 6.2 mmol/l compared with those with FPG < 4.8 mmol/l [99]. In another study of 28477 non-diabetic individuals, baseline fasting blood glucose over 5.6 mmol/l was associated with a 24% increased risk of stroke or transient ischemic attacks as compared with fasting blood glucose < 5.6 mmol/l (multivariable adjusted HR 1.24 (1.05-1.46)) [103]. The study in the Northern Manhattan (NOMAS) including 2372 subjects found distinct ethnic difference regarding the FPG-stroke relationship. In a multivariate adjusted model, FPG is a better predictor for ischemic stroke in African-American, but not in Hispanic and White Americans, the corresponding HRs were 1.38(1.09-1.74), 0.97(0.70-1.34) and 0.81(0.47-1.40), respectively [98]. Data from 3246 British women aged 60-79 years free of baseline CHD, stroke and diabetes did not, however, show a positive relationship between linear form of FPG and the incidence of stroke [102].

In the DECODE study including 13 European cohorts of 21706 participants without a prior history of diabetes, the multivariate adjusted HRs for stroke mortality corresponding to one SD increase in 2hPG (mmol/l) was 1.21(1.06-1.38) for men and 1.31(1.06-1.61) for women; whereas the corresponding figures for FPG for stroke mortality was not significant for men, with a HR of 1.02(0.83-1.25) in men and 1.52(1.22-1.88) in women [55]. In the United Kingdom General Post Office study, the elevated 2hPG levels was, however, not significantly associated with increased stroke mortality, with the HRs of 1.06(0.83-1.35) for men and 1.25(0.97-1.61) for women corresponding to a one SD increase in 2hPG (mmol/l) [104].

As regard to the stroke risk in individuals with IFG, the West of Scotland Prevention Study including 6447 men aged 55 years failed to show an increased stroke mortality among participants with IFG defined by either a FPG of 6.1-6.9 mmol/l or 5.6-6.9 mmol/l during a 15-years follow-up [105]. The Strong Heart Study based on 4549 American-Indians participants aged 45 to 74 years did not revealed a higher stroke incidence in subjects with IFG or IGT defined by the 1998 World Health Organization (WHO) criteria as compared with nomorglycemic subjects after adjusting for co-variables [85]. In the Hisayama Study consisting of 2421 subjects aged 40 to 79 years who underwent a 75 g OGTT, neither IFG (FPG: 6.1-6.9 mmol/l and 2hPG<7.8 mmol/l) nor IGT (FPG<7.0 mmol/l and 2hPG 7.8-11.1 mmol/l) had increased risk of ischemic stroke in both genders, as compared with participants with both normal fasting and normal 2h plasma glucose [106].

HbA1c has been shown to be associated with atherosclerosis in adults with diabetes in a cross-sectional study [107] and able to predict future cardiovascular disease in individuals with or without diabetes [24, 34, 108]. HbA1c was also found to increase the risk of stroke in non-diabetic subjects. In the ARIC Study including 11092 Black and White adults free of a history of diabetes or CVD, both HbA1c and fasting glucose concentrations increased with increasing risk of ischemic stroke with a RR of 1.34(1.22-1.48) for a 1% increase in HbA1c concentration and of 1.07(1.03-1.10) for a 10 mg/dl (0.56 mmol/l) increase in fasting glucose concentration. However, when the two were fitted in the same model simultaneously the prediction of the FPG became non-significant (RR=0.95, 95%CI: 0.89-1.01) while that for the HbA1c remained significant (RR=1.55, 95%CI: 1.28-1.88) [35], suggesting that raised HbA1c could be an independent risk factor for stroke in individuals without diagnosed diabetes.

To summarize the previous reports on the relationship between hyperglycemia and stroke risk, a meta-analysis based on 710958 participants aged 25-89 years from 9 prospective studies with FPG measures and 68852 participants from 5 prospective studies with 2hPG measures was conducted, and the results of the meta-analysis are shown in Figs. **11** and **12**. A total of 6558 stroke events for studying FPG and 2525 for studying 2hPG were recorded. The estimated overall RRs for stroke were 1.21(1.19-1.23) for men, 1.29 (1.14-1.47) for women and 1.16(1.08-1.24) for both genders combined corresponding to a one SD increase in the FPG levels (mmol/l or mg/dl); and 1.20(1.11-1.29), 1.27(1.12-1.45) and 1.19(1.13-1.25), respectively, for a one SD increase in the 2hPG levels (mmol/l) (Figs. **11** and **12**). The effect sizes for FPG were, however, heterogeneous among studies as shown by the large I-square value and the small p value. This is similar to the findings for the FPG-CHD relationship (Figs. **7** and **8**).

The pathogenesis of hyperglycemia on risk of the ischemic stroke is still unclear. Hyperglycemia is known to be associated with inflammation reaction and oxidative stress [109, 110]. The elevated blood glucose triggers a series of inflammation reaction to decrease the concentration of proteins, which keeps the integrity of the blood-brain barrier, resulting in edema with the leakage of plasma proteins and inflammatory cells. Thus, hyperglycemia may increase the cerebral damage by disrupting the microcirculation and upregulating the inflammatory and thrombotic/fibrinolytic markers in the brain [110, 111]. Animal studies have consistently shown the correlation between hyperglycemia and acidosis [112, 113]. Acidosis may increase ischemic damage by accelerating free radical production, perturbing intracellular signal transduction and activating pH-dependent endonuclease [114]. Another hypothesis is that the hyperglycemia may activate excitatory amino acids [115]. This activation leads to an excessive influx of calcium through ion channels, mitochondrial injury, and eventually cell death.

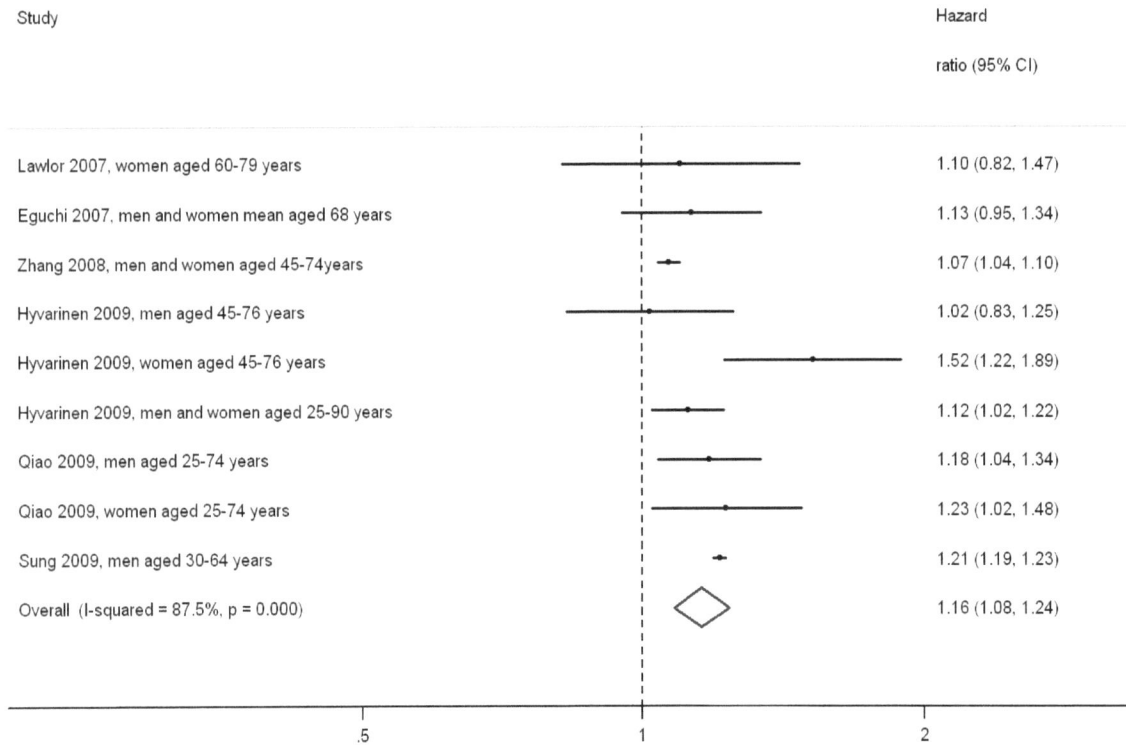

Figure 11: Hazard ratio (dot) and 95% confidence interval (bar) corresponding to a one standard deviation increase in fasting plasma glucose concentration (mmol/l or mg/dl) in relation to first fatal and non-fatal stroke events in participants without a history of diabetes.

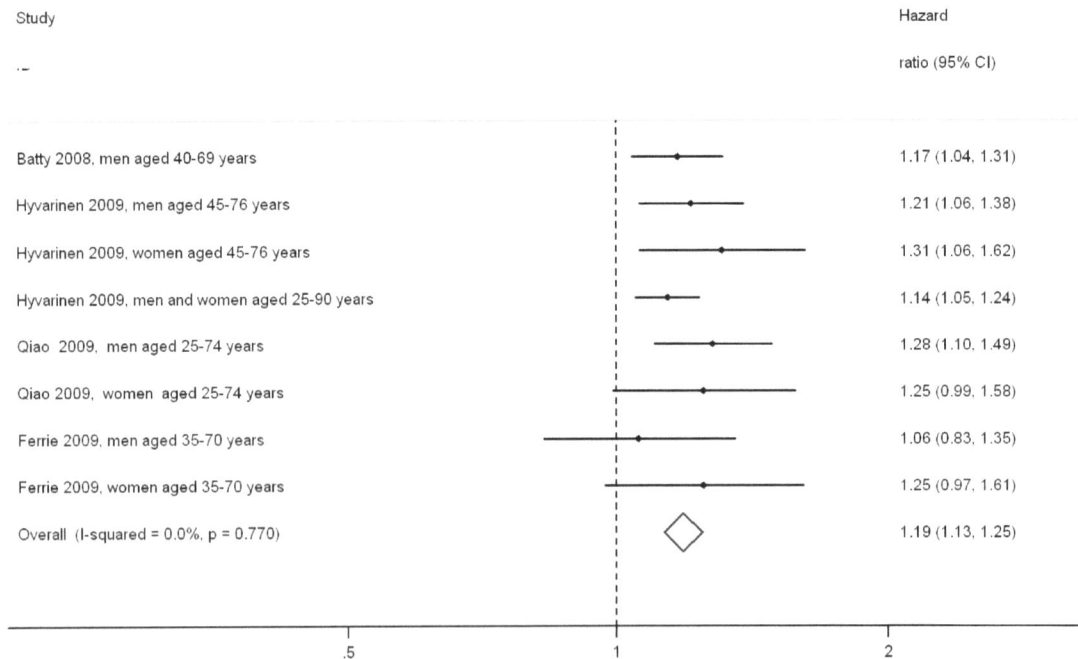

Figure 12: Hazard ratio (dot) and 95% confidence interval (bar) corresponding to a one standard deviation increase in 2-hour plasma glucose concentration (mmol/l or mg/dl) in relation to first fatal and non-fatal stroke events in participants without a history of diabetes.

8.3. HYPERTENSION IN RELATION TO GLYCEMIC LEVELS

The prevalence of diabetes is leading to increased rates of heart failure, MI and cardiovascular death. Hypertension is the leading global risk for mortality, responsible for 12.8% (7.5 million) of total deaths worldwide, according to a new report issued by the WHO [116]. Both diabetes and high Blood Pressure (BP) affect the same major target organs. They occur together so frequently that they are officially considered to be "comorbidities" [117-119]. Hypertension is known to be highly prevalent among patients with diabetes and associated with an increased risk of cardiovascular damage [120, 121]. Notably, hypertensive individuals are more predisposed to the development of diabetes than are normotensive persons. In a large prospective cohort study that included 12550 adults, the development of type 2 diabetes was almost 2.5 times as likely in persons with hypertension than in their normotensive counterparts [119]. In addition, IGT or IFG also greatly increased the CVD risk in prehypertensive people [122].

The common denominator of hypertensive/diabetic target organ disease is the vascular tree. Left ventricular hypertrophy and coronary artery disease are much more common in diabetic hypertensive patients than in patients suffering from hypertension or diabetes alone [123]. The combined presence of hypertension and diabetes concomitantly accelerates the decline in renal function [124-126], the development of diabetic retinopathy [127, 128] and the development of cerebral diseases [129-131]. Lowering BP to less than 130/80 mmHg is the primary goal for the management of hypertension in patients with diabetes [132, 133]. Randomized controlled trials that have included large diabetic populations including the United Kingdom Prospective Diabetes Study (UKPDS) [134], Hypertension Optimal Treatment (HOT) Trial [135], Systolic Hypertension in Europe (SHEP) trial [136], the Systolic Hypertension in Europe (Syst-EUR) trial [137], the Heart Outcomes Prevention Evaluation (HOPE) study [138], the Losartan Intervention For Endpoint reduction in hypertension study (LIFE) [139] and the Antihypertensive and Lipid-Lowering Treatment to Prevent Heart Attack Trial (ALLHAT) [140], have demonstrated that adequate BP control improves CVD outcomes, especially stroke, when aggressive BP targets are achieved.

8.3.1. Definition of Hypertension in Patients with Diabetes

Epidemiological studies and therapeutic trials have often used different criteria to define hypertension in diabetic patients. Studies in the general population indicate an increased risk of CVD with increasing level of BP. An increase in Systolic (SBP) or Diastolic Blood Pressure (DBP) of 5 mmHg is associated with a concomitant increase in CVD of 20-30% [141]. Previous studies in diabetic patients have shown a markedly higher frequency of the progression of diabetic retinopathy when DBP is over 70 mmHg [142]. Most early epidemiological studies have used a categorical definition of hypertension, using levels of 160 mmHg for SBP and 90 mmHg for DBP. Based on the current evidence from clinical trials showing significant benefits of treating hypertension in diabetic individuals, these values, however, are considered too high to serve as a threshold for the definition of hypertension in diabetic patients. Evidence obtained from clinical trials in diabetic patients suggests a continuum of risk and clinically significant benefit in outcomes with reductions of BP below 140 mmHg for SBP and 80 mmHg for DBP [143, 144]. Epidemiological studies indicate that there is a benefit to reducing SBP still further to 130 mmHg or below [145, 146]. Therefore, the Joint National Committee on Prevention, Detection, Evaluation, and Treatment of High Blood Pressure (JNC) VII report [133], the guidelines from the American Diabetes Association (ADA) [147] and the guidelines from the National Kidney Foundation (NKF) [148] have consistently recommended that BP in diabetic patients be controlled to levels of 130/80 mmHg or lower.

8.3.2. Prevalence and Risk Factors of Hypertension in Patients with Diabetes

Data from several epidemiologic studies have suggested that the prevalence of hypertension in patients with diabetes is approximately 1.5-3.0 times greater than in an appropriately matched nondiabetic population [149-154]. For example, a large cross-sectional survey of over 250000 patients from general practices across the United Kingdom reported that 56.2% of pharmacologically treated and 47.2% of diet-treated patients with diabetes had hypertension, as compared to 10.3% in those without diabetes [155]. In patients with type 1 diabetes, hypertension is generally not present at the time of diagnosis [156], the appearance of hypertension in type 1 diabetes is usually related to the presence and progress of kidney damage. In contrast, many patients with type 2 diabetes are already hypertensive at the time of diagnosis.

The major risk factors for high BP include older age [157-159], family history [160-162], overweight or obesity [163, 164], unhealthy lifestyle habits (too much sodium intake [165], lack of potassium intake [166], Vitamin D deficiency [167], excessive alcohol drinking [168-170], physical inactivity [171-173] and smoking [174] and stress [175, 176]. Since the prevalence of type 2 diabetes is high in obese subjects and it increases with age, the co-existence of diabetes and hypertension is particularly high in obese and/or elderly patients. In addition, compared to Caucasians and other ethnic groups, African-Americans are much more likely to have high BP [177]. It may account for over 40% of all-cause deaths in this ethnic group. High BP tends to start at a younger age among African-Americans, is often more severe, and causes greater risks for premature death from heart attack, stroke, heart failure, and kidney failure[177, 178] . Most studies in the United Kingdom and United States also report a higher prevalence and lower awareness of hypertension in black than in white people [179, 180]. Racial and ethnic differences in occurrence of BP may attribute to a complex relationship of gene and environment interactions [181, 182].

8.3.3. Pathophysiology of Hypertension in Patients with Diabetes

Epidemiologic studies provide evidence for co-existence of hypertension and diabetes and possibly point towards common genetic and environmental factors promoting the both conditions. Insulin resistance, increased tissue inflammation and Reactive Oxygen Species (ROS) production resulting in endothelial dysfunction and increased tissue Renin-Angiotensin-Aldosterone System (RAAS) have all been implicated in this complex pathophysiology of diabetes and hypertension [183-185]. Other possible causes of hypertension with diabetes include activation of the Sympathetic Nervous System (SNS), increased renal tubular sodium retention, elevated intracellular calcium concentration and vascular smooth muscle cell proliferation and impaired Nitric Oxide (NO) metabolism in skeletal muscle [186, 187]. Some studies even suggest that excess levels of insulin can interfere with compliance of the great vessels and decrease the ability of the aorta to reflect aortic waves [188].

8.3.3.1. Insulin Resistance

It is estimated that up to 50% of persons with hypertension are hyperinsulinemic or insulin resistant [183, 189]. The relationship of insulin resistance, diabetes and hypertension is complex and interrelated. Untreated patients with essential hypertension have higher fasting and postprandial insulin levels than age-and sex-matched normotensive persons, regardless of body mass index [183, 190, 191]. Interestingly, the relationship between hyperinsulinemia and hypertension is not seen in secondary hypertension [191]. This indicates that insulin resistance and hyperinsulinemia might not be the consequences of hypertension, but rather a genetic predisposition that acts as a fertile soil for both diabetes and hypertension. This is supported by the observation that there is impaired glucose regulation in the offspring of hypertensive patients [191, 192].

It is possible that insulin resistance and compensatory hyperinsulinemia have major roles in the regulation of BP in subjects predisposed to hypertension by hereditary susceptibility or environmental factors [187]. Enhanced sympathetic activity and diminished adrenal medullary activity would be important links between the defect in insulin action and the development of hypertension [193]. In hypertension, the main site of insulin resistance is represented by skeletal muscle, one of the major sites for glucose consumption involving the conversion of glucose to glycogen independent of blood flow [194]. The degree of resistance is related to the severity of hypertension. It has been suggested that hyperinsulinemia and insulin resistance may also contribute to the maintenance of an elevated BP because insulin is known to promote sodium retention and enhance sympathetic nervous system activity, leading to hypertension in individuals with obesity and other insulin-resistant states, such as type 2 diabetes [195].

8.3.3.2. Upregulation of Renin-Angiotensin-Aldosterone System (RAAS)

There is also a strong association between upregulation of RAAS, diabetes, and hypertension [184, 196]. This up-regulation of RAAS results enhanced generation of ROS and may explain impaired glucose utilisation as well as hypertension associated with insulin resistance and type 2 diabetes [197]. It has been suggested that increased autocrine/paracrine activity of angiotensin II(ANG II) results in diminished action of insulin and insulin growth factor-1 (IGF-1) signalling, inducing inhibition of mechanisms involved in the vasodilator and glucose transport properties of insulin and IGF-1 [197, 198].

Activation of the RAAS also results in increased aldosterone secretion from the adrenal gland and resultant salt retention and plasma volume expansion and consequent hypertension. Further, aldosterone also contributes to hypertension by enhancing sympathetic nervous system activity, decreasing parasympathetic activity, and reducing baroreceptor sensitivity [199]. Other effects of aldosteronein kidney including increased extracellular matrix deposition by glomerular cells also lead to glomerulosclerosis and hypertension [199].

8.3.3.3. Endothelial Dysfunction and Oxidative Stress

It is known that the endothelium mediates the ability of the blood vessels to modify their architecture in response to hemodynamic changes [185, 200, 201]. The normal endothelium reduces the vascular tonus by producing relaxation of the vascular wall and inhibiting the growth of the smooth muscle, adhesion and aggregation of platelets and leukocytes and thus preventing thrombosis [202], a process mediated by NO-originally described as endothelium-derived relaxing factor. NO is released from endothelial cells in response to shear stress produced by blood flow, and in response to activation of a variety of receptors. Diabetic patients show an elevated oxidative stress producing a larger amount of free radicals that inactivates the NO, and damage the coupling of the vasodilator to the endothelium receptor [203, 204]. The coexistence of hypertension and diabetes enhances the loss of the endothelium-mediated vasodilation, which could be explained by a low production of NO or by a reduction in the response to the NO in the vascular smooth muscle [205]. An alteration of the inhibitory function of the vascular endothelium that often seen in diabetic patients usually leads to vasoconstriction with an increase of the peripheral vascular resistance and raising in blood pressure, stimulation of the growth of the vascular smooth muscle and elevation of the adhesion and platelet aggregation [206], finally leading to cardiovascular events.

8.3.3.4. Abnormalities of Lipids

The consequence of insulin resistance in diabetes is a decrease of the synthesis and activity of the adipocyte lipoprotein lipase (LPL) since insulin acts as its major regulator and increases the activity of the liver lipase. This accelerates the synthesis and secretion of hepatic Very-Low-Density Lipoprotein (VLDL) rich in triglycerides, producing hypertriglyceridemia, reduction of HDL cholesterol, changes in the composition of the LDL generating small and dense LDL particles and accumulation of VLDL remnants and chylomycrons [207, 208]. All of these factors contribute to the genesis and persistence of hypertension in patients with diabetes. It has been demonstrated that hypercholesterolemia promotes an increased endothelial production of oxygen free radicals, which rapidly degrade NO molecules [209]. In addition, hypercholesterolemia reduces the synthesis of NO in endothelial cells *via* transcriptional inhibition of the endothelial NO synthase (NOS) gene, post-transcriptional mRNA destabilisation and competitive inhibition of NO generation by NOS [64, 210].

8.3.4. Management of Hypertension in Diabetes

Hypertension by itself is a powerful risk factor for cardiovascular morbidity and mortality as established by data from the Framingham study [211]. The presence of hypertension in diabetic patients substantially increases the risks of coronary heart disease, stroke, nephropathy and retinopathy [190, 212-214]. The higher the BP, the greater the chance of heart attack, heart failure, stroke and kidney diseases [133]. A meta-analysis from observational studies involving more than 1 million individuals have indicated that death from both ischemic heart disease and stroke increases progressively and linearly from levels as low as 115 mmHg SBP and 75 mmHg DBP upward [215]. In addition, longitudinal data obtained from the Framingham Heart Study have indicated that BP values between 130-139/85-89 mmHg are associated with a more than two-folds increase in relative risk from CVD as compared with those with BP levels below 120/80 mmHg [216]. In diabetic patients, BP is an important determinant of the risks of macro-vascular and micro-vascular complications of type 2 diabetes. However, in 4733 patients with type 2 diabetes at high risk for cardiovascular events, targeting a SBP of less than 120 mmHg, as compared with less than 140 mmHg, did not reduce the rate of a composite outcome of fatal and nonfatal major cardiovascular events, according to the Action to Control Cardiovascular Risk in Diabetes (ACCORD) blood pressure trial (ACCORD BP) [217].

The JNC VII recommends a target BP of <130/80 mmHg in order to prevent death and disability associated with high BP for individuals with diabetes [133]. Once hypertension is detected, both pharmacological and non-pharmacological interventions should be implemented. Lifestyle modification is paramount, along with medical therapy at the earliest detection of the pre-hypertensive patient.

8.3.4.1. Lifestyle Intervention

Lifestyle changes are critical in the management of hypertension among patients with diabetes. These changes should include reduced salt intake, improved diet, regular physical activity, weight management and smoking cessation. Weight loss has shown to be an effective therapy in hypertension management. Moreover, studies have shown that modest weight loss can lower or even eliminate the need for antihypertensive medication [218]. Patients should be advised to adopt the Dietary Approach to Stop Hypertension (DASH) eating plan, consisting of a low sodium, high potassium, low calorie (800-1500 kcal/day) and high fibre diet, as it is shown to be effective in lowering BP [219]. Coupled with diet, increased physical activity, such as walking for 30-45minutes at least five days a week, has been shown to improve BP, prevent or delay the incidence of hypertension, enhance antihypertensive drug efficacy and decrease cardiovascular risk [219, 220]. Smoking cessation and moderation of alcohol intake are also recommended by JNC VII and are clearly appropriate for all patients with diabetes [221].

8.3.4.2. Pharmacologic Treatment

Diabetic patients with blood pressures >130 mmHg systolic or >80 mmHg diastolic are candidates for antihypertensive treatment aimed at lowering BP to <130/80 mmHg. A large number of drugs are currently available for reducing BP. Regarding the selection of medications, clinical trials with diuretics, Angiotensin-Converting Enzyme Inhibitors (ACE-I), Angiotensin Receptor Blockers (ARBs), Beta blockers, and calcium antagonists have a demonstrated benefit in the treatment of hypertension in both type 1 and type 2 diabetes [134, 135, 137, 140]. More than two-thirds of hypertensive individuals cannot be controlled on one drug and usually require two or more antihypertensive agents selected from different drug classes [135, 139, 222, 223].

8.3.4.3. Angiotensin-Converting Enzyme Inhibitors (ACE-I)

A systematic review of the use of ACE-I in patients with diabetic nephropathy showed that treatment at maximum tolerable dosages was associated with a significant reduction in the risk of all-cause mortality [223]. It has been shown that interruption of the RAAS could provide cardio-protective properties [224]. Data from several studies, such as the Captopril Prevention Project (CAPPP) and the MICRO-HOPE study, a sub-study of the Heart Outcomes Prevention Evaluation (HOPE) trial, have demonstrated the cardiovascular benefits of ACE-I [224-226]. The HOPE trial [226] randomized patients with diabetes and at least one other cardiovascular risk factor to 10 mg of ramipril daily or placebo. Patients in the treatment arm had significantly lower all-cause mortality rates (10.8% *versus* 14.0%) and a lower risk of death from the combined outcome of MI, stroke or other cardiovascular events (15.3% *versus* 19.8%). ACE-I are also known to improve insulin sensitivity, retard the progression of diabetes and even prevent the development of diabetes in hypertensive patients by inhibiting RAAS [225, 227]. Notably, ACE-I have also been shown to slow progression of nephropathy in microalbuminuric, normotensive type 2 diabetes compared with other antihypertensive drugs [228, 229].

The NKF recommends ACE-I or ARBs as preferred agents for the treatment of hypertension in patients with diabetes and chronic kidney disease (stages 1, 2, 3, or 4) [148]. However, initiation of an ACE-I or ARB may cause a transient reduction in Glomerular Filtration Rate (GFR) and an increase in serum creatinine levels [230]. An acute increase in the serum creatinine level of greater than 30% or the development of hyperkalemia implies a requirement of dosage reduction or discontinuation of the drug [230, 231]. In contrast, transient elevations of less than 30% above baseline are associated with subsequent preservation of renal function and should not be considered grounds for cessation of therapy [230, 231].

8.3.4.3.1. Angiotensin Receptor Blockers (ARB)

ARBs can also prevent progression of diabetic kidney disease. In a randomized controlled trial of patients with type 2 diabetes and early nephropathy, telmisartan demonstrated non-inferiority compared with enalapril in preventing reductions in GFR [232]. No patient developed end-stage renal disease during the five-year study. The antihypertensive action of ARBs is roughly equivalent to ACE-I, but does have an improved side effect profile when compared with ACE-I. Therefore, it is considered as a first-line alternative for patients intolerant of ACE-I. Similar to ACE-I, ARBs have beneficial effects in reducing the progression of diabetes and carry other cardiovascular and renal benefits [224].

Several clinical trials demonstrate that ARBs have beneficial effects on glucose metabolism that are likely independent of bradykinin-mediated mechanisms [233, 234]. In the LIFE study, losartan reduced the relative risk of developing type 2 diabetes by 25% compared with the beta-blocker atenolol [235]. Similar reduction in the relative risk of developing diabetes was reported for candesartan and valsartan, respectively in the Candesartan in Heart failure: Assessment of Reduction in Mortality and morbidity (CHARM) study [234] and in the Valsartan Antihypertensive Long-term Use Evaluation (VALUE) trial [236]. Results from the Telmisartan Alone and in combination with Ramipril Global Endpoint Trial (ONTARGET), a double-blinded controlled trial set up to investigate the role of an ARB and an ACE-I, alone or in combination, in prevention the incidence of type 2 diabetes, showed that telmisartan was equivalent to ramipril in high-risk patients for diabetes and was associated with less angioedema. The combination of the two drugs was associated with more adverse events but without an increase in benefit [237].

Some recent studies have investigated to what extent does inhibition of the RAAS can reduce the incidence of new onset diabetes in patients with impaired glucose tolerance. The Diabetes Reduction Assessment with Ramipril and Rosiglitazone Medications (DREAM) trial is a large international multicentre randomized, prospective double-blind controlled trial involving 4, 000 people, randomized to receive either ramipril and/or rosiglitazone using a 2*2 factorial design and assessed for new onset diabetes. The use of ramipril for 3 years does not significantly reduce the incidence of diabetes or death but significantly increases regression to normoglycemia [238]. The Nateglinide and Valsartan in Impaired Glucose Tolerance Outcomes Research (NAVIGATOR) is another study that evaluates the effects of an oral antidiabetic drug, nateglinide, and an ARB, valsartan, on prevention of type 2 diabetes and CVD in patients with impaired glucose tolerance. The results of the NAVIGATOR study are largely negative. Neither drug (nor the combination) reduced the two co-primary cardiovascular outcomes. The only positive result was a weak, albeit statistically significant, reduction in the incidence of diabetes with valsartan. The relative reduction of 14% and the absolute reduction of 3.7 percentage points in incident diabetes with valsartan, as compared with placebo, over a mean follow-up of 5 years [239].

8.3.4.3.2. Beta Blockers

Beta blockers are an important component of antihypertensive regimens in patients who have diabetes, CAD, and stable angina [133, 240]. They usually act as a useful adjunct when combination therapy is needed to achieve target blood pressure in patients with diabetes [133]. The effectiveness of beta blockers was demonstrated in the UKPDS study, where atenolol was comparable with captopril in reducing the incidence of micro-vascular complications, MI, diabetes-related and all-cause mortality [241]. In addition, beta blockers significantly decrease post-MI mortality rates and mortality associated with heart failure [221, 240]. Although these agents have been associated with adverse effects on glucose metabolism, insulin sensitivity and lipid profiles [119, 242], they are not absolute contraindication for use in diabetic patients. Data from the UKPDS have not shown differences in the rates of minor or major hypoglycemic episodes in patients treated with atenolol compared with those treated with captopril [134]. Moreover, these changes are usually of little clinical significance and can be adequately managed through adjustment of the diabetes therapy, if necessary. In fact, carvedilol, which has both α-and β-receptor blocking properties, is less likely than traditional beta blockers to worsen insulin sensitivity in patients with diabetes [242]. However, it is not known if the neutral metabolic effects can lead to reduced morbidity and mortality rates.

8.3.4.3.3. Calcium Channel Blockers (CCB)

It has been shown that non-dihydropyridine CCBs, such as verapamil and diltiazem, can decrease proteinuria in diabetic patients receiving combination therapy with ACE-I [229]. The Syst-Eur trial with netrendipine demonstrated that intensive antihypertensive therapy for older patients with type 2 diabetes and isolated systolic hypertension eliminated the additional risk for CVD events and stroke associated with diabetes [243]. In the Hypertension Optimal Treatment (HOT) trial, there was a reduction in major CVD events with diastolic BP control in patients with diabetes when felodipine was used as first-line therapy [135]. Two large randomized controlled trials found a significantly greater risk of fatal and nonfatal MI in patients with type 2 diabetes who were treated with a dihydropyridine CCB compared with those treated with an ACE inhibitor [244, 245]. The ALLHAT study [140] found no significant difference in the incidence of nonfatal MI, fatal CHD, and all-cause mortality in patients treated with amlodipine compared with those treated with a diuretic; however, amlodipine was associated with a higher rate of heart failure (hazard ratio = 1.39; 95% confidence interval, 1.22 to 1.59).

Dihydropyridine and non-dihydropyridine CCBs are less effective than ACE-I and ARBs in slowing progression of diabetic kidney disease [148]. In one large randomized controlled trial, amlodipine was less effective than irbesartan, and no more effective than placebo in reducing progression to end-stage renal disease [246]. Because CCBs may be inferior to ARBs or ACE-I in some patient-oriented outcomes in those with diabetes, they should be reserved for patients who cannot tolerate preferred agents or those who need additional agents to achieve target blood pressure [148]. Thus, CCBs are not contraindicated in hypertensive patients with diabetes and the combination of an ACE-I/ARB and a calcium antagonistis effective for the management of hypertension in diabetic patients [247].

8.3.4.3.4. Thiazide Diuretics

Thiazide diuretics, either as monotherapy or as part of acombination regimen, are beneficial in the treatment of hypertension in patients with diabetes [133]. Thiazide diuretics have been shown to improve cardiovascular outcomes and may address the volume or salt-sensitive components of hypertension, complementing the mechanisms of action of other drugs, so these are appropriate choices for a second or third drug and can be used for initial therapy in patients without additional cardiovascular risk factors or proteinuria. In the SHEP study, chlorthalidone reduced cardiovascular and cerebrovascular events in patients with type 2 diabetes and isolated systolic hypertension [143]. The Antihypertensive and Lipid-lowering Treatment to Prevent Heart Attack Trial (ALLHAT), which compared chlorthalidone with amlodipine or an ACE-I (lisinopril), found that the thiazide was less expensive and superior to the ACE-I or CCB in lowering the incidence of CVD in hypertensive individuals [140]. Treating volume expansion with thiazide diuretics can increase the activity of the RAAS. Thus, combining a diuretic with an ACE-I or an ARB can be an effective BP lowering combination. The effect of thiazide diuretics on the progression of diabetic nephropathy compared with other drugs is unknown.

Thiazide diuretics are less effective in patients with diminished renal function; patients with a GFR of less than 50 mL per min per 1.73 m^2 may require a loop diuretic [147]. Metabolic alterations are a potential concern with the use of thiazide diuretics. High dosages have been linked to elevations in cholesterol and triglycerides levels and loss of glycemic control; however, these dosages are not routinely used in clinical practice [248]. When used in low to moderate dosages (*i.e.*, up to 25 mg of hydrochlorothiazide per day), the risk of clinically significant alterations in glucose metabolism is minimal.

8.3.4.3.5. Combination Therapy

When the target blood pressure is not achieved with lifestyle modifications, ACE inhibitors are recommended as first-line therapy for patients with diabetes and hypertension [148, 249]. ARBs may be used in patients who cannot tolerate ACE-I. Most patients with diabetes require combination therapy to attain a blood pressure of less than 130/80 mmHg [133, 148, 249]. If the use of ACE-I or ARB does not provide satisfactory blood pressure reduction, the addition of a thiazide diuretic is the next step [249]. In patients with significant renal insufficiency, a loop diuretic may be used instead; however, there is not sufficient data from clinical trials to support this recommendation. For most patients, beta blockers or CCBs are third-line agents [148]. If BP is not controlled with the addition of a beta blocker, a CCB should be added (or *vice versa*). Antihypertensive medications with different mechanisms of action should be used. Many fixed-dose combinations are available and should be considered if more than one agent is needed to control blood pressure [250].

In general, the combination of a beta blocker and a nondihydropyridine CCB should be avoided because of the risk of bradycardia and heart block. Alternative agents, such as alpha blockers and hydralazine, may be considered in patients with resistant hypertension. These patients should be evaluated for adherence, and referral to a subspecialist should be considered [221, 249]. Finally, treatment decisions should, of course, be individualized based on the clinical characteristics of the patient, including comorbidities as well as tolerability, personal preference and cost.

8.4. INTENSIVE GLUCOSE CONTROL AND CVD RISK

The UKPDS is the first randomized controlled clinical trial among 3867 patients with newly diagnosed type 2 diabetes recruited between 1977 and 1991 to evaluate the effect of intensive *versus* the conventional glucose control on the risk of micro-vascular and macro-vascular complications of diabetic patients. In 1997, with a median trial period of 10 years, the study has unequivocally shown that patients in the intensive glucose control arm (sulfonylurea and insulin treatment) had a 25% (p=0.0099) lower risk to have diabetic retinopathy and nephropathy, and a 16% (p=0.052) lower risk to get MI than the patients in the conventional glucose control arm [251]. At the trial end in 1997, patients were returned to usual physician care for their diabetes management, and no attempt was made to influence their therapy or to maintain them in randomized groups. The trial participants were, however, monitored regarding their clinical outcomes for 10-years from 1997 to 2007 [252]. The study found that 10 years after the trial, patients in the intensive treatment group with sulfonylurea and insulin remained a lower risk for MI (15%, p=0.01) and for any cause death (13%, p=0.007) as compared with conventional-therapy group (Fig. **13**) [252].

Following the UKPDS, other randomized controlled clinical trials have been conducted to examine the effect of intensive glucose control on the CVD outcomes among either patients with type 2 diabetes [253-256] or individuals with IGT [239, 257]. The ACCORD [120, 253, 254], the ADVANCE (Action in Diabetes and Vascular Disease: Preterax and Diamicron Modified Release Controlled Evaluation) [254], the VADT [125, 258] (Veterans Affairs Diabetes Trial) [255, 258] and the PROactive (PROspective pioglitAzone Clinical Trial In macroVascular Events) [256, 259, 260], all showed a reduction in either single or composite CVD events in the intensive treatment groups as compared with control treatment groups but the risk reduction was borderline significant or not significant in most of the individual trials. Meta-analysis based on all 5 trials showed a significant risk reduction in non-fatal MI (-17%) and in CHD (-15%), but not in stroke and all-cause deaths (Figs. **14-17**) [261].

It should be pointed out that the inclusion criteria, therapeutic regimens and glucose target goals varied across the trials. Different combinations of diet, metformin or insulin therapies were applied to achieve different target levels of intensive glucose control (FPG < 6.0 mmol/l for the UKPDS trial, HbA1c < 6.0% for the ACCORD and the VADT or HbA1c ≤ 6.5% for the ADVANCE and the PROactive) with the trial durations ranging from 3.5 to 10.7 years. Thus, some potential factors, such as long duration of diabetes, history of hypoglycemia or atherosclerosis and advanced age, might diminish the effect of intensive glycemic control on the end events [262]. Nevertheless, intensive glucose-lowering therapies were noted to be associated with a wide range of unexpected adverse consequences, such as weight gain, heart failure and hypoglycemia [251, 255, 263, 264]. Severe hypoglycemia was associated with a significant increase in the risks of major macro-vascular disease (death from a cardiovascular cause, nonfatal MI, or nonfatal stroke) and death from any cause in the ADVANCE trial with a median follow-up of 5 years, with HRs of 2.88(2.01-4.12) and 2.69(1.97-3.67), respectively [263]. Determining the causes of the excess deaths will inform the design of future studies to examine the association between intensive glycemic control and cardiovascular risk.

In conclusion, accumulative epidemiological evidences have unequivocally shown that elevated glycemic levels are risk factors for both fatal and non-fatal CVD events. But the results from randomized controlled clinical trials have not provided with convincing evidences showing the effect of intensive glucose control on CVD risk reduction. Only a modest risk reduction in the CHD morbidity and mortality has been obtained with the intensive glucose control but not in stroke and all-cause mortality. Well designed clinical trials and observational studies are still required to investigate the relationship between hyperglycemia and CVD risk, particularly the impact of age, gender and ethnicities on the relationship.

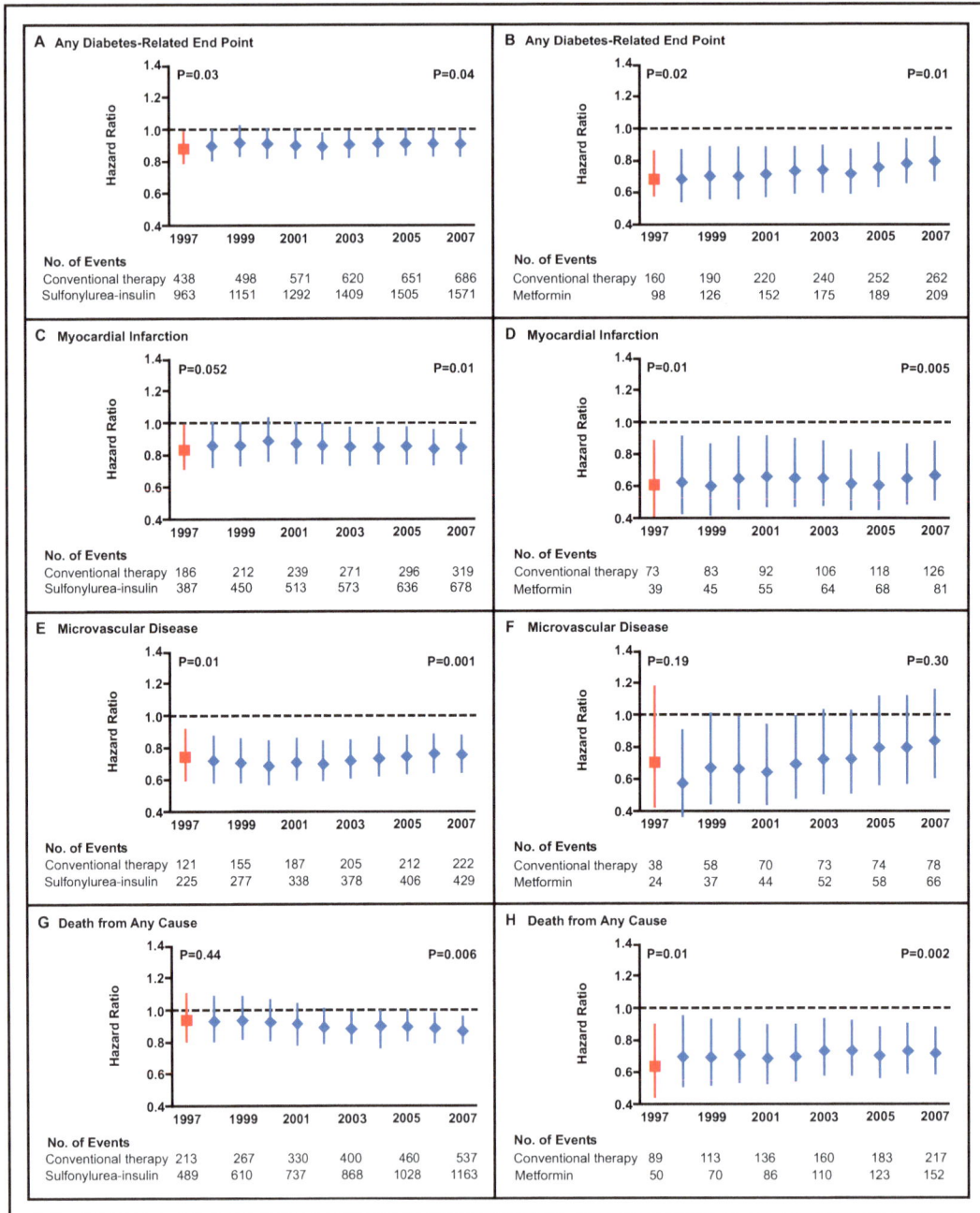

Figure 13: Hazard ratios for four prespecified aggregate clinical outcomes. Hazard ratios for patients in the United Kingdom Prospective Diabetes Study who had any diabetes-related end point (Panels A and B), myocardial infarction (Panels C and D), or micro-vascular disease (Panels E and F) or who died from any cause (Panels G and H) are shown for the sulfonylurea-insulin group *versus* the conventional-therapy group and for the metformin group *versus* the conventional-therapy group. The overall values at the end of the study in 1997, are shown (red squares), along with the annual values during the 10-year post-trial monitoring period (blue diamonds). Hazard ratios below unity indicate a favorable outcome from sulfonylurea or metformin therapy. Numbers of first events in an aggregate outcome that accumulated in each group are shown at 2-year intervals. The vertical bars represent 95% confidence intervals. This figure was adapted from [252].

	Intensive treatment/ standard treatment		Weight of study size	Odds ratio (95%CI)	Odds ratio (95%CI)
	Participants	Events			
UKPDS[4.7]	3071/1549	221/141	21.8%		0.78(0.62-0.98)
PROactive[18-20]	2605/2633	119/144	18.0%		0.83(0.64-1.06)
ADVANCE[5]	5571/5569	153/156	21.9%		0.98(0.78-1.23)
VADT[21,22]	892/899	64/78	9.4%		0.81(0.58-1.15)
ACCORD[8]	5128/5123	186/235	28.9%		0.78(0.64-0.95)
Overall	17267/15773	743/754	100%		**0.83(0.75-0.93)**

0.4   0.6   0.8   1.0   1.2   1.4 1.6 1.8 2.0

Intensive treatment better   Standard treatment better

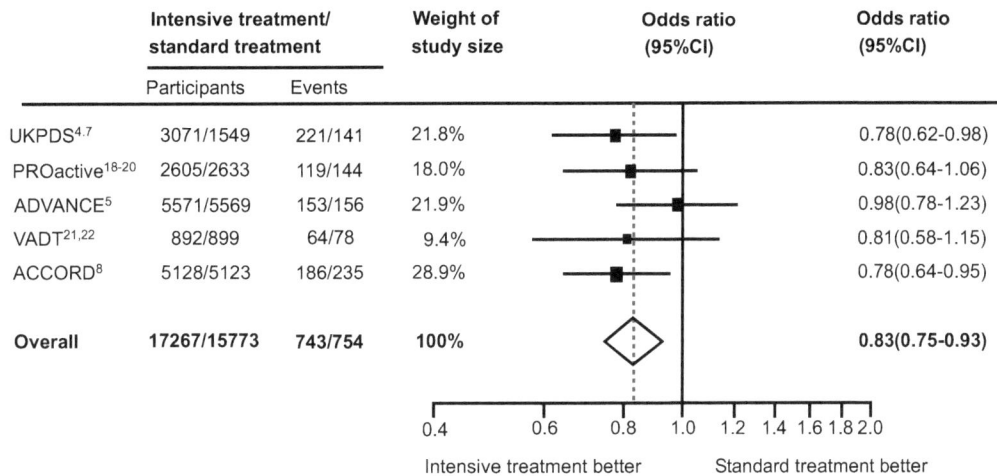

Figure 14: Probability of events of non-fatal myocardial infarction with intensive glucose-lowering *versus* standard treatment. This figure was adapted from [261].

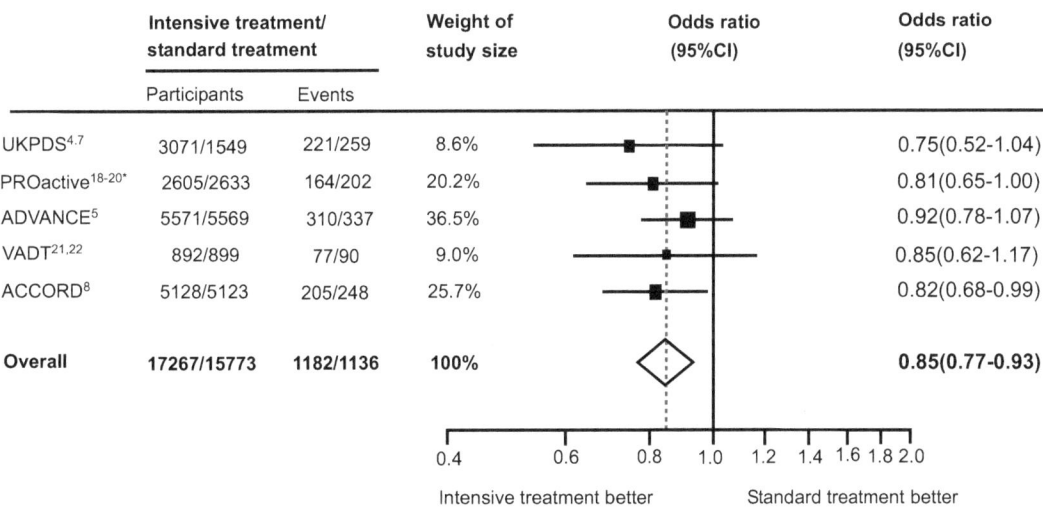

	Intensive treatment/ standard treatment		Weight of study size	Odds ratio (95%CI)	Odds ratio (95%CI)
	Participants	Events			
UKPDS[4.7]	3071/1549	221/259	8.6%		0.75(0.52-1.04)
PROactive[18-20*]	2605/2633	164/202	20.2%		0.81(0.65-1.00)
ADVANCE[5]	5571/5569	310/337	36.5%		0.92(0.78-1.07)
VADT[21,22]	892/899	77/90	9.0%		0.85(0.62-1.17)
ACCORD[8]	5128/5123	205/248	25.7%		0.82(0.68-0.99)
Overall	17267/15773	1182/1136	100%		**0.85(0.77-0.93)**

0.4   0.6   0.8   1.0   1.2   1.4 1.6 1.8 2.0

Intensive treatment better   Standard treatment better

Figure 15: Probability of events of coronary heart disease with intensive glucose-lowering *versus* standard Treatment. *Included non-fatal myocardial infarction and death from all-cardiac mortality. This figure was adapted from [261].

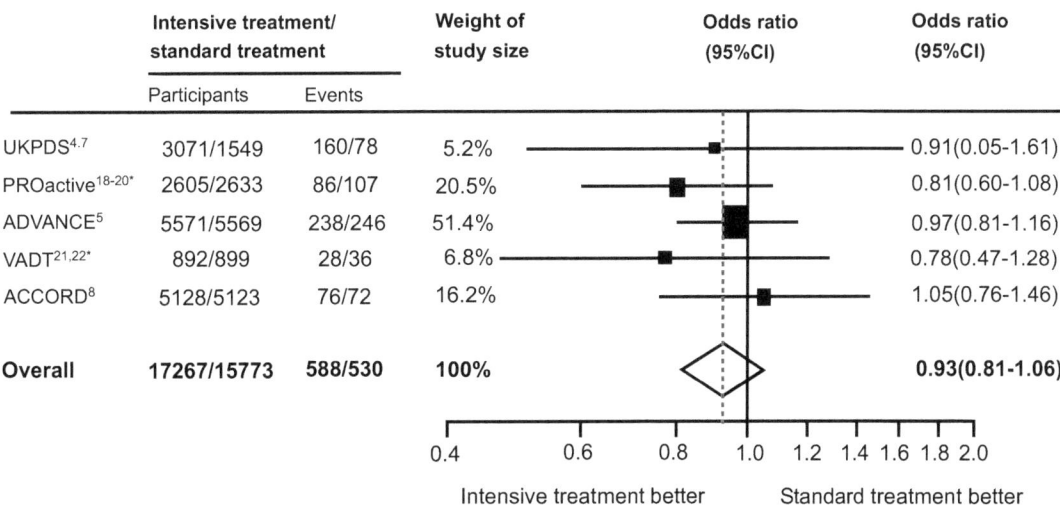

	Intensive treatment/ standard treatment		Weight of study size	Odds ratio (95%CI)	Odds ratio (95%CI)
	Participants	Events			
UKPDS[4.7]	3071/1549	160/78	5.2%		0.91(0.05-1.61)
PROactive[18-20*]	2605/2633	86/107	20.5%		0.81(0.60-1.08)
ADVANCE[5]	5571/5569	238/246	51.4%		0.97(0.81-1.16)
VADT[21,22*]	892/899	28/36	6.8%		0.78(0.47-1.28)
ACCORD[8]	5128/5123	76/72	16.2%		1.05(0.76-1.46)
Overall	17267/15773	588/530	100%		**0.93(0.81-1.06)**

0.4   0.6   0.8   1.0   1.2   1.4 1.6 1.8 2.0

Intensive treatment better   Standard treatment better

Figure 16: Probability of events of stroke with intensive glucose-lowering *versus* standard treatment *Included only non-fatal strokes. This figure was adapted from [261].

Intensive treatment/ standard treatment		Weight of study size	Odds ratio (95%CI)	Odds ratio (95%CI)
Participants	Events			
UKPDS[4,7] 3071/1549	539/302	10.1%		0.79(0.53-1.20)
PROactive[18-20] 2605/2633	177/186	21.5%		0.96(0.77-1.19)
ADVANCE[5] 5571/5569	498/533	29.4%		0.93(0.82-1.05)
VADT[21,22] 892/899	102/95	15.5%		1.09(0.81-1.47)
ACCORD[8] 5128/5123	257/203	23.6%		1.28(1.06-1.54)
Overall **17267/15773**	**1573/1319**	**100%**		**1.02(0.87-1.19)**

0.4   0.6   0.8   1.0   1.2 1.4 1.6 1.8 2.0

Intensive treatment better   Standard treatment better

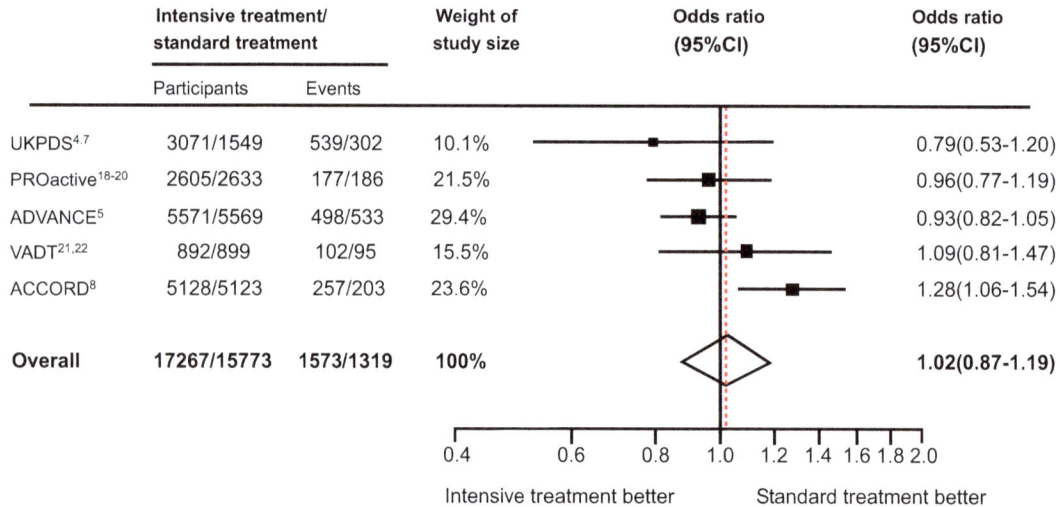

Figure 17: Probability of events of all-cause mortality with intensive glucose-lowering *versus* standard Treatment. This figure was adapted from [261].

In spite of the strong epidemiological evidence that shows individuals with IGT have increased CVD risk, the NAVIGATOR trial is the first and the only randomized controlled clinical trial to investigate the effect of intensive treatment of postprandial hyperglycemia on CVD outcomes [239, 257, 265]. The NAVIGATOR trial recruited 9306 participants from 806 centers of 40 countries with IGT who had concurrent CVD or CVD risk factors at enrolment. Lifestyle modification was administrated to all participants. Participants were randomized into one of the four arms: Valsartan/Nateglinide, Valsartan/placebo, Nateglinide/placebo and placebo/placebo. Primary CVD events include extended cardiovascular outcome (cardiovascular death, nonfatal MI, nonfatal stroke, hospitalization for heart failure, arterial revascularization, or unstable angina) and core cardiovascular outcome (cardiovascular death, nonfatal MI, nonfatal stroke, or hospitalization for heart failure). After a median follow-up of 6.5-years, neither the extended cardiovascular outcome nor the core cardiovascular outcome has been reduced in either the Nateglinide (Figs. **18** and **19**) or the Valsartan (Figs. **20** and **21**) groups as compared with the placebo group. The NAVIGATOR trial failed to show that control of postprandial hyperglycemia can reduce the cardiovascular outcomes in IGT individuals who had unfavorable CVD risk profiles [239, 257]. Factors that might have diluted the outcome of the NAVIGATOR include using other antihypertensive medications and high drop-out rate in both arms, and higher weight in the intervention arm than in the control arm (0.35 kg in the Nateglinide group and 0.28 kg in the Valsartan group, p<0.001 for both) [239, 257].

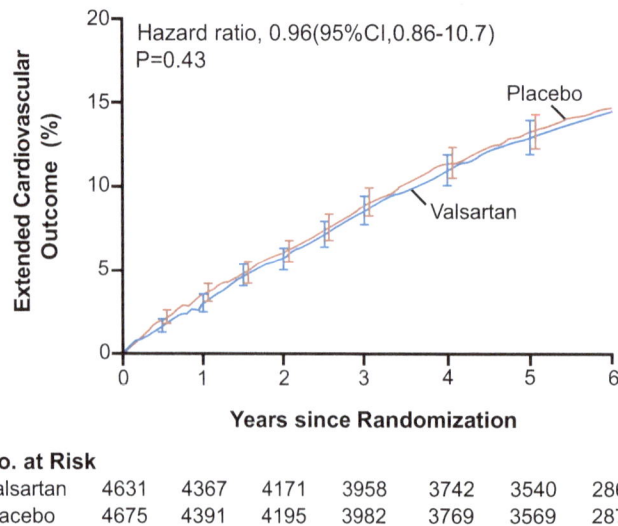

Hazard ratio, 0.96(95%CI,0.86-10.7)
P=0.43

No. at Risk							
Valsartan	4631	4367	4171	3958	3742	3540	2864
Placebo	4675	4391	4195	3982	3769	3569	2872

Figure 18: Kaplan-Meier Curves for the coprimary extended cardiovascular outcomes in the Nateglinide and placebo groups. This figure was adapted from [239].

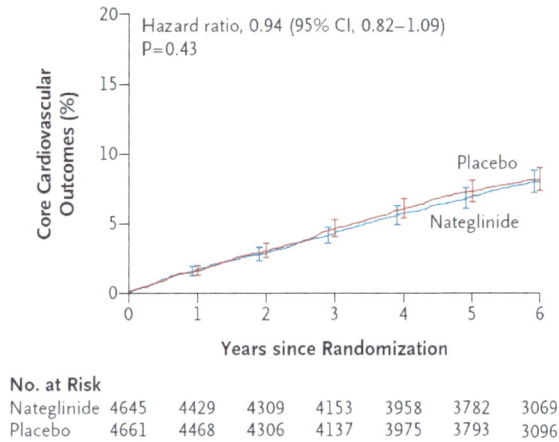

Figure 19: Kaplan-Meier Curves for the coprimary core cardiovascular outcomes in the Nateglinide and placebo groups. This figure was adapted from [239].

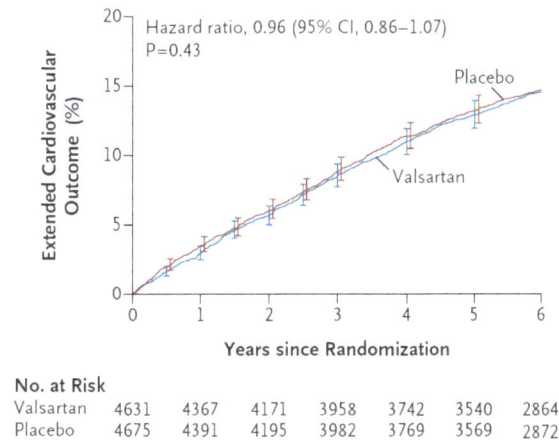

Figure 20: Kaplan-Meier Curves for the coprimary extended cardiovascular outcomes in the Valsartan and placebo groups. This figure was adapted from [257].

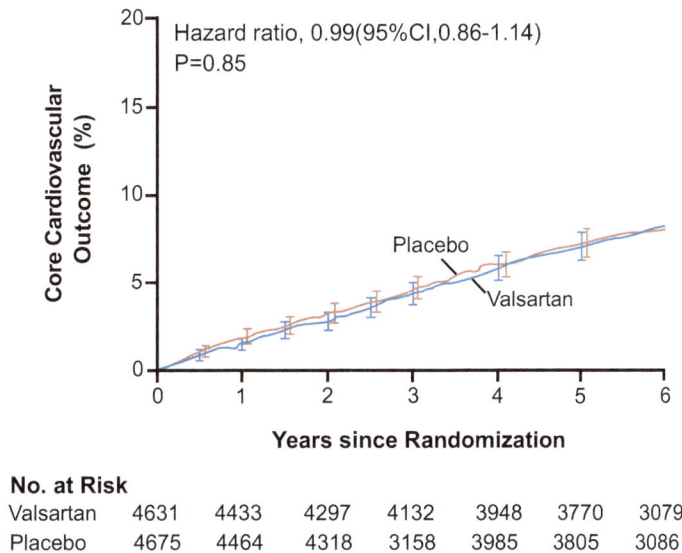

Figure 21: Kaplan-Meier Curves for the coprimary core cardiovascular outcomes in the Valsartan and placebo groups. This figure was adapted from [257].

REFERENCES

[1] Howard BV, Lee ET, Fabsitz RR, *et al.* Diabetes and coronary heart disease in American Indians: The Strong Heart Study. Diabetes 1996; 45 (Suppl 3): S6-13.

[2] Magliano DJ, Söderberg S, Zimmet PZ, *et al.* Mortality, all-cause and CVD, over 15 years in multi-ethnic Mauritius: the impact of diabetes and intermediate forms of glucose tolerance. Diabetes Care 2010; 33:1983-9.

[3] Qiao Q, Tuomilehto J, Moltchanova E, Balkau B, Borch-Johnsen K. The DECODE study group. Is the current definition for diabetes relevant to mortality risk from all causes and cardiovascular and noncardiovascular diseases? Diabetes Care 2003; 26: 688-96.

[4] Qiao Q, Tuomilehto J. The DECODE study group. Glucose tolerance and cardiovascular mortality: comparison of fasting and 2-hour diagnostic criteria. Arch Intern Med 2001;161:397-405.

[5] Fujishima M, Kiyohara Y, Kato I, *et al.* Diabetes and cardiovascular disease in a prospective population survey in japan: The Hisayama Study. Diabetes 1996; 45:14S-16S.

[6] Huxley R, Barzi F, Woodward M. Excess risk of fatal coronary heart disease associated with diabetes in men and women: meta-analysis of 37 prospective cohort studies. BMJ 2006; 332:73-8.

[7] Sarwar N, Gao P, Seshasai SR, *et al.* Emerging Risk Factors Collaboration. Diabetes mellitus, fasting blood glucose concentration, and risk of vascular disease: a collaborative meta-analysis of 102 prospective studies. Lancet 2010; 375:2215-22.

[8] Haffner SM, Lehto S, Rönnemaa T, Pyörälä K, Laakso M. Mortality from Coronary Heart Disease in Subjects with Type 2 Diabetes and in Nondiabetic Subjects with and without Prior Myocardial Infarction. N Engl J Med 1998; 339: 229-34.

[9] Malmberg K, Yusuf S, Gerstein HC, *et al.* Impact of diabetes on long-term prognosis in patients with unstable angina and non-q-wave myocardial infarction : results of the oasis (organization to assess strategies for ischemic syndromes) registry. Circulation 2000; 102:1014-9.

[10] Hu FB, Stampfer MJ, Solomon CG, *et al.* The impact of Diabetes Mellitus on mortality from all causes and coronary heart disease in women: 20 years of follow-up. Arch Intern Med 2001; 161:1717-23.

[11] Vaccaro O, Eberly LE, Neaton JD, *et al.* Impact of diabetes and previous myocardial infarction on long-term survival: 25-year mortality follow-up of primary screenees of the multiple risk factor intervention trial. Arch Intern Med 2004; 164:1438-43.

[12] Lee CD, Folsom AR, Pankow JS, Brancati FL for the Atherosclerosis Risk in Communities (ARIC) Study Investigators. Cardiovascular events in diabetic and nondiabetic adults with or without history of myocardial infarction. Circulation 2004; 109: 855-60.

[13] Cho E, Rimm EB, Stampfer MJ, Willett WC, Hu FB. The impact of diabetes mellitus and prior myocardial infarction on mortality from all causes and from coronary heart disease in men. J Am Coll Cardiol 2002; 40: 954-60.

[14] Bulugahapitiya U, Siyambalapitiya S, Sithole J, Idris I. Is diabetes a coronary risk equivalent? Systematic review and meta-analysis. Diabet Med 2009; 26:142-8.

[15] Nakagami T. Hyperglycemia and mortality from all causes and from cardiovascular disease in five populations of Asian origin. Diabetologia 2004; 47:385-94.

[16] Qiao Q, Tuomilehto J, Borch-Johnsen K. Post-challenge hyperglycemia is associated with premature death and macrovascular complications. Diabetologia2003; 46 (Suppl 1): M17-21.

[17] Niskanen L, Turpeinen A, Penttilä I, Uusitupa MI. Hyperglycemia and compositional lipoprotein abnormalities as predictors of cardiovascular mortality in type 2 diabetes: a 15-years follow-up from the time of diagnosis. Diabetes Care 1998; 21:1861-9.

[18] Crouse JR, Goldbourt U, Evans G, *et al.* Risk factors and segment-specific carotid arterial enlargement in the atherosclerosis risk in communities (ARIC) cohort. Stroke 1996; 27: 69-75.

[19] Crouse J, Toole J, McKinney W, *et al.* Risk factors for extracranial carotid artery atherosclerosis. Stroke 1987; 18: 990-6.

[20] Poli A, Tremoli E, Colombo A, Sirtori M, Pignoli P, Paoletti R. Ultrasonographic measurement of the common carotid artery wall thickness in hypercholesterolemic patients A new model for the quantitation and follow-up of preclinical atherosclerosis in living human subjects. Atherosclerosis 1988; 70: 253-61.

[21] O'Leary DH, Polak JF, Kronmal RA, Manolio TA, Burke GL, Wolfson SK. Carotid-artery intima and media thickness as a risk factor for myocardial infarction and stroke in older adults. N Engl J Med 1999; 340: 14-22.

[22] Lorenz MW, Markus HS, Bots ML, Rosvall M, Sitzer M. Prediction of clinical cardiovascular events with carotid intima-media thickness: a systematic review and meta-analysis. Circulation 2007; 115: 459-67.

[23]   Brohall G, Oden A and Fagerberg B. Carotid artery intima-media thickness in patients with Type 2 diabetes mellitus and impaired glucose tolerance: a systematic review. Diabet Med 2006; 23: 609-16.

[24]   Levitan EB, Song Y, Ford ES, Liu S. Is nondiabetic hyperglycemia a risk factor for cardiovascular disease? A meta-analysis of prospective studies. Arch Intern Med 2004; 164: 2147-55.

[25]   Barr EL, Boyko EJ, Zimmet PZ, Wolfe R, Tonkin AM, Shaw JE. Continuous relationships between non-diabetic hyperglycemia and both cardiovascular disease and all-cause mortality: the Australian Diabetes, Obesity, and Lifestyle (AusDiab) study. Diabetologia 2009; 52: 415-24.

[26]   Wandell PE, Theobald H. The association between low fasting blood glucose value and mortality. Curr Diabetes Rev 2007; 3: 274-9.

[27]   Wei M, Gibbons LW, Mitchell TL, Kampert JB, Stern MP, Blair SN. Low fasting plasma glucose level as a predictor of cardiovascular disease and all-cause mortality. Circulation 2000; 101: 2047-52.

[28]   Coutinho M, Gerstein HC, Wang Y and Yusuf S. The relationship between glucose and incident cardiovascular events. A metaregression analysis of published data from 20 studies of 95, 783 individuals followed for 12.4 years. Diabetes Care 1999; 22: 233-40.

[29]   The International Collaborative Group. Asymptomatic hyperglycemia and coronary heart disease. A series of papers by the International Collaborative Group, based on studies in fifteen populations. Introduction. J Chronic Dis 1979; 32: 683-91.

[30]   Epstein FH. Hyperglycemia as a risk factor for coronary heart disease. Monogr Atheroscler 1985; 13: 92-7.

[31]   Higgins JP, Thompson SG. Quantifying heterogeneity in a meta-analysis. Stat Med 2002; 21:1539-58.

[32]   American Diabetes Association. Executive Summary: Standards of Medical Care in Diabetes-2010. Diabetes Care 2010; 33: S4-S10.

[33]   Park S, Barrett-Connor E, Wingard DL, Shan J, Edelstein S. GHb is a better predictor of cardiovascular disease than fasting or postchallenge plasma glucose in women without diabetes. The Rancho Bernardo Study. Diabetes Care 1996; 19: 450-6.

[34]   Khaw K, Wareham N, Bingham S, Luben R, Welch A, Day N. Association of hemoglobin A1c with cardiovascular disease and mortality in adults: the european prospective investigation into cancer in Norfolk. Ann Intern Med 2004; 141: 413-20.

[35]   Selvin E, Steffes MW, Zhu H, *et al.* Glycated hemoglobin, diabetes, and cardiovascular risk in nondiabetic adults. N Engl J Med 2010; 362: 800-11.

[36]   Florkowski CM, Scott RS, Moir CL, Graham PJ. Lipid but not glycemic parameters predict total mortality from type 2 diabetes mellitus in Canterbury, New Zealand. Diabet Med 1998; 15: 386-92.

[37]   Mattock MB, Barnes DJ, Viberti G, *et al.* Microalbuminuria and coronary heart disease in NIDDM: an incidence study. Diabetes 1998; 47: 1786-92.

[38]   Stratton IM, Adler AI, Neil HAW, *et al.* Association of glycemia with macrovascular and micro-vascular complications of type 2 diabetes (UKPDS 35): prospective observational study. BMJ 2000; 321: 405-12.

[39]   Sarwar N, Aspelund T, Eiriksdottir G, *et al.* Markers of dysglycemia and risk of coronary heart disease in people without diabetes: Reykjavik prospective study and systematic review. PLoS Med 2010;7:e1000278.

[40]   Barr EL, Zimmet PZ, Welborn TA, *et al.* Risk of cardiovascular and all-cause mortality in individuals with diabetes mellitus, impaired fasting glucose, and impaired glucose tolerance: the Australian Diabetes, Obesity, and Lifestyle Study (AusDiab). Circulation 2007; 116: 151-7.

[41]   Levitzky YS, Pencina MJ, D'Agostino RB, *et al.* Impact of impaired fasting glucose on cardiovascular disease: the framingham heart study. J Am Coll Cardiol 2008; 51: 264-70.

[42]   Jarrett RJ, McCartney P, Keen H. The Bedford survey: ten year mortality rates in newly diagnosed diabetics, borderline diabetics and normoglycemic controls and risk indices for coronary heart disease in borderline diabetics. Diabetologia 1982; 22: 79-84.

[43]   Tominaga M, Eguchi H, Manaka H, Igarashi K, Kato T, Sekikawa A. Impaired glucose tolerance is a risk factor for cardiovascular disease, but not impaired fasting glucose. The Funagata Diabetes Study. Diabetes Care 1999; 22: 920-4.

[44]   Qiao Q, Jousilahti P, Eriksson J, Tuomilehto J. Predictive properties of impaired glucose tolerance for cardiovascular risk are not explained by the development of overt diabetes during follow-up. Diabetes Care 2003; 26: 2910-4.

[45]   Zhang YF, Hong J, Zhan WW, *et al.* Hyperglycemia after glucose loading is a major predictor of preclinical atherosclerosis in nondiabetic subjects. Clin Endocrinol (Oxf) 2006; 64: 153-7.

[46]   Mohan V, Gokulakrishnan K, Sandeep S, Srivastava BK, Ravikumar R, Deepa R. Intimal media thickness, glucose intolerance and metabolic syndrome in Asian Indians-the Chennai Urban Rural Epidemiology Study (CURES-22). Diabet Med 2006; 23: 845-50.

[47]   Wagenknecht LE, D'Agostino RB, Haffner SM, Savage PJ, Rewers M. Impaired glucose tolerance, Type 2 Diabetes, and carotid wall thickness: the insulin resistance atherosclerosis study. Diabetes Care 1998; 21: 1812-8.

[48]   Tuomilehto J, Qiao Q, Salonen R, Nissinen A, Salonen JT. Ultrasonographic manifestations of carotid atherosclerosis and glucose intolerance in elderly eastern Finnish men. Diabetes Care 1998; 21: 1349-52.

[49]   Brohall G, Schmidt C, Behre CJ, Hulthe J, Wikstrand J, Fagerberg B. Association between impaired glucose tolerance and carotid atherosclerosis: a study in 64-years-old women and a meta-analysis. Nutr Metab Cardiovasc Dis 2009; 19: 327-33.

[50]   Stern MP, Williams K, Haffner SM. Identification of persons at high risk for type 2 diabetes mellitus: do we need the oral glucose tolerance test? Ann Intern Med 2002; 136:575-81.

[51]   Barrett-Connor E, Wingard DL, Criqui MH, Suarez L. Is borderline fasting hyperglycemia a risk factor for cardiovascular death? J Chronic Dis 1984; 37: 773-9.

[52]   Cederberg H, Saukkonen T, Laakso M, et al. Postchallenge glucose, HbA1c, and fasting glucose as predictors of type 2 diabetes and cardiovascular disease. Diabetes Care 2010; 33: 2077-83.

[53]   Smith NL, Barzilay JI, Shaffer D, et al. Fasting and 2-hours postchallenge serum glucose measures and risk of incident cardiovascular events in the elderly: the cardiovascular health study. Arch Intern Med 2002; 162: 209-16.

[54]   Tuomilehto J, Qiao Q, Borch-Johnsen K, Balkau B. The DECODE study group. Glucose tolerance and mortality: comparison of WHO and American Diabetes Association diagnostic criteria. European Diabetes Epidemiology Group. Diabetes Epidemiology: Collaborative analysis Of Diagnostic criteria in Europe. Lancet 1999; 354: 617-21.

[55]   Hyvarinen M, Qiao Q, Tuomilehto J, et al. Hyperglycemia and stroke mortality: comparison between fasting and 2-h glucose criteria. Diabetes Care 2009; 32: 348-54.

[56]   Meigs JB, Nathan DM, D'Agostino RB, Wilson PWF. Fasting and postchallenge glycemia and cardiovascular disease risk. Diabetes Care 2002; 25: 1845-50.

[57]   Laakso M, Zilinskaite J, Hansen T, et al. Insulin sensitivity, insulin release and glucagon-like peptide-1 levels in persons with impaired fasting glucose and/or impaired glucose tolerance in the EUGENE2 study. Diabetologia 2008; 51: 502-11.

[58]   Nathan DM, Davidson MB, DeFronzo RA, et al. Impaired fasting glucose and impaired glucose tolerance. Diabetes Care 2007; 30:753-759.

[59]   Festa A, D'Agostino R, Hanley AJG, Karter AJ, Saad MF, Haffner SM. Differences in insulin resistance in nondiabetic subjects with isolated impaired glucose tolerance or isolated impaired fasting glucose. Diabetes 2004; 53: 1549-55.

[60]   Meyer C, Pimenta W, Woerle HJ, et al. Different mechanisms for impaired fasting glucose and impaired postprandial glucose tolerance in humans. Diabetes Care 2006; 29: 1909-14.

[61]   Dignat-George F, Sampol J. Circulating endothelial cells in vascular disorders: new insights into an old concept. Eur J Haematol 2000; 65: 215-20.

[62]   Bakker W, Eringa EC, Sipkema P, van Hinsbergh VW. Endothelial dysfunction and diabetes: roles of hyperglycemia, impaired insulin signaling and obesity. Cell Tissue Res 2009; 335: 165-89.

[63]   Goldfine AB, Beckman JA, Betensky RA, et al. Family history of diabetes is a major determinant of endothelial function. J Am Coll Cardiol 2006; 47: 2456-61.

[64]   Boger RH, Bode-Boger SM, Szuba A, et al. Asymmetric dimethylarginine (ADMA): a novel risk factor for endothelial dysfunction: its role in hypercholesterolemia. Circulation 1998; 98: 1842-7.

[65]   Balletshofer BM, Rittig K, Enderle MD, et al. Endothelial dysfunction is detectable in young normotensive first-degree relatives of subjects with type 2 diabetes in association with insulin resistance. Circulation 2000; 101: 1780-4.

[66]   Hanley AJG, McKeown-Eyssen G, Harris SB, et al. Cross-sectional and prospective associations between proinsulin and cardiovascular disease risk factors in a population experiencing rapid cultural transition. Diabetes Care 2001; 24: 1240-7.

[67]   Haffner SM, Mykkänen L, Stern MP, Valdez RA, Heisserman JA, Bowsher RR. Relationship of proinsulin and insulin to cardiovascular risk factors in nondiabetic subjects. Diabetes 1993; 42: 1297-302.

[68]   Yudkin JS, Denver AE, Mohamed-Ali V, et al. The relationship of concentrations of insulin and proinsulin-like molecules with coronary heart disease prevalence and incidence. A study of two ethnic groups. Diabetes Care 1997; 20: 1093-100.

[69]   Goh S, Cooper ME. The role of advanced glycation end products in progression and complications of diabetes. J Clin Endocrinol Metab 2008; 93: 1143-52.

[70]   Yamagishi S, Nakamura K, Imaizumi T. Advanced glycation end products (AGEs) and diabetic vascular complications. Curr Diabetes Rev 2005;1:93-106.

[71] Nilsson-Berglund LM, Zetterqvist AV, Nilsson-Ohman J, *et al.* Nuclear factor of activated t cells regulates osteopontin expression in arterial smooth muscle in response to diabetes-induced hyperglycemia. Arterioscler Thromb Vasc Biol 2010; 30: 218-24.

[72] Klein R. Hyperglycemia and micro-vascular and macrovascular disease in diabetes. Diabetes Care 1995; 18: 258-68.

[73] Abdul-Ghani MA, Williams K, DeFronzo R, Stern M. Risk of progression to type 2 diabetes based on relationship between postload plasma glucose and fasting plasma glucose. Diabetes Care 2006; 29: 1613-8.

[74] Succurro E, Marini MA, Grembiale A, *et al.* Differences in cardiovascular risk profile based on relationship between post-load plasma glucose and fasting plasma levels. Diabetes Metab Res Rev 2009;25:351-6.

[75] Ning F, Tuomilehto J, Pyorala K, Onat A, Soderberg S, Qiao Q for the DECODE Study Group. Cardiovascular disease mortality in Europeans in relation to fasting and 2-h plasma glucose levels within a normoglycemic range. Diabetes Care 2010; 33: 2211-6.

[76] O'Malley G, Santoro N, Northrup V, *et al.* High normal fasting glucose level in obese youth: a marker for insulin resistance and beta cell dysregulation. Diabetologia 2010; 53: 1199-209.

[77] Piche ME, Lemieux S, Perusse L, Weisnagel SJ. High normal 2-hours plasma glucose is associated with insulin sensitivity and secretion that may predispose to type 2 diabetes. Diabetologia 2005; 48: 732-40.

[78] Bonora E, Kiechl S, Willeit J, *et al.* Plasma glucose within the normal range is not associated with carotid atherosclerosis: prospective results in subjects with normal glucose tolerance from the Bruneck Study. Diabetes Care 1999; 22: 1339-46.

[79] Barrett-Connor E, Khaw KT. Diabetes mellitus: an independent risk factor for stroke? Am J Epidemiol 1988; 128: 116-23.

[80] Kuusisto J, Mykkanen L, Pyorala K, Laakso M. Non-insulin-dependent diabetes and its metabolic control are important predictors of stroke in elderly subjects. Stroke 1994; 25: 1157-64.

[81] Tuomilehto J, Rastenyte D, Jousilahti P, Sarti C, Vartiainen E. Diabetes mellitus as a risk factor for death from stroke : prospective study of the middle-aged finnish population. Stroke 1996; 27: 210-5.

[82] Berger K, Schulte H, Stogbauer F, Assmann G. Incidence and risk factors for stroke in an occupational cohort : the PROCAM study. Stroke1998; 29: 1562-6.

[83] Wannamethee SG, Perry IJ, Shaper AG. Nonfasting serum glucose and insulin concentrations and the risk of stroke. Stroke 1999; 30: 1780-6.

[84] Kissela BM, Khoury J, Kleindorfer D, *et al.* Epidemiology of ischemic stroke in patients with diabetes. Diabetes Care 2005; 28: 355-9.

[85] Zhang Y, Galloway JM, Welty TK, *et al.* Incidence and risk factors for stroke in American Indians: the strong heart study. Circulation 2008; 118: 1577-84.

[86] Pyorala K, Laakso M, Uusitupa M. Diabetes and atherosclerosis: an epidemiologic view. Diabetes Metab Rev1987; 3: 463-524.

[87] Stokes J 3rd, Kannel WB, Wolf PA, Cupples LA, D'Agostino RB. The relative importance of selected risk factors for various manifestations of cardiovascular disease among men and women from 35 to 64 years old: 30 years of follow-up in the Framingham Study. Circulation 1987; 75:V65-73.

[88] Kokubo Y, Okamura T, Watanabe M, *et al.* The combined impact of blood pressure category and glucose abnormality on the incidence of cardiovascular diseases in a Japanese urban cohort: the Suita Study. Hypertens Res 2010; 33: 1238-43.

[89] Hyvarinen M, Tuomilehto J, Mahonen M, *et al.* Hyperglycemia and incidence of ischemic and hemorrhagic stroke-comparison between fasting and 2-hour glucose criteria. Stroke 2009; 40: 1633-7.

[90] Lee WL, Cheung AM, Cape D, Zinman B. Impact of diabetes on coronary artery disease in women and men: a meta-analysis of prospective studies. Diabetes Care 2000; 23: 962-8.

[91] Hart CL, Hole DJ, Smith GD. Comparison of risk factors for stroke incidence and stroke mortality in 20 years of follow-up in men and women in the renfrew/paisley study in Scotland. Stroke 2000; 31: 1893-6.

[92] Almdal T, Scharling H, Jensen JS, Vestergaard H. The independent effect of type 2 diabetes mellitus on ischemic heart disease, stroke, and death: a population-based study of 13, 000 men and women with 20 years of follow-up. Arch Intern Med 2004; 164: 1422-6.

[93] Hyvarinen M, Qiao Q, Tuomilehto J, Soderberg S, Eliasson M, Stehouwer CD. The difference between acute coronary heart disease and ischemic stroke risk with regard to gender and age in Finnish and Swedish populations. Int J Stroke 2010; 5: 152-6.

[94] Reeves MJ, Bushnell CD, Howard G, *et al.* Sex differences in stroke: epidemiology, clinical presentation, medical care, and outcomes. Lancet Neurol 2008; 7: 915-926.

[95] Wassertheil-Smoller S, Hendrix S, Limacher M, *et al.* Effect of estrogen plus progestin on stroke in postmenopausal women. JAMA 2003; 289: 2673-84.

[96] Hendrix SL, Wassertheil-Smoller S, Johnson KC, *et al.* Effects of conjugated equine estrogen on stroke in the women's health initiative. Circulation 2006; 113: 2425-34.

[97] Carroll BJ, Barrett JE. Anteromedial Temporal-Prefrontal Connectivity: A Functional Neuroanatomical System Implicated in Schizophrenia. Psychopathology and the brain 1991; 25.

[98] Eguchi K, Boden-Albala B, Jin Z, *et al.* Usefulness of fasting blood glucose to predict vascular outcomes among individuals without diabetes mellitus (from the Northern Manhattan Study). Am J Cardiol 2007; 100:1404-9.

[99] Cremer P, Nagel D, Mann H, *et al.* Ten-years follow-up results from the Goettingen Risk, Incidence and Prevalence Study (GRIPS). I. Risk factors for myocardial infarction in a cohort of 5790 men. Atherosclerosis 1997; 129: 221-230.

[100] Danaei G, Lawes CM, Vander Hoorn S, Murray CJ, Ezzati M. Global and regional mortality from ischemic heart disease and stroke attributable to higher-than-optimum blood glucose concentration: comparative risk assessment. Lancet 2006; 368: 1651-9.

[101] Haheim L, Holme I, Hjermann I, Leren P. Risk factors of stroke incidence and mortality. A 12-years follow-up of the Oslo Study. Stroke1993; 24: 1484-9.

[102] Lawlor DA, Fraser A, Ebrahim S, Smith GD. Independent associations of fasting insulin, glucose, and glycated hemoglobin with stroke and coronary heart disease in older women. PLoS Med 2007; 4: e263.

[103] Nielson C, Fleming RM. Blood glucose and cerebrovascular disease in nondiabetic patients. Angiology 2007; 58: 625-9.

[104] Ferrie JE, Singh-Manoux A, Kivimäki M, *et al.* Cardiorespiratory risk factors as predictors of 40-years mortality in women and men. Heart 2009; 95: 1250-7.

[105] Preiss D, Welsh P, Murray HM, *et al.* Fasting plasma glucose in non-diabetic participants and the risk for incident cardiovascular events, diabetes, and mortality: results from WOSCOPS 15-year follow-up. Eur Heart J 2010; 31: 1230-6.

[106] Doi Y, Ninomiya T, Hata J, *et al.* Impact of glucose tolerance status on development of ischemic stroke and coronary heart disease in a general Japanese population: the hisayama study. Stroke 2010; 41: 203-9.

[107] Selvin E, Coresh J, Golden SH, Boland LL, Brancati FL, Steffes MW. Glycemic control, atherosclerosis, and risk factors for cardiovascular disease in individuals with diabetes. Diabetes Care 2005; 28: 1965-73.

[108] Selvin E, Marinopoulos S, Berkenblit G, *et al.* Meta-analysis: glycosylated hemoglobin and cardiovascular disease in diabetes mellitus. Ann Intern Med 2004; 141: 421-31.

[109] Ling PR, Mueller C, Smith RJ, Bistrian BR. Hyperglycemia induced by glucose infusion causes hepatic oxidative stress and systemic inflammation, but not STAT3 or MAP kinase activation in liver in rats. Metabolism 2003; 52: 868-74.

[110] Garg R, Chaudhuri A, Munschauer F, Dandona P. Hyperglycemia, insulin, and acute ischemic stroke: a mechanistic justification for a trial of insulin infusion therapy. Stroke 2006; 37: 267-73.

[111] Tuttolomondo A, Pinto A, Corrao S, *et al.* Immuno-inflammatory and thrombotic/fibrinolytic variables associated with acute ischemic stroke diagnosis. Atherosclerosis 2009; 203: 503-8.

[112] Anderson RE, Tan WK, Martin HS, Meyer FB, Hurn PD. Effects of glucose and pao2 modulation on cortical intracellular acidosis, nadh redox state, and infarction in the ischemic penumbra. Editorial comment. Stroke 1999; 30: 160-70.

[113] Hoxworth JM, Xu K, Zhou Y, Lust WD, LaManna JC. Cerebral metabolic profile, selective neuron loss, and survival of acute and chronic hyperglycemic rats following cardiac arrest and resuscitation. Brain Res 1999; 821: 467-79.

[114] Siesjo BK, Katsura KI, Kristian T, Li PA, Siesjo P. Molecular mechanisms of acidosis-mediated damage. Acta Neurochir Suppl 1996; 66: 8-14.

[115] Lee JM, Zipfel GJ, Choi DW. The changing landscape of ischemic brain injury mechanisms. Nature 1999; 399: A7-14.

[116] Mathers C, Stevens G, Mascarenhas M. Global health risks: mortality and burden of disease attributable to selected major risks. World Health Organisation, Geneva: Switzerland 2009.

[117] Franjic B, Marwick TH. The diabetic, hypertensive heart: epidemiology and mechanisms of a very high-risk situation. J Hum Hypertens 2009; 23: 709-17.

[118] Fisman EZ, Tenenbaum A. Cardiovascular diabetology: clinical, metabolic and inflammatory facets. Adv Cardiol 2008; 45: 82-106.

[119] Gress TW, Nieto FJ, Shahar E, Wofford MR, Brancati FL. Hypertension and antihypertensive therapy as risk factors for type 2 diabetes mellitus. Atherosclerosis Risk in Communities Study. N Engl J Med 2000; 342: 905-12.

[120] Bunnag P, Plengvidhya N, Deerochanawong C, *et al.* Thailand diabetes registry project: prevalence of hypertension, treatment and control of blood pressure in hypertensive adults with type 2 diabetes. J Med Assoc Thai 2006; 89 (Suppl 1): S72-7.

[121] Dhobi GN, Majid A, Masoodi SR, Bashir MI, Wani AI, Zargar AH. Prevalence of hypertension in patients with new onset type 2 diabetes mellitus. J Indian Med Assoc 2008; 106: 92, 94-8.

[122] Zhang Y, Lee ET, Devereux RB, *et al.* Prehypertension, diabetes, and cardiovascular disease risk in a population-based sample: the Strong Heart Study. Hypertension 2006; 47: 410-4.

[123] Messerli FH, Grossman E, Michalewicz L. Combination therapy and target organ protection in hypertension and diabetes mellitus. Am J Hypertens 1997;10:198S-201S.

[124] Tsaih SW, Korrick S, Schwartz J, *et al.* Lead, diabetes, hypertension, and renal function: the normative aging study. Environ Health Perspect 2004; 112: 1178-82.

[125] Ellis PA, Cairns HS. Renal impairment in elderly patients with hypertension and diabetes. QJM 2001; 94: 261-5.

[126] Mogensen CE. Renal dysfunction and hypertension, focus on Type 2 Diabetes. John Wiley & Sons, Inc. 2005; pp.245-270.

[127] Fong DS, Aiello L, Gardner TW, *et al.* Diabetic retinopathy. Diabetes Care 2003; 26 (Suppl 1):S99-102.

[128] Manaviat MR, Afkhami M, Shoja MR. Retinopathy and microalbuminuria in type II diabetic patients. BMC Ophthalmol 2004; 4: 9.

[129] Hu G, Sarti C, Jousilahti P, *et al.* The impact of history of hypertension and type 2 diabetes at baseline on the incidence of stroke and stroke mortality. Stroke 2005; 36: 2538-43.

[130] Kissela BM, Khoury J, Kleindorfer D, *et al.* Epidemiology of ischemic stroke in patients with diabetes: the greater Cincinnati/Northern Kentucky Stroke Study. Diabetes Care 2005; 28: 355-9.

[131] Jafar TH. Blood pressure, diabetes, and increased dietary salt associated with stroke--results from a community-based study in Pakistan. J Hum Hypertens 2006; 20: 83-5.

[132] Mancia G, Laurent S, Agabiti-Rosei E, *et al.* Reappraisal of European guidelines on hypertension management: a European Society of Hypertension Task Force document. J Hypertens 2009; 27: 2121-58.

[133] Chobanian AV, Bakris GL, Black HR, *et al.* The seventh report of the joint national committee on prevention, detection, evaluation, and treatment of high blood pressure: the jnc 7 report. JAMA 2003; 289: 2560-72.

[134] Turner R. UK Prospective Diabetes Study Group. Tight blood pressure control and risk of macrovascular and micro-vascular complications in type 2 diabetes: UKPDS 38. UK Prospective Diabetes Study Group. BMJ 1998; 317: 703-13.

[135] Hansson L, Zanchetti A, Carruthers SG, *et al.* Effects of intensive blood-pressure lowering and low-dose aspirin in patients with hypertension: principal results of the Hypertension Optimal Treatment (HOT) randomised trial. HOT Study Group. Lancet 1998; 351:1755-62.

[136] Staessen JA, Thijs L, Fagard R, *et al.* Predicting cardiovascular risk using conventional *vs.* ambulatory blood pressure in older patients with systolic hypertension. Systolic Hypertension in Europe Trial Investigators. JAMA 1999; 282: 539-46.

[137] Mann JF, Gerstein HC, Pogue J, Bosch J, Yusuf S. Renal insufficiency as a predictor of cardiovascular outcomes and the impact of ramipril: the HOPE randomized trial. Ann Intern Med 2001; 134: 629-36.

[138] Yusuf S, Sleight P, Pogue J, Bosch J, Davies R, Dagenais G. Effects of an angiotensin-converting-enzyme inhibitor, ramipril, on cardiovascular events in high-risk patients. The Heart Outcomes Prevention Evaluation Study Investigators. N Engl J Med 2000; 342: 145-53.

[139] Dahlof B, Devereux RB, Kjeldsen SE, *et al.* Cardiovascular morbidity and mortality in the Losartan Intervention For Endpoint reduction in hypertension study (LIFE): a randomised trial against atenolol. Lancet 2002; 359: 995-1003.

[140] Furberg CD, Wright JT, Davis BR, *et al.* ALLHAT Officers and Coordinators for the ALLHAT Collaborative Research Group. The Antihypertensive and Lipid-Lowering Treatment to Prevent Heart Attack Trial. Major outcomes in high-risk hypertensive patients randomized to angiotensin-converting enzyme inhibitor or calcium channel blocker *vs.* diuretic: The Antihypertensive and Lipid-Lowering Treatment to Prevent Heart Attack Trial (ALLHAT). JAMA 2002; 288: 2981-97.

[141] MacMahon S, Peto R, Cutler J, *et al.* Blood pressure, stroke, and coronary heart disease. Part 1, Prolonged differences in blood pressure: prospective observational studies corrected for the regression dilution bias. Lancet 1990; 335:765-74.

[142] Janka HU, Warram JH, Rand LI, Krolewski AS. Risk factors for progression of background retinopathy in long-standing IDDM. Diabetes 1989; 38: 460-4.

[143] Curb JD, Pressel SL, Cutler JA, *et al.* Effect of diuretic-based antihypertensive treatment on cardiovascular disease risk in older diabetic patients with isolated systolic hypertension. Systolic Hypertension in the Elderly Program Cooperative Research Group. JAMA 1996; 276: 1886-92.

[144] Tuomilehto J, Rastenyte D, Birkenhager WH, *et al.* Effects of calcium-channel blockade in older patients with diabetes and systolic hypertension. Systolic Hypertension in Europe Trial Investigators. N Engl J Med 1999; 340:677-84.

[145] Adler AI, Stratton IM, Neil HA, *et al.* Association of systolic blood pressure with macrovascular and micro-vascular complications of type 2 diabetes (UKPDS 36): prospective observational study. BMJ 2000; 321:412-9.

[146] Nishimura R, LaPorte RE, Dorman JS, Tajima N, Becker D, Orchard TJ. Mortality trends in type 1 diabetes. The Allegheny County (Pennsylvania) Registry 1965-1999. Diabetes Care 2001; 24: 823-7.

[147] American Diabetes Association. Standards of medical care in diabetes--2009. Diabetes Care 2009; 32 (Suppl 1): S13-61.

[148] KDOQI. KDOQI clinical practice guidelines and clinical practice recommendations for diabetes and chronic kidney disease. Am J Kidney Dis 2007; 49: S12-154.

[149] Wayne VM, Doren F, Ann B, *et al.* Prevalence of hypertension in patients with type ii diabetes in referral *versus* primary care clinics. J Diabetes Complications 1998; 12: 302-306.

[150] Turner RC, Holman RR, Matthews DR, *et al.* UKPDS Study Group. Hypertension in Diabetes Study (HDS): I. Prevalence of hypertension in newly presenting type 2 diabetic patients and the association with risk factors for cardiovascular and diabetic complications. J Hypertens 1993; 11: 309-17.

[151] Simonson DC. Etiology and prevalence of hypertension in diabetic patients. Diabetes Care 1988; 11: 821-7.

[152] Shrestha UK, Singh DL, Bhattarai MD. The prevalence of hypertension and diabetes defined by fasting and 2-h plasma glucose criteria in urban Nepal. Diabet Med 2006; 23:1130-5.

[153] Skliros E, Sotiropoulos A, Vasibossis A, *et al.* Poor hypertension control in Greek patients with diabetes in rural areas. The VANK study in primary care. Rural Remote Health 2007;7:583.

[154] Mubarak FM, Froelicher ES, Jaddou HY, Ajlouni KM. Hypertension among 1000 patients with type 2 diabetes attending a national diabetes center in Jordan. Ann Saudi Med 2008; 28:346-51.

[155] Hippisley-Cox J, Pringle M. Prevalence, care, and outcomes for patients with diet-controlled diabetes in general practice: cross sectional survey. Lancet 2004; 364: 423-8.

[156] Kropp S, Grohmann R, Hauser U, Ruther E, Degner D. Hyperglycemia associated with antipsychotic treatment in a multicenter drug safety project. Pharmacopsychiatry 2004; 37 (Suppl 1):S79-83.

[157] Franklin S, Gustin W, Wong N, Larson M, Weber M, Kannel W. Hemodynamic patterns of age-related changes in blood pressure. The Framingham Heart Study. Circulation 1997; 96: 308-19.

[158] Wang W, Lee ET, Fabsitz RR, *et al.* A Longitudinal Study of Hypertension Risk Factors and Their Relation to Cardiovascular Disease. Hypertension 2006; 47: 403-9.

[159] Kosugi T, Nakagawa T, Kamath D, Johnson R. Uric acid and hypertension: an age-related relationship? J Hum Hypertens 2009; 23: 75-76.

[160] Al-Mahroos F, Al-Roomi K and McKeigue PM. Relation of high blood pressure to glucose intolerance, plasma lipids and educational status in an Arabian Gulf population. Int J Epidemiol 2000; 29: 71-6.

[161] Luma G, Spiotta R. Hypertension in children and adolescents. Am Fam Physician 2006; 73: 1558-68.

[162] Dickson M, Sigmund C. Genetic basis of hypertension: revisiting angiotensinogen. Hypertension 2006; 48: 14-20.

[163] Rahmouni K, Correia M, Haynes W, Mark A. Obesity-associated hypertension: new insights into mechanisms. Hypertension 2005; 45: 9-14.

[164] Segura J, Ruilope L. Obesity, essential hypertension and renin-angiotensin system. Public Health Nutr 2007; 10:1151-5.

[165] Lackland DT, Egan BM. Dietary salt restriction and blood pressure in clinical trials. Curr Hypertens Rep 2007; 9: 314-9.

[166] Kyrou I, Chrousos GP, Tsigos C. Stress, visceral obesity, and metabolic complications. Ann N Y Acad Sci 2006; 1083: 77-110.

[167] Lee JH, O'Keefe JH, Bell D, Hensrud DD, Holick MF. Vitamin D deficiency an important, common, and easily treatable cardiovascular risk factor? J Am Coll Cardiol 2008; 52:1949-56.

[168] MacMahon S.Alcohol consumption and hypertension. Hypertension 1987; 9: 111-21.

[169] Stranges S, Wu T, Dorn JM, *et al.* Relationship of alcohol drinking pattern to risk of hypertension: a population-based study. Hypertension 2004; 44: 813-9.

[170] Fuchs FD, Chambless LE, Whelton PK, Nieto FJ, Heiss G. Alcohol consumption and the incidence of hypertension: The Atherosclerosis Risk in Communities Study. Hypertension 2001;37:1242-50.

[171] Sobngwi E, Mbanya JC, Unwin NC, *et al.* Physical activity and its relationship with obesity, hypertension and diabetes in urban and rural Cameroon. Int J Obes Relat Metab Disord 2002; 26:1009-16.

[172] Duncan DT, Quarells RC, Din-Dzietham R, Arroyo C, Davis SK. Physical activity and incident hypertension among blacks: no relationship? Prev Chronic Dis 2006; 3:A109.

[173] Foy CG, Foley KL, D'Agostino.Jr RB, Goff Jr DC, Mayer-Davis E, Wagenknecht LE. Physical activity, insulin sensitivity, and hypertension among US adults: findings from the Insulin Resistance Atherosclerosis Study. Am J Epidemiol 2006; 163: 921-8.

[174] Groppeli A, DM. G, Omboni S, Parati G, Mancia G. Persistent blood pressure increase induced by heavy smoking. J Hypertens 1992; 10: 495-9.

[175] Markovitz JH, Matthews KA, Kannel WB, Cobb JL, D'Agostino RB. Psychological predictors of hypertension in the Framingham Study. Is there tension in hypertension? JAMA 1993; 270: 2439-43.

[176] Lucini D, Di Fede G, Parati G, Pagani M. Impact of chronic psychosocial stress on autonomic cardiovascular regulation in otherwise healthy subjects. Hypertension 2005; 46:1201-6.

[177] Wang X, Poole JC, Treiber FA, Harshfield GA, Hanevold CD, Snieder H. Ethnic and gender differences in ambulatory blood pressure trajectories: results from a 15-year longitudinal study in youth and young adults. Circulation 2006; 114: 2780-7.

[178] Jones DW, Chambless LE, Folsom AR, *et al.* Risk factors for coronary heart disease in African Americans: the atherosclerosis risk in communities study, 1987-1997. Arch Intern Med 2002; 162: 2565-71.

[179] Agyemang C, Bhopal R. Is the blood pressure of people from African origin adults in the UK higher or lower than that in European origin white people? A review of cross-sectional data. J Hum Hypertens 2003;17:523-34.

[180] Brown MJ. Hypertension and ethnic group. BMJ 2006; 332: 833-6.

[181] Minor DS, Wofford MR, Jones DW. Racial and ethnic differences in hypertension. Curr Atheroscler Rep 2008; 10:121-7.

[182] Jones DW, Hall JE. Racial and ethnic differences in blood pressure: biology and sociology. Circulation 2006; 114:2757-9.

[183] Zavaroni I, Mazza S, Dall'Aglio E, Gasparini P, Passeri M, Reaven GM. Prevalence of hyperinsulinemia in patients with high blood pressure. J Intern Med 1992; 231:235-40.

[184] Ogihara T, Asano T, Ando K, *et al.* Angiotensin II-induced insulin resistance is associated with enhanced insulin signaling. Hypertension 2002; 40:872-9.

[185] Perticone F, Ceravolo R, Pujia A, *et al.* Prognostic significance of endothelial dysfunction in hypertensive patients. Circulation 2001; 104:191-6.

[186] Sowers JR. Treatment of hypertension in patients with diabetes. Arch Intern Med 2004; 164:1850-7.

[187] DeFronzo RA, Ferrannini E. Insulin resistance. A multifaceted syndrome responsible for NIDDM, obesity, hypertension, dyslipidemia, and atherosclerotic cardiovascular disease. Diabetes Care 1991;14:173-94.

[188] Westerbacka J, Vehkavaara S, Bergholm R, Wilkinson I, Cockcroft J, Yki-Jarvinen H. Marked resistance of the ability of insulin to decrease arterial stiffness characterizes human obesity. Diabetes 1999; 48: 821-7.

[189] Lima NK, Abbasi F, Lamendola C, Reaven GM. Prevalence of insulin resistance and related risk factors for cardiovascular disease in patients with essential hypertension. Am J Hypertens 2009; 22:106-11.

[190] Sowers JR, Epstein M, Frohlich ED. Diabetes, hypertension, and cardiovascular disease: an update. Hypertension 2001;37:1053-9.

[191] Sechi LA, Melis A, Tedde R. Insulin hypersecretion: a distinctive feature between essential and secondary hypertension. Metabolism 1992; 41: 1261-6.

[192] Grunfeld B, Balzareti M, Romo M, Gimenez M, Gutman R. Hyperinsulinemia in normotensive offspring of hypertensive parents. Hypertension 1994;23:I12-5.

[193] Landsberg L. Role of the sympathetic adrenal system in the pathogenesis of the insulin resistance syndrome. Ann N Y Acad Sci 1999; 892: 84-90.

[194] Solini A, Di Virgilio F, Chiozzi P, Fioretto P, Passaro A, Fellin R. A defect in glycogen synthesis characterizes insulin resistance in hypertensive patients with type 2 diabetes. Hypertension 2001; 37: 1492-6.

[195] Steinberger J, Daniels SR. Obesity, insulin resistance, diabetes, and cardiovascular risk in children: an American Heart Association scientific statement from the Atherosclerosis, Hypertension, and Obesity in the Young Committee (Council on Cardiovascular Disease in the Young) and the Diabetes Committee (Council on Nutrition, Physical Activity, and Metabolism). Circulation 2003;107:1448-53.

[196] Brenner BM, Cooper ME, de Zeeuw D, *et al.* Effects of losartan on renal and cardiovascular outcomes in patients with type 2 diabetes and nephropathy. N Engl J Med 2001; 345: 861-9.

[197] Sowers JR. Insulin resistance and hypertension. Am J Physiol Heart Circ Physiol 2004; 286: H1597-1602 .

[198] Sloniger JA, Saengsirisuwan V, Diehl CJ, *et al.* Defective insulin signaling in skeletal muscle of the hypertensive TG(mREN2)27 rat. Am J Physiol Endocrinol Metab 2005; 288:E1074-81.

[199] McFarlane SI, Sowers JR. Cardiovascular endocrinology 1: aldosterone function in diabetes mellitus: effects on cardiovascular and renal disease. J Clin Endocrinol Metab 2003; 88:516-23.

[200] Panza JA, Quyyumi AA, Brush JE, Jr, Epstein SE. Abnormal endothelium-dependent vascular relaxation in patients with essential hypertension. N Engl J Med 1990; 323:22-7.

[201] Linder L, Kiowski W, Buhler FR, Luscher TF. Indirect evidence for release of endothelium-derived relaxing factor in human forearm circulation *in vivo*. Blunted response in essential hypertension. Circulation 1990; 81: 1762-7.

[202] Sudano I, Spieker LE, Hermann F, *et al.* Protection of endothelial function: targets for nutritional and pharmacological interventions. J Cardiovasc Pharmacol 2006; 47 (Suppl 2):S136-50; discussion S172-6.

[203] Pan HZ, Zhang H, Chang D, Li H, Sui H. The change of oxidative stress products in diabetes mellitus and diabetic retinopathy. Br J Ophthalmol 2008; 92: 548-51.

[204] Evans JL, Goldfine ID, Maddux BA, Grodsky GM. Oxidative stress and stress-activated signaling pathways: a unifying hypothesis of type 2 diabetes. Endocr Rev 2002; 23: 599-622.

[205] Patel ST, Kent KC. Risk factors and their role in the diseases of the arterial wall. Semin Vasc Surg 1998; 11:156-68.

[206] Keaney JF, Jr, Loscalzo J. Diabetes, oxidative stress, and platelet activation. Circulation 1999; 99: 189-91.

[207] Semenkovich CF. Insulin resistance and atherosclerosis. J Clin Invest 2006; 116: 1813-22.

[208] Bakogianni MC, Kalofoutis CA, Skenderi KI, Kalofoutis AT. Clinical evaluation of plasma high-density lipoprotein subfractions (HDL2, HDL3) in non-insulin-dependent diabetics with coronary artery disease. J Diabetes Complications 2001;15:265-9.

[209] Guzik TJ, West NE, Black E, *et al.* Vascular superoxide production by NAD(P)H oxidase: association with endothelial dysfunction and clinical risk factors. Circ Res 2000; 86: E85-90.

[210] Uehara Y, Urata H, Sasaguri M, *et al.* Increased chymase activity in internal thoracic artery of patients with hypercholesterolemia. Hypertension 2000; 35: 55-60.

[211] Kannel WB, Wolf PA. Framingham Study insights on the hazards of elevated blood pressure. JAMA 2008; 300: 2545-7.

[212] Sowers JR, Haffner S. Treatment of cardiovascular and renal risk factors in the diabetic hypertensive. Hypertension 2002; 40: 781-8.

[213] Funatsu H, Yamashita H. Pathogenesis of diabetic retinopathy and the renin-angiotensin system. Ophthalmic Physiol Opt 2003; 23: 495-501.

[214] Matthews DR, Stratton IM, Aldington SJ, Holman RR, Kohner EM. Risks of progression of retinopathy and vision loss related to tight blood pressure control in type 2 diabetes mellitus: UKPDS 69. Arch Ophthalmol 2004; 122: 1631-40.

[215] Lewington S, Clarke R, Qizilbash N, Peto R, Collins R. Age-specific relevance of usual blood pressure to vascular mortality: a meta-analysis of individual data for one million adults in 61 prospective studies. Lancet 2002; 360: 1903-13.

[216] Vasan RS, Larson MG, Leip EP, *et al.* Impact of high-normal blood pressure on the risk of cardiovascular disease. N Engl J Med 2001; 345:1291-7.

[217] Cushman WC, Evans GW, Byington RP, *et al.* The ACCORD Study Group. Effects of intensive blood-pressure control in type 2 diabetes mellitus. N Engl J Med 2010; 362:1575-85.

[218] Gordon NF, Salmon RD, Franklin BA, *et al.* Effectiveness of therapeutic lifestyle changes in patients with hypertension, hyperlipidemia, and/or hyperglycemia. Am J Cardiol 2004; 94:1558-61.

[219] Sacks FM, Svetkey LP, Vollmer WM, *et al.* Effects on blood pressure of reduced dietary sodium and the Dietary Approaches to Stop Hypertension (DASH) diet. DASH-Sodium Collaborative Research Group. N Engl J Med 2001; 344: 3-10.

[220] Whelton SP, Chin A, Xin X, He J. Effect of aerobic exercise on blood pressure: a meta-analysis of randomized, controlled trials. Ann Intern Med 2002; 136: 493-503.

[221] Arauz-Pacheco C, Parrott MA, Raskin P. Hypertension management in adults with diabetes. Diabetes Care 2004; 27 (Suppl 1): S65-7.

[222] Black HR, Elliott WJ, Grandits G, *et al.* Principal results of the Controlled Onset Verapamil Investigation of Cardiovascular End Points (CONVINCE) trial. JAMA 2003; 289: 2073-82.

[223] Strippoli GF, Bonifati C, Craig M, Navaneethan SD, Craig JC. Angiotensin converting enzyme inhibitors and angiotensin II receptor antagonists for preventing the progression of diabetic kidney disease. Cochrane Database Syst Rev 2006;CD006257.

[224] Scheen AJ. Renin-angiotensin system inhibition prevents type 2 diabetes mellitus. Part 1. A meta-analysis of randomised clinical trials. Diabetes Metab 2004; 30: 487-96.

[225] Niklason A, Hedner T, Niskanen L, Lanke J. Development of diabetes is retarded by ACE inhibition in hypertensive patients--a subanalysis of the Captopril Prevention Project (CAPPP). J Hypertens 2004; 22: 645-52.

[226] Gerstein H C, Yusuf S, Mann JFE, et al. Heart Outcomes Prevention Evaluation Study Investigators. Effects of ramipril on cardiovascular and micro-vascular outcomes in people with diabetes mellitus: results of the HOPE study and MICRO-HOPE substudy. Lancet 2000; 355: 253-9.

[227] Whaley-Connell A, Sowers JR. Hypertension management in type 2 diabetes mellitus: recommendations of the Joint National Committee VII. Endocrinol Metab Clin North Am 2005; 34: 63-75.

[228] Ravid M, Lang R, Rachmani R, Lishner M. Long-term renoprotective effect of angiotensin-converting enzyme inhibition in non-insulin-dependent diabetes mellitus. A 7-years follow-up study. Arch Intern Med 1996; 156: 286-9.

[229] Bakris GL, Smith AC, Richardson DJ, et al. Impact of an ACE inhibitor and calcium antagonist on microalbuminuria and lipid subfractions in type 2 diabetes: a randomised, multi-centre pilot study. J Hum Hypertens 2002;16:185-91.

[230] Bakris GL, Weir MR. Angiotensin-converting enzyme inhibitor-associated elevations in serum creatinine: is this a cause for concern? Arch Intern Med 2000; 160: 685-93.

[231] Kidney Disease Outcomes Quality Initiative (K/DOQI). K/DOQI clinical practice guidelines on hypertension and antihypertensive agents in chronic kidney disease. Am J Kidney Dis 2004; 43: S1-290.

[232] Barnett AH, Bain SC, Bouter P, et al. Angiotensin-receptor blockade versus converting-enzyme inhibition in type 2 diabetes and nephropathy. N Engl J Med 2004; 351:1952-61.

[233] Lindholm LH, Persson M, Alaupovic P, Carlberg B, Svensson A, Samuelsson O. Metabolic outcome during 1 year in newly detected hypertensives: results of the Antihypertensive Treatment and Lipid Profile in a North of Sweden Efficacy Evaluation (ALPINE study). J Hypertens 2003; 21:1563-74.

[234] Pfeffer MA, Swedberg K, Granger CB, et al. Effects of candesartan on mortality and morbidity in patients with chronic heart failure: the CHARM-Overall programme. Lancet 2003; 362:759-66.

[235] Lindholm LH, Ibsen H, Borch-Johnsen K, et al. Risk of new-onset diabetes in the Losartan Intervention For Endpoint reduction in hypertension study. J Hypertens 2002; 20:1879-86.

[236] Julius S, Kjeldsen SE, Weber M, et al. Outcomes in hypertensive patients at high cardiovascular risk treated with regimens based on valsartan or amlodipine: the VALUE randomised trial. Lancet 2004; 363: 2022-31.

[237] Yusuf S, Teo KK, Pogue J, et al. Telmisartan, ramipril, or both in patients at high risk for vascular events. N Engl J Med 2008; 358:1547-59.

[238] Bosch J, Yusuf S, Gerstein HC, et al. Effect of ramipril on the incidence of diabetes. N Engl J Med 2006; 355: 1551-62.

[239] Holman RR, Haffner SM, McMurray JJ, et al. The NAVIGATOR study group. Effect of nateglinide on the incidence of diabetes and cardiovascular events. N Engl J Med 2010; 362:1463-76.

[240] Rosendorff C, Black HR, Cannon CP, et al. Treatment of hypertension in the prevention and management of ischemic heart disease: a scientific statement from the American Heart Association Council for High Blood Pressure Research and the Councils on Clinical Cardiology and Epidemiology and Prevention. Circulation 2007; 115: 2761-88.

[241] Holman R, Turner R, Stratton I, et al. UK Prospective Diabetes Study Group. Efficacy of atenolol and captopril in reducing risk of macrovascular and micro-vascular complications in type 2 diabetes: UKPDS 39. BMJ 1998; 317: 713-20.

[242] Kveiborg B, Christiansen B, Major-Petersen A, Torp-Pedersen C. Metabolic effects of beta-adrenoceptor antagonists with special emphasis on carvedilol. Am J Cardiovasc Drugs 2006; 6: 209-17.

[243] Birkenhager WH, Staessen JA, Gasowski J, de Leeuw PW. Effects of antihypertensive treatment on endpoints in the diabetic patients randomized in the Systolic Hypertension in Europe (Syst-Eur) trial. J Nephrol 2000; 13: 232-7.

[244] Estacio RO, Jeffers BW, Hiatt WR, Biggerstaff SL, Gifford N, Schrier RW. The effect of nisoldipine as compared with enalapril on cardiovascular outcomes in patients with non-insulin-dependent diabetes and hypertension. N Engl J Med 1998; 338: 645-52.

[245] Lindholm LH, Hansson L, Ekbom T, et al. Comparison of antihypertensive treatments in preventing cardiovascular events in elderly diabetic patients: results from the Swedish Trial in Old Patients with Hypertension-2. STOP Hypertension-2 Study Group. J Hypertens 2000; 18: 1671-5.

[246] Lewis EJ, Hunsicker LG, Clarke WR, et al. Renoprotective effect of the angiotensin-receptor antagonist irbesartan in patients with nephropathy due to type 2 diabetes. N Engl J Med 2001; 345: 851-60.

[247] Poulter NR. Calcium antagonists and the diabetic patient: a response to recent controversies. Am J Cardiol 1998; 82: 40R-41R.

[248] Luna B, Feinglos MN. Drug-induced hyperglycemia. JAMA 2001; 286: 1945-8.

[249] American Diabetes Association. Standards of medical care in diabetes--2010. Diabetes Care 2010; 33 (Suppl 1):S11-61.

[250] Arauz-Pacheco C, Parrott MA, Raskin P. The treatment of hypertension in adult patients with diabetes. Diabetes Care 2002; 25:134-47.

[251] Turner RC, Holman RR, Cull CA, et al. UK Prospective Diabetes Study (UKPDS) Group. Intensive blood-glucose control with sulphonylureas or insulin compared with conventional treatment and risk of complications in patients with type 2 diabetes (UKPDS 33). Lancet 1998; 352:837-53.

[252] Holman RR, Paul SK, Bethel MA, Matthews DR, Neil HA. 10-Years Follow-up of Intensive Glucose Control in Type 2 Diabetes. N Engl J Med 2008; 359: 1577-89.

[253] Gerstein HC, Miller ME, Byington RP, et al. The action to control cardiovascular risk in diabetes study group. Effects of intensive glucose lowering in Type 2 Diabetes. N Engl J Med 2008; 358: 2545-59.

[254] Patel A, MacMahon S, Chalmers J, et al. The ADVANCE collaborative group. Intensive blood glucose control and vascular outcomes in patients with Type 2 Diabetes. N Engl J Med 2008; 358: 2560-72.

[255] Duckworth W, Abraira C, Moritz T, et al. Glucose Control and Vascular Complications in Veterans with Type 2 Diabetes. N Engl J Med 2009; 360: 129-39.

[256] Wilcox R, Kupfer S, Erdmann E, PROactive Study investigators. Effects of pioglitazone on major adverse cardiovascular events in high-risk patients with type 2 diabetes: results from PROspective pioglitAzone Clinical Trial In macro Vascular Events (PROactive 10). Am Heart J 2008; 155: 712-7.

[257] McMurray JJ, Holman RR, Haffner SM, et al. The NAVIGATOR study group. Effect of valsartan on the incidence of diabetes and cardiovascular events. N Engl J Med 2010; 362:1477-90.

[258] Abraira C, Duckworth W, McCarren M, et al. Design of the cooperative study on glycemic control and complications in diabetes mellitus type 2: Veterans Affairs Diabetes Trial. J Diabetes Complications 2003; 17: 314-22.

[259] Charbonnel B, Dormandy J, Erdmann E, Massi-Benedetti M, Skene A. The prospective pioglitazone clinical trial in macrovascular events (PROactive). Diabetes Care 2004; 27: 1647-53.

[260] Dormandy JA, Charbonnel B, Eckland DJ, et al. Secondary prevention of macrovascular events in patients with type 2 diabetes in the PROactive Study (PROspective pioglitAzone Clinical Trial In macroVascular Events): a randomised controlled trial. Lancet 2005; 366: 1279-89.

[261] Ray KK, Seshasai SR, Wijesuriya S, et al. Effect of intensive control of glucose on cardiovascular outcomes and death in patients with diabetes mellitus: a meta-analysis of randomised controlled trials. Lancet 2009; 373: 1765-72.

[262] Skyler JS, Bergenstal R, Bonow RO, et al. Intensive glycemic control and the prevention of cardiovascular events: implications of the ACCORD, ADVANCE, and VA Diabetes Trials: a position statement of the american diabetes association and a scientific statement of the american college of cardiology foundation and the american heart association. Circulation 2009; 119:351-7.

[263] Zoungas S, Patel A, Chalmers J, et al. Severe hypoglycemia and risks of vascular events and death. N Engl J Med 2010; 363: 1410-8.

[264] Gerstein HC, Miller ME, Byington RP, et al. The action to control cardiovascular risk in diabetes study group. Effects of intensive glucose lowering in Type 2 Diabetes. N Engl J Med 2008; 358: 2545-59.

[265] Califf RM, Boolell M, Haffner SM, et al. Prevention of diabetes and cardiovascular disease in patients with impaired glucose tolerance: rationale and design of the Nateglinide And Valsartan in Impaired Glucose Tolerance Outcomes Research (NAVIGATOR) Trial. Am Heart J 2008;156: 623-32.

INDEX

www.ingramcontent.com/pod-product-compliance
Lightning Source LLC
Chambersburg PA
CBHW041713210326
41598CB00007B/638